T0314280

Pediatric Neurovascular Disease

Surgical, Endovascular, and Medical Management

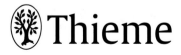

Pediatric Neurovascular Disease
Surgical, Endovascular, and Medical Management

Michael J. Alexander, M.D.
Director
Duke Neurovascular Center
Division of Neurosurgery
Duke University Medical Center
Durham, North Carolina

Robert F. Spetzler, M.D.
Director
Barrow Neurological Institute
J.N. Harber Chairman of Neurological Surgery
Phoenix, Arizona
Professor
Section of Neurosurgery
University of Arizona
Tucson, Arizona

Thieme
New York • Stuttgart

Thieme Medical Publishers, Inc.
333 Seventh Ave.
New York, NY 10001

Associate Editor: David Price
Consulting Editor: Esther Gumpert
Vice-President, Production and Electronic Publishing: Anne T. Vinnicombe
Production Editor: Becky Dille
Sales Director: Ross Lumpkin
Associate Marketing Director: Verena Diem
Chief Financial Officer: Peter van Woerden
President: Brian D. Scanlan
Compositor: Compset Inc.
Printer: Maple-Vail Book Manufacturing Group

Library of Congress Cataloging-in-Publication Data

Alexander, Michael J., 1962-
Pediatric neurovascular disease : surgical, endovascular, and medical management/Michael J. Alexander,
Robert F. Spetzler.
    p. ; cm.
    Includes bibliographical references and index.
    ISBN 1-58890-368-0 (alk. paper)—ISBN 3-13-126611-2 (alk. paper)
    1. Neurovascular diseases.   2. Children—Diseases—Treatment.
    [DNLM: 1. Cerebrovascular Disorders—surgery—Child. 2. Nervous System Diseases—surgery—
Child. 3. Neurosurgical Procedures—Child. 4. Vascular Surgical Procedures—Child. WL 355 A377p
2006] I. Spetzler, Robert F. (Robert Friedrich), 1944— II. Title.
RC367A44 2006
618.92'81—dc22   2005021931

Important note: Medical knowledge is ever-changing. As new research and clinical experience broaden our
knowledge, changes in treatment and drug therapy may be required. The authors and editors of the material
herein have consulted sources believed to be reliable in their efforts to provide information that is complete
and in accord with the standards accepted at the time of publication. However, in the view of the possibility of
human error by the authors, editors, or publisher of the work herein or changes in medical knowledge,
neither the authors, editors, or publisher, nor any other party who has been involved in the preparation of this
work, warrants that the information contained herein is in every respect accurate or complete, and they are
not responsible for any errors or omissions or for the results obtained from use of such information. Readers
are encouraged to confirm the information contained herein with other sources. For example, readers are
advised to check the product information sheet included in the package of each drug they plan to administer
to be certain that the information contained in this publication is accurate and that changes have not been
made in the recommended dose or in the contraindications for administration. This recommendation is of
particular importance in connection with new or infrequently used drugs.

Some of the product names, patents, and registered designs referred to in this book are in fact registered
trademarks or proprietary names even though specific reference to this fact is not always made in the text.
Therefore, the appearance of a name without designation as proprietary is not to be construed as a represen-
tation by the publisher that it is in the public domain.

Printed in the United States of America

5 4 3 2 1

TMP ISBN 1-58890-368-0
GTV ISBN 3 13 126611 2

To my lovely wife Joann, whose compassion and care for children inspired me to organize this book. And to my girls Julia, Emily, and Kathryn, who are daily reminders of what a precious gift children are.

Every good and perfect gift is from above. *(James 1: 17)*

Michael J. Alexander, M.D.

Contents

Foreword

It is a pleasure and a privilege to write a foreword to *Pediatric Neurovascular Disease*, a specialized textbook on cerebrovascular pediatric diseases edited by Drs. Michael Alexander and Robert Spetzler. My task has been made easier by my personal knowledge of the personal and professional integrity of Drs. Spetzler and Alexander. Through their active and intense participation in teaching and improvement of their specialties, they have demonstrated a commitment to disseminating the state of the art on the therapeutic management of cerebrovascular diseases and in this particular book on pediatric cerebrovascular diseases.

This excellent textbook brings concise and modern information on imaging and the use of combined therapeutic modalities to treat the most challenging pediatric cerebrovascular diseases. The selection of the chapters and their respective authors reflects the editors' desire to bring together in one book a thorough review of the subject including the embryology and anatomy of the cerebrovascular system, its pathophysiology, and therapeutic management of pediatric cerebrovascular diseases.

The chapters on the etiology and medical and surgical management of pediatric ischemic stroke are excellent. Also included and well done are chapters on pediatric thrombolysis and craniocervical angioplasty, and on endovascular, radiosurgical, and surgical therapeutic management of hemorrhagic stroke related to aneurysms, Galenic and non-Galenic arteriovenous fistulae, dual and pial arteriovenous malformations, and spinal vascular malformations.

This textbook, written by renowned authorities in the field, allows the reader to compare the three main therapeutic approaches—surgical, radiosurgical, and endovascular—to pediatric cerebrovascular diseases. It also emphasizes the concept that the modern therapeutic management of pediatric cerebrovascular diseases requires the cooperation of a group of specialized physicians in neo-ICU environments, in which the neonatologist, pediatric anesthesiologist, and pediatric neurosurgeon play essential pivotal roles. The interventional neuroradiologists need to be experienced in using specialized intracranial navigational systems as well as embolic materials to minimize cerebral or systemic iatrogenia in these patients.

Congratulations to the editors and authors for bringing this excellent and much needed comprehensive review of modern diagnostic and therapeutic management of pediatric cerebrovascular diseases to print.

Fernando Vinuela, M.D.

Preface

Neurovascular disease is a multifaceted area that most clinicians associate with adult pathologies, such as atherosclerotic disease, stroke, or cerebral hemorrhage. These are high acuity problems that typically require a neurovascular specialist at a tertiary care hospital. Pediatric neurovascular disease is more rare than in adults, and as such, the acuity level increases. Many pediatric neurosurgeons or other pediatric specialists are not accustomed to dealing with neurovascular pathologies, and many neurovascular specialists are not accustomed to dealing with pediatric patients. It is my hope that this book will give some additional insight into dealing with these complex patients.

The pediatric neurovascular field has seen tremendous advances in the past few decades with refinements in microsurgery, endovascular therapy, radiosurgery, and medical management. My interest in neurovascular disease developed early in my medical training, working under Alfred Luessenhop at Georgetown University and Thoralf Sundt at the Mayo Clinic. Both were established neurovascular surgeons who pioneered microvascular and endovascular techniques. The former pioneered cerebral ateriovenous malformation (AVM) embolization, the latter pioneered intracranial angioplasty for atherosclerotic disease. I was fortunate to complete my neurosurgery residency at UCLA Medical Center in the early 1990s, where I learned microvascular techniques from Neil Martin and John Frazee and helped manage the care of some of the very first patients treated with GDC coils. It was here I developed a subspecialty interest in pediatric neurovascular disease, treating patients with Moyamoya disease, vein of Galen malformations, cerebral and spinal AVMs, and so on. I was able to further this interest by completing post-graduate clinical fellowships in cerebrovascular surgery with Robert Spetzler and Joe Zabramski at the Barrow Neurological Institute and in endovascular therapy at UCLA Medical Center with Fernando Vinuela, Gary Duckwiler, Pierre Gobin, and Guido Guglielmi. Over the past five years at Duke University, I have enjoyed working with Allan Friedman, Taka Fukushima, Dave Enterline, and Tony Smith, as well as several dedicated, hard-working clinical fellows. I have learned and benefited from their expertise and creativity, and I hope we continue to push the field forward to benefit our patients and their families.

We have attempted to choose topics and authors for these chapters to provide a balanced view of contemporary management of pediatric neurovascular disease. As such, many of the disease topics will have mirror chapters in surgical and endovascular management. As a vascular neurosurgeon, who performs microsurgery, endovascular treatment, and stereotactic radiosurgery (the so-called "triple threat"), I believe the best way to minimize the morbidity for the patient and to obtain the best outcome is to employ multi-modal management. A neurovascular team is more apt to deal best with the multiple issues presented in the child with a neurovascular problem.

Michael J. Alexander, M.D.

Contributors

Felipe C. Albuquerque, M.D.
Division of Neurological Surgery
Barrow Neurological Institute
Phoenix, Arizona

Michael J. Alexander, M.D.
Director
Duke Neurovascular Center
Division of Neurosurgery
Duke University Medical Center
Durham, North Carolina

Mir Jafer Ali, M.D.
Resident
Department of Otolaryngology—Head and Neck Surgery
University of California, San Francisco
San Francisco, California

H. Hunt Batjer, M.D.
Michael J. Marchese Professor and Chair
Department of Neurological Surgery
Northwestern University Feinberg School
    of Medicine
Chicago, Illinois

Bernard R. Bendok, M.D.
Assistant Professor
Departments of Neurological Surgery
    and Radiology
Northwestern University School Feinberg School
    of Medicine
Chicago, Illinois

Kerry R. Crone, M.D.
Associate Professor of Pediatric Neurosurgery
Department of Neurosurgery
University of Cincinnati School of Medicine
Director
Division of Pediatrics
Cincinnati Children's Hospital Medical Center
Cincinnati, Ohio

Jeffrey Florman, M.D.
Neurosurgery Associates Scarborough, Maine

William A. Friedman, M.D.
Chairman
Department of Neurological Surgery
University of Florida
Gainesville, FL

Masashi Fukui, M.D.
Department of Neurosurgery
Kyushu University
Higashi-ku, Fukuoka, Japan

Christopher C. Getch, M.D.
Associate Professor
Department of Neurological Surgery
Northwestern University Feinberg School of Medicine
Chicago, Illinois

Van V. Halbach, M.D.
Department of Radiology
University of California at San Francisco
San Francisco, CA

Manraj K.S. Heran, M.D.
Department of Radiology
Vancouver General Hospital
Vancouver, British Columbia, Canada

Michael A. Horgan, M.D.
Assistant Professor of Neurosurgery
Division of Neurosurgery
University of Vermont
Burlington, Vermont

Stephen Lawrence Huhn, M.D.
Associate Professor
Division of Neurosurgery
Stanford University School of Medicine
Palo Alto, CA

Tooru Inoue, M.D.
Department of Neurosurgery
National Kyushu Medical Center
Higashi-ku, Fukuoka, Japan

David M. Johnson, M.D.
Department of Radiology
Mount Sinai Medical Center
New York, NY

Yasuo Kuwabara, M.D.
Department of Radiology
Kyushu University
Higashi-ku, Fukuoka, Japan

Jeff A. Lee, M.D.
Department of Neurosurgery
Kaiser San Diego Medical Center
San Diego, California

James E. Lefler, M.D.
Department of Radiology
Tampa General Hospital
Tampa, Florida

G. Michael Lemole Jr., M.D.
Assistant Professor
Department of Neurosurgery
University of Illinois at Chicago College of Medicine
Chicago, Illinois

David S. Liebeskind, M.D.
Assistant Professor
Associate Neurology Director of the
    UCLA Stroke Center
Department of Neurology
University of California, Los Angeles
Los Angeles, California

Cormac O. Maher, M.D.
Shillito Staff Associate
Department of Neurosurgery Children's
    Hospital Boston
Harvard Medical School
Boston, Massachusetts

Cameron G. McDougall, M.D.
Division of Neurological Surgery
Barrow Neurological Institute
Phoenix, Arizona

Toshio Matsushima, M.D.
Chief
Department of Neurosurgery
Hamanomachi Hospital
Fukuoka
Japan

Fredric B. Meyer, M.D.
Professor and Chair
Department of Neurologic Surgery
Mayo Clinic College of Medicine
Rochester, Minnesota

Ronnie I. Mimran, M.D.
Department of Neurological Surgery
University of Florida
Gainesville, FL

Thomas P. Naidich, M.D.
Department of Neurosurgery
Mount Sinai Medical Center
New York, New York

Aman Patel, M.D.
Department of Neurosurgery
Mount Sinai Medical Center
New York, New York

Howard A. Riina, M.D.
Department of Neurological Surgery
Weill/Cornell Medical College
New York Presbyterian Hospital
New York, New York

E. Steve Roach, M.D.
Department of Neurology
Wake Forest University School of Medicine
Winston-Salem, North Carolina

Cesar C. Santos, M.D.
Wake Forest University School
    of Medicine
Winston-Salem, North Carolina

Jeffrey L. Saver, M.D.
Professor
Neurology Director of the UCLA Stroke Center
Department of Neurology
University of California, Los Angeles
Los Angeles, California

Tony P. Smith, M.D.
Professor
Department of Radiology
Duke University Medical Center
Durham, North Carolina

Robert F. Spetzler, M.D.
Director
Barrow Neurological Institute
J.N. Harber Chairman of Neurological Surgery
Phoenix, Arizona
Professor
Section of Neurosurgery
University of Arizona
Tucson, Arizona

Gary K. Steinberg, M.D., Ph.D.
Professor and Chairman
Department of Neurosurgery
Stanford University School of Medicine
Palo Alto, California

Rabih G. Tawk, M.D.
Clinical Assistant Professor and Medical Resident
Department of Neurosurgery
University of Buffalo/Millard Fillmore Hospital
Buffalo, New York

Karel G. TerBrugge, M.D., F.R.C.P.(C.)
Professor of Radiology and Surgery
Department of Medical Imaging
University of Toronto
Toronto Western Hospital
Toronto, Ontario Canada

David Yeh, M.D.
Resident
Department of Neurosurgery
University of Cincinnati School of Medicine
Cincinnati Ohio

Osama O. Zaidat, M.D., M.Sc.
Department of Neurosurgery and Neurology
University of Wisconsin-Milwaukee
Milwaukee, Wisconsin

Medical and Diagnostic Evaluation and Issues

1

Development of the Cerebral Vasculature

DAVID M. JOHNSON, THOMAS P. NAIDICH, AND AMAN B. PATEL

The standard model and numerous variations of the cerebrovascular system all stem from its complicated embryogenesis. This chapter reviews the formation of the arterial and venous systems of the head and neck through five main sections: early embryogenesis, vasculogenesis, formation of the aortic arches, the cerebral arterial system, and the cerebral venous system. The description relies on the pioneering work of Streeter,[1] Padget,[2–4] and Congdon,[5] as well as more recent work by many others.[6–12]

■ Early Embryogenesis

The early embryo takes the form of a bilaminar disk. The superficial cell layer is designated the epiblast, whereas the deep, subjacent cell layer is designated the hypoblast. All of the future embryo derives from the epiblast. The hypoblast develops into the related extraembryonic tissues, such as the placenta.

By day 15, the primitive streak and the primitive node (Hensen's node) form in the midline toward the caudal end of the bilaminar disk (**Fig. 1–1**).[9,13] Beginning around day 16, epiblastic cells proliferate, migrate toward the primitive streak, ingress into the streak, and reach the potential space between the epiblast and hypoblast. This ingression (gastrulation) forms the future endoderm and mesoderm. The first ingressing epiblastic cells displace the hypoblast laterally and become the definitive endoderm.[9] Subsequent epiblastic cells ingress at the primitive streak and pass laterally between the two cell layers to both sides forming a new third layer, the mesoderm. From medial to lateral the mesoderm is considered in three longitudinally oriented zones: the paraxial mesoderm, the narrow intermediate mesoderm, and the broad lateral mesoderm. By day 17, epiblastic cells ingress at the primitive streak and ascend in the midline to form the notochordal process and later the notochord. The remaining epiblastic cells then spread out over the surface to become the definitive ectoderm.

Ultimately, the paraxial mesoderm forms the axial skeleton and musculature. The intermediate mesoderm forms the genitourinary system. The lateral mesoderm splits into superficial and deep layers to form the superficial dorsolateral *somatopleuric* mesoderm and the subjacent ventromedial *splanchnopleuric* mesoderm. The splanchnopleuric mesoderm is believed to be the precursor of the hematopoietic system and the blood vessels, as well as of the mesothelial coverings of the viscera (**Fig. 1–2**).[13]

On day 18, the neural plate appears as a thickening of the midline ectoderm. On day 22, the neural plate buckles at the future mesencephalic flexure. At around the same time, the neural plate begins to fold along its long axis and roll up into the neural tube. This process is designated neurulation. On day 24, the rostral opening of the neural tube, designated the cranial or anterior neuropore, closes. The caudal (posterior) neuropore closes a few days later.

As the neural folds approximate each other, cells delaminate from the dorsal edges of each fold and migrate ventrolaterally to form the neural crest.[9] Cephalic neural crest cells will contribute to the cranial nerve ganglia and will give rise to all of the craniofacial mesenchyme and the developing mesenchymal cores of the pharyngeal arches. Neural crest cells also contribute to the meninx primitiva and, therefore, to the future leptomeninges (pia-arachnoid).[14]

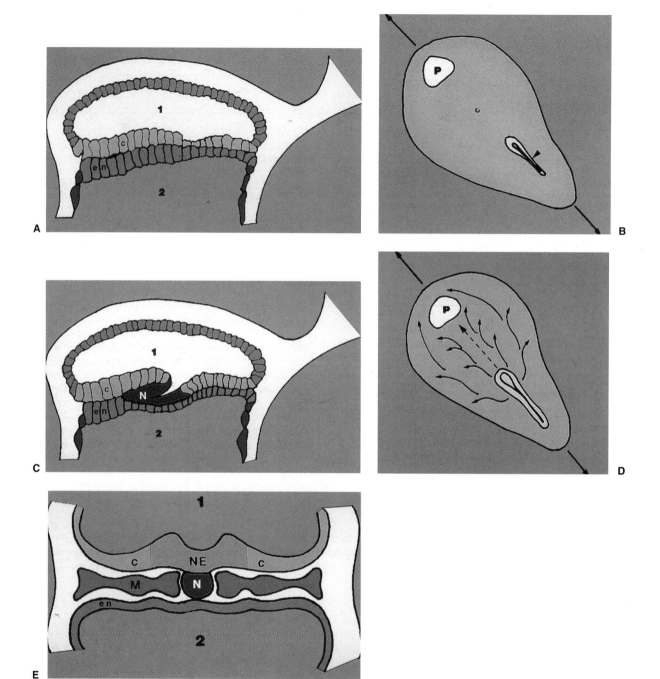

FIGURE 1–1 (A,B,D) Bilaminar disk. The early embryo is a two-layered disk formed by the epiblastic cell layer (e), which faces the amnion (1) and the hypoblastic cell layer (h), which faces the yolk sac (2). The epiblast forms all of the future embryo. The hypoblast will form the extra-embryonic tissues. The disk is marked by the prochordal plate (p) at the future cephalic end of the embryo, and the primitive streak (arrowhead) in the caudal half of the disk. Hensen's node lies at the cephalic end of the primitive streak. **(C–E)** Trilaminar disk. Cells from the epiblast (e) migrate to the primitive streak (arrowhead), enter, and descend through it to form the future endoderm and mesoderm (gastrulation). The first cells to enter displace the hypoblast laterally and become the deep cell layer designated endoderm. The next-migrating cells pass between the epiblast and the new endoderm to form (from medial to lateral) the future paraxial mesoderm, inter-mediate mesoderm, and lateral mesoderm. The last-entering epiblastic cells ascend in the midline toward the prochordal plate to form the notochordal process (n) that will become the notochord. The epiblastic cells then spread out to become the ectoderm. By these processes, the bilaminar disk is converted to the trilaminar disk. Thereafter, under the influence of signaling, differentiation occurs into the central plate of the neural ectoderm (ne) overlying the notochord and the cutaneous ectoderm (c) laterally (see Color Plate 1–1). (Reprinted with permission from Naidich TP, Blaser SI, Delman BN, et al. Congenital anomalies of the spine and spinal cord: embryology and malformations. In: Atlas SW, ed. Magnetic Resonance Imaging of the Brain and Spine. Philadelphia: Lippincott Williams and Wilkins; 2002:1527–1537, Figs. 27.1 and 27.2, pp. 1528 and 1529.)

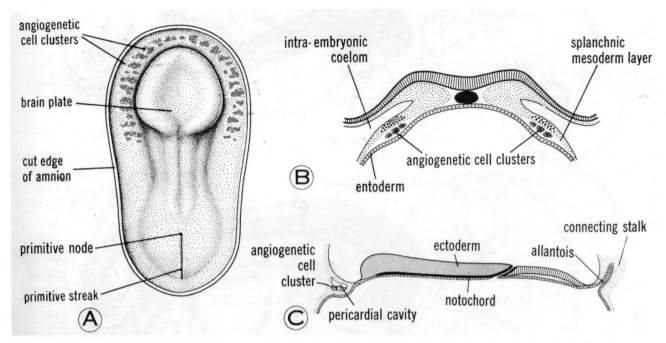

FIGURE 1–2 The angioblastic cells originating in the splanchnopleuric mesoderm. (Reprinted with permission from Langman J. Medical Embryology. Baltimore: Williams and Wilkins; 1975, Fig. 12–3, p. 203.)

■ Vasculogenesis

The metabolic needs of the developing, *open* neural tube are met by diffusion from the amniotic fluid. This period of amniotic fluid diffusion ends when the neural tube closes at ~26 days. At that time, the neural tube is surrounded by the meninx primitiva. The metabolic needs of the closed neural tube are then met by diffusion from the meninx primitiva and the vascular plexi developing within it.[8] Within the meninx primitiva, hemangioblastic cells from the splanchnopleuric mesoderm condense into blood islands. The inner cells of these blood islands evolve into hematopoietic stem cells. The outer cells of the blood islands become angioblasts. During vasculogenesis, the angioblasts differentiate into endothelial cells. The endothelial cells grow into tubes that interconnect to form a rich, multilayered capillary plexus that envelops the neural tube. The more superficial layers of the plexus join to form the major arteries, whereas the deeper layers form the veins.

As the metabolic needs of the developing brain increase, intraneural vascularization begins.[15] By the end of the seventh week of gestation (wg), capillaries begin to penetrate the cerebral surface (**Fig. 1–3**).[16] During the eighth and ninth wg, these vessels form intracortical branches that align parallel to the cortical and ventricular surfaces (designated the parallel vessels). During the ninth and tenth wg, a second group of vessels arises from the pial vasculature. These pial vessels may anastamose with branches from the parallel vessels or invade the mantle together with penetrating branches arising from the parallel vessels. During the eleventh and twelfth wg, the penetrating branches reach into the germinal layer and form a rete within the germinal matrix.

> **PEARL** Early in development, vessels grow toward the angiogenic stimulus (VEGF) secreted by the periventricular matrix.

This extensive vasculogenesis depends upon rapid endothelial cell proliferation coordinated through signaling systems. In mice, vascular endothelial growth factor (VEGF) and its receptors (VEGFR-1 and VEGFR-2) are necessary for normal vascular development.[17] In developing murine neuroectoderm, VEGFRs are expressed on the penetrating endothelial cells, whereas VEGF messenger ribonucleic acid (mRNA) is expressed in the periventricular matrix zone.[18,19] This system coordinates capillary ingrowth with the proper target tissue, so the vessels grow toward the angiogenic stimulus (VEGF) secreted by the periventricular matrix. Later, angiopoietin-1 mediates the interaction between maturing endothelial cells and pericytes/smooth muscle cells, which they enlist to invest them.[20]

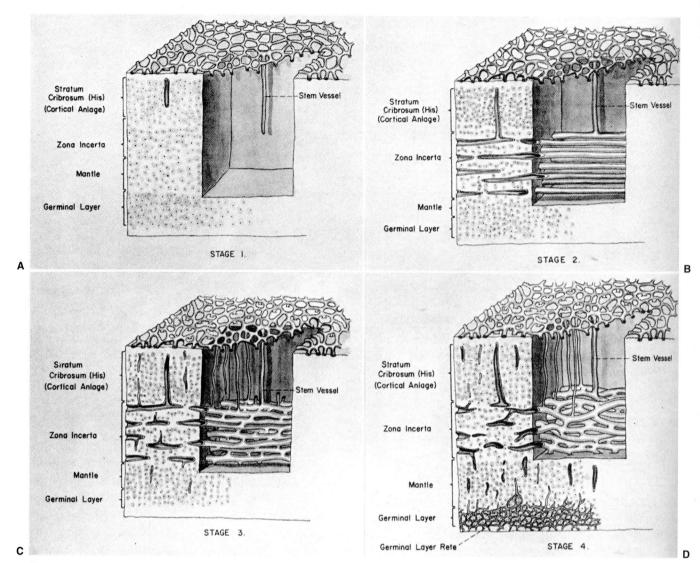

FIGURE 1–3 (A–D) The four major stages of internal vascularization of the cerebral hemispheres, as described in the text. (Reprinted with permission from Duckett S. The establishment of the internal vascularization in the human telencephalon. Acta Anat 1971;80:107–113, Fig. 7, p. 110.)

■ Formation of the Aortic Arches

Stepping back in time, around day 19, paired longitudinal endocardial tubes develop in the splanchnopleuric mesoderm of the cardiogenic region. Paired dorsal aortae form on both sides of the notochord and connect with the developing endocardial tubes. In the third wg, the embryo begins cephalic and lateral folding, which bring the endocardial tubes into close apposition in the thoracic region.[14] This folding draws the dorsal aortae ventrally, forming the first pair of aortic arches. Fusion of the paired endocardial tubes forms the primitive heart tube. During the fourth and fifth weeks, four additional pairs of aortic arches develop in relation to the developing pharyngeal arches (**Fig. 1–4**).[17] By days 22 to 24, the first pair of aortic arches becomes visible in the first pharyngeal arches. The first pair of aortic arches consists of transient structures that, by day 28, have largely regressed. Their remnants (still attached to the dorsal aortae) become the paired mandibular arteries. By day 29, the second pair of aortic arches has similarly formed and regressed. Their remnants (similarly attached to the dorsal aortae) become the hyoid arteries.

By the end of the fifth week, the third pair of aortic arches will become the common carotid arteries. The paired internal carotid arteries (ICAs) develop from cranial extensions of the paired dorsal aortae. The ventral pharyngeal plexi arise in the pharyngeal arches and help form the external carotid arteries.

The definitive aorta and brachiocephalic vessels develop from the aortic sac, asymmetric portions of the paired fourth and sixth aortic arches, and the paired

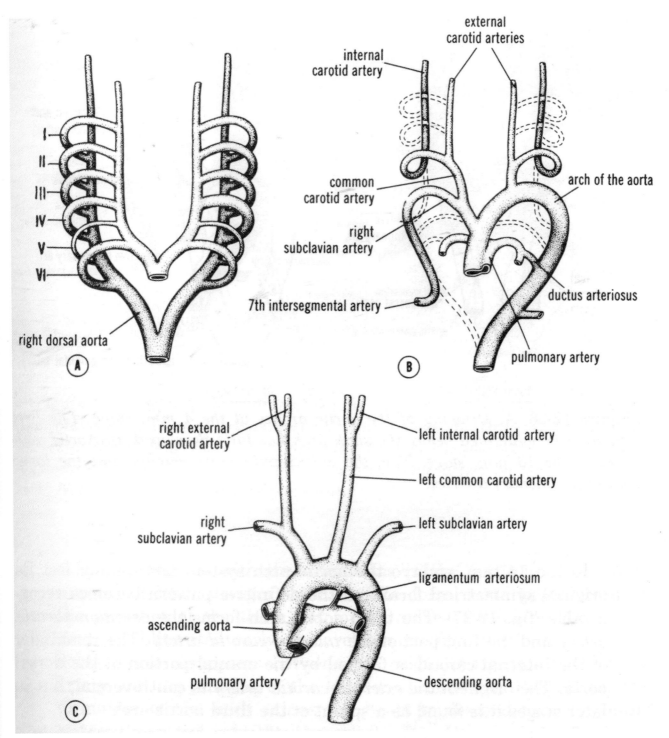

FIGURE 1–4 Formation of the aortic arch and great vessels. **(A)** Pattern of the aortic arches and dorsal aortae prior to their transformation into the adult pattern. **(B)** Pattern of the aortic arches and dorsal aortae following their transformation to the adult pattern. The dashed lines indicate those components that become obliterated. **(C)** Definitive form of the aorta and great vessels. (Reprinted with permission from Langman J. Medical Embryology. Baltimore: Williams and Wilkins; 1975, Fig. 12–35, p. 235.)

dorsal aortae, as follows. The aortic sac gives rise to the proximal aortic arch and the brachiocephalic artery. The left fourth aortic arch forms the apex of the aortic arch. The left dorsal aorta forms the distal arch. The paired dorsal aortae fuse at approximately the fourth thoracic segment to form the descending aorta. The right subclavian artery forms from the right fourth aortic arch and portions of the right dorsal aorta and

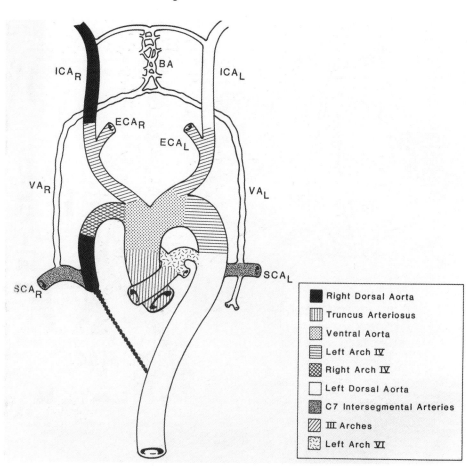

FIGURE 1–5 Formation of the aortic arch and great vessels. The diagram summarizes the complex embryology of these vessels and depicts the embryonic origins of each portion, as listed in the legend. Compare with Fig. 1–3. (Reprinted with permission from Osborn AG. Diagnostic Neuroradiology. St. Louis: Mosby; 1999, Fig. 1–4, p. 11.)

Legend:
- Right Dorsal Aorta
- Truncus Arteriosus
- Ventral Aorta
- Left Arch IV
- Right Arch IV
- Left Dorsal Aorta
- C7 Intersegmental Arteries
- III Arches
- Left Arch VI

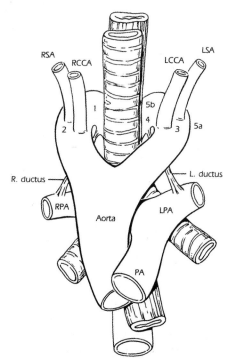

FIGURE 1–6 Hypothetical double aortic arch of Edwards. The diagram summarizes the points at which the numbered "breaks" of the primitive dual arch could give rise to the diverse variations in the formation of the aortic arch. A single break at point 1 would give the typical "normal" aortic arch. A single break at 2 would give rise to the left aortic arch with aberrant left subclavian artery. A single break at 3 would give rise to a right aortic arch with aberrant left subclavian artery. A single break at 4 would give rise to a right aortic arch with mirror-image branching pattern. Dual breaks at 5a and 5b would give rise to a right aortic arch with isolation of the left subclavian artery. Other dual breaks could lead to other exceedingly rare isolated vessels. (Reprinted with permission from Kirks DR. Practical Pediatric Radiology: Diagnostic Imaging of Infants and Children. Philadelphia: Lippincott-Raven; 1998, Fig. 6–65, p. 581.)

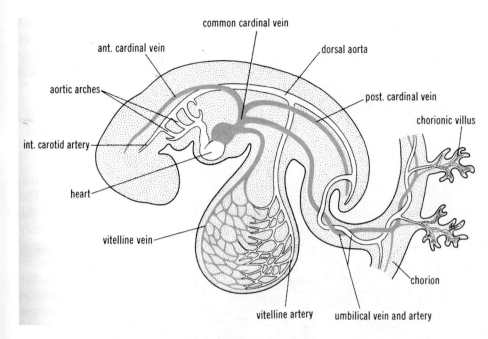

FIGURE 1–7 Formation of the great vessels. The diagram depicts the major components of the venous system seen in a 4 mm embryo toward the end of the fourth week of gestation. (Reprinted with permission from Langman J. Medical Embryology. Baltimore: Williams and Wilkins; 1975, Fig. 12–43, p. 243.)

seventh intersegmental artery. The left sixth aortic arch becomes the ductus arteriosus. The right sixth arch regresses without known remnant (**Figs. 1–5, 1–6**).[10,21]

By the third to fourth wg, two pairs of cardinal veins form: the paired anterior (superior) cardinal veins and the paired posterior (inferior) cardinal veins. The paired anterior cardinal veins drain the developing head and neck and will form the paired internal jugular veins. The paired posterior cardinal veins drain the body wall. Ultimately, the anterior cardinal vein and posterior cardinal vein of each side join to form a short, common cardinal vein that drains into the primitive heart (**Fig. 1–7**).[20]

■ The Cerebral Arterial System

Dorcas Padget classified the development of the cerebral arteries into seven stages by correlating embryo size, measured as the crown to rump length (CRL), and estimated gestational age (EGA) with a specific set of vascular features/events that typify that particular stage of development.[2,3] These seven stages represent "snapshot summaries" of events that actually occur as a continuous progression (**Fig. 1–8**).[2]

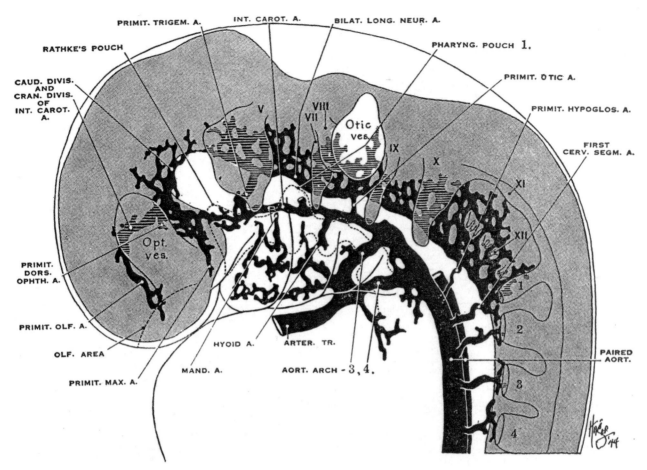

A Arterial Stage 1

FIGURE 1–8 The cerebral arterial system. **(A–G)** The seven sequential stages of arterial formation detailed in the text. **(H)** The arterial system of a newborn. (Reprinted with permission from Padget DH. The development of the cranial arteries in the human embryo. Contrib Embryol 1948;32:205–261, Figs. 2–11, pp. 213–229.)

Arterial Stage 1

In stage 1 (CRL 4 mm, EGA 28 days), the first and second aortic arches begin to involute, leaving the precursors for the mandibular and hyoid arteries. Blood is now supplied to the developing brain via the third aortic arches and the cranial portions of the dorsal aortae, which form the common and ICAs, respectively. The ICAs bifurcate at the level of the trigeminal ganglia. The *anterior* divisions of the ICAs course toward Rathke's pouch and anastamose with each other in the region of the future anterior communicating artery. In stage 1, the most anterior extensions of the ICAs are the primitive maxillary arteries. These extend to the optic vesicles.

The *posterior* divisions of the ICAs are designated the primitive trigeminal arteries. These extend dorsally to join an arterial plexus of the hindbrain designated the paired longitudinal neural arteries. Initially, the paired longitudinal neural arteries receive their major supply from the trigeminal arteries. Later, they will also receive supply from the first cervical segmental arteries and (transiently) from the primitive otic, primitive hypoglossal, and primitive proatlantal arteries. These primitive caroticobasilar anastamoses develop during the period in which their associated ganglia grow rapidly.[6] Failure of these primitive connections to regress leads to the infrequent persistent trigeminal, otic, hypoglossal, and proatlantal arteries.[2,3,6,22–25]

> **PEARL** Failure of the primitive caroticobasilar connections to regress leads to the infrequent persistent trigeminal, otic, hypoglossal, and proatlantal arteries.

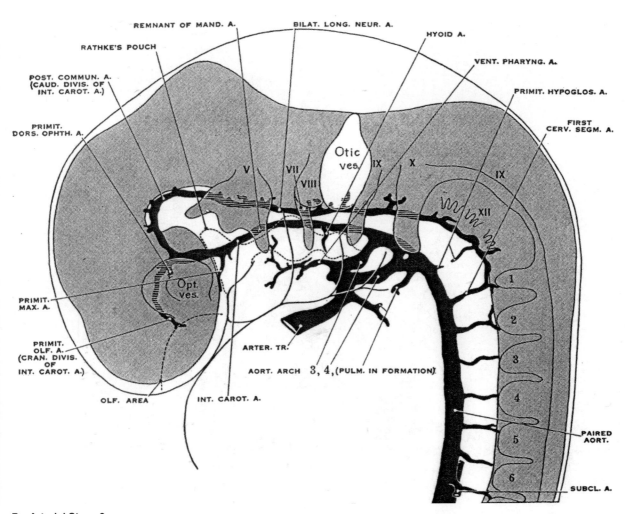

B Arterial Stage 2

FIGURE 1–8 *(Continued)*

Arterial Stage 2

In stage 2 (CRL 5 to 6 mm, EGA 32 days), the mandibular arteries have largely regressed. Paired ventral pharyngeal arteries have developed in the first and second pharyngeal arches. These extend from the aortic sac to the mandibular divisions of the trigeminal nerves and will contribute to both the stapedial arteries and the branches of the external carotid arteries. In stage 2, the anterior divisions of the ICAs now give rise to long dorsal ophthalmic arteries that extend through the superior orbital fissures to the optic vesicles. Posterior communicating arteries develop and carry flow to the longitudinal neural arteries, so the primitive trigeminal arteries begin to regress. The longitudinal neural arteries also begin to coalesce to form the basilar artery. Incomplete coalescence leaves zones of persistent "duplication" designated basilar artery fenestrations. Such vascular fenestrations may be associated with aneurysms.[26,27]

Arterial Stage 3

In stage 3 (CRL 7 to 12 mm, EGA 37 days), the anterior divisions of the ICAs show stems for the middle cerebral and anterior cerebral arteries. The primitive ventral ophthalmic arteries arise opposite the anterior choroidal arteries and course through the optic canals to the developing orbits. In stage 3, the anterior divisions of the ICAs end in the primitive olfactory arteries. The anterior choroidal and posterior choroidal arteries supply the diencephalon and the mesencephalon en route to the choroid plexi. Paired superior cerebellar arteries arise to supply the developing metencephalon. Regression of the cervical segmental arteries leads to formation of the paired vertebral arteries. Asymmetric regression of the cervical segmental arteries may lead to one hypoplastic vertebral artery that ends in the ipsilateral posterior inferior cerebellar artery. Incomplete regression of the cervical segmental arteries may lead to vertebral artery fenestration.

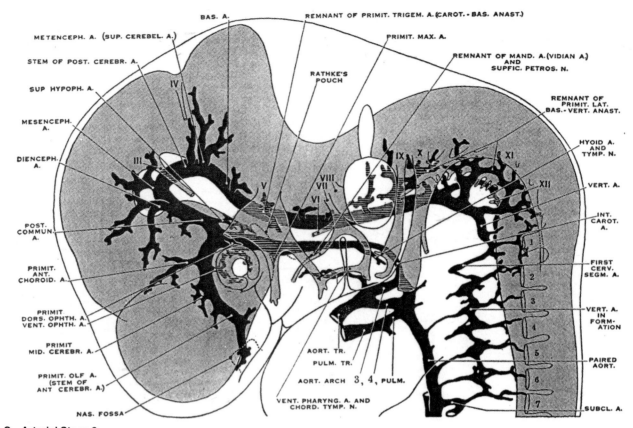

C Arterial Stage 3

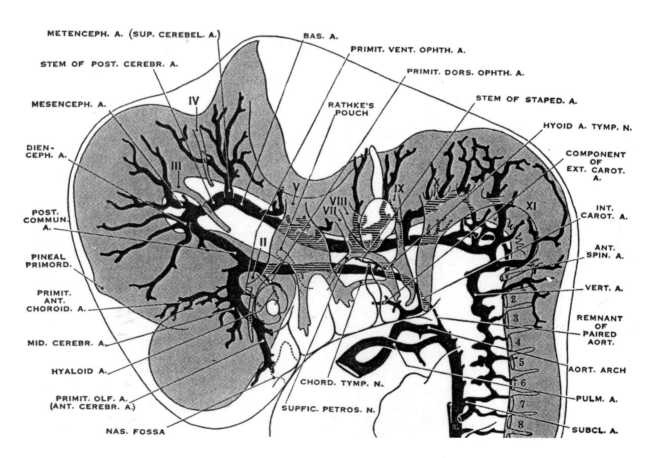

FIGURE 1–8 (Continued)

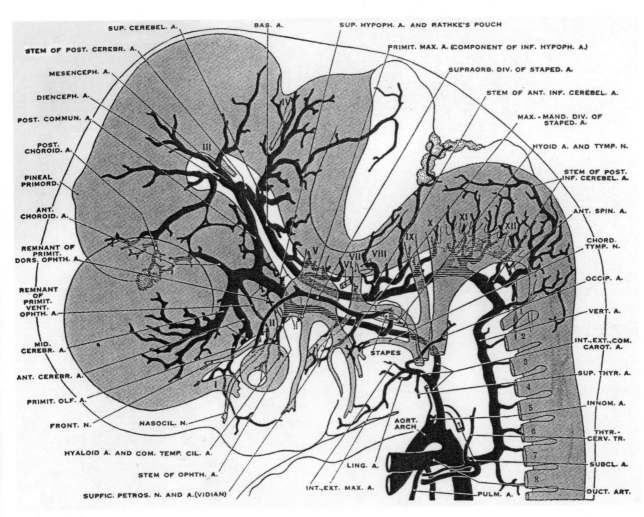

E Arterial Stage 5

FIGURE 1–8 *(Continued)*

Arterial Stage 4

In stage 4 (CRL 12 to 14 mm, EGA 41 days), collateral branches of the hyoid arteries course through the primordia of the stapes into the mandibular substance. These will join remnants of the ventral pharyngeal arteries to form the maxillomandibular branches of the stapedial arteries. In stage 4, the distal ICAs still end in the primitive olfactory arteries, but these arteries now have two branches. The original primitive olfactory arteries, now designated the "lateral branches," course to the nasal fossae. The new mesial branches pass to the roots of the olfactory nerves and will later carry the anterior cerebral arteries cephalically. The paired anterior cerebral arteries may join through a plexiform anastomosis, the future anterior communicating artery. A persistent trigeminal artery may now be seen. If so, the ipsilateral posterior communicating artery will be either small or entirely absent.

Arterial Stage 5

In stage 5 (CRL 16 to 18 mm, EGA 44 to 48 days), the common carotid arteries elongate as the heart descends into the chest. Two branches of each stapedial artery are now visible: the maxillomandibular arteries and the supraorbital arteries. The proximal internal maxillary arteries extend from the external carotid arteries to the maxillomandibular branches of the stapedial arteries (foreshadowing the future annexation of the middle meningeal arteries by the internal maxillary arteries). The supraorbital branches of the stapedial arteries course lateral to the geniculate ganglia, through the superior orbital fissures to supply the orbits.

The permanent stems of the ophthalmic arteries now give rise to the primitive ventral and primitive dorsal ophthalmic arteries. These two arteries anastomose within the orbit to form a loop around the optic nerve. The primitive dorsal ophthalmic arteries occasionally

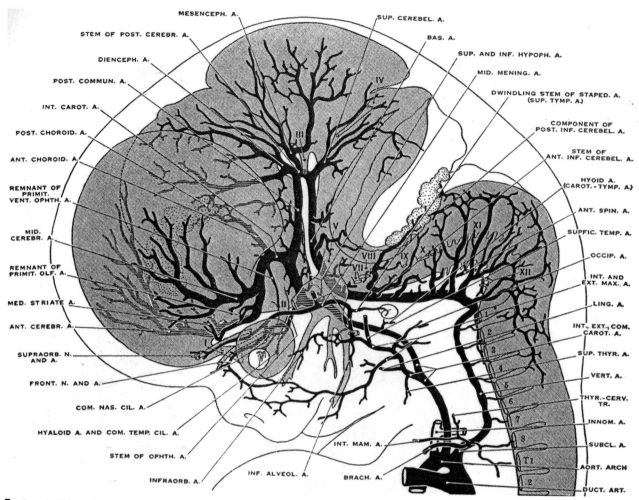

F   Arterial Stage 6

FIGURE 1–8 *(Continued)*

form the origins of the ophthalmic arteries. The ophthalmic arteries then arise from the cavernous segments of the ICAs and course through the superior orbital fissures. The proximal segments of the posterior cerebral arteries may now arise from the distal basilar artery.

Arterial Stage 6

In stage 6 (CRL 20 to 24 mm, EGA 51 days), the embryonic head begins to develop mature features and to lift away from the chest. The anterior communicating artery is now recognizable, completing the circle of Willis. A small branch arising from the anterior communicating artery extends to the commissural plate as the median artery of the corpus callosum. This branch usually regresses as the anterior cerebral arteries mature and begin to supply the corpus callosum. The median artery of the corpus callosum, however, may persist as an accessory anterior cerebral artery or even as an azygous anterior cerebral artery (when there is bilateral anterior cerebral artery aplasia).[2]

The stapedial arteries now undergo significant change: the supraorbital branches of the stapedial arteries give rise to orbital branches, which join the arterial rings previously formed around the optic nerves by the primitive ventral and dorsal ophthalmic arteries. The internal maxillary arteries have annexed the proximal portions of the maxillomandibular branches of the stapedial arteries. As a result, the future middle meningeal arteries will arise from the internal maxillary arteries.[2,7] Thus proximal portions of the maxillomandibular arteries form the stems of the middle meningeal arteries, whereas the dorsal aspects of the supraorbital arteries form the distal continuation of the middle meningeal arteries. Near the stapes, the stapedial arteries begin to dwindle. The more proximal remnants of the stapedial arteries remain as the superior tympanic arteries. The remnants of the hyoid arteries, which were, transiently, the stems for the stapedial arteries, remain as the caroticotympanic branches of the ICAs.

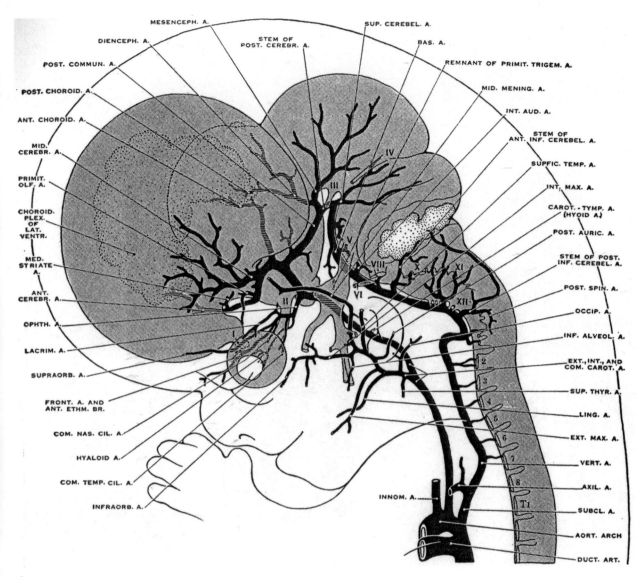

G   Arterial Stage 7

FIGURE 1–8 *(Continued)*

Arterial Stage 7

In stage 7 (CRL 40 mm, EGA 9 wks), the ophthalmic arteries have attained adult configuration. The intraorbital portions of the supraorbital arteries lose their connection to the stapedial arteries and are now supplied by the ophthalmic arteries. The circle of Willis also attains adult configuration. The size of the posterior communicating arteries varies inversely with the size of the P1 segments of the posterior cerebral arteries. Large "posterior communicating arteries" that give rise to the posterior cerebral arteries may be designated the persistent fetal origin of the posterior cerebral arteries or the "direct origin" of the posterior cerebral arteries. Cerebellar development is associated with marked reciprocal variations in the calibers and territories of the evolving cerebellar arteries.

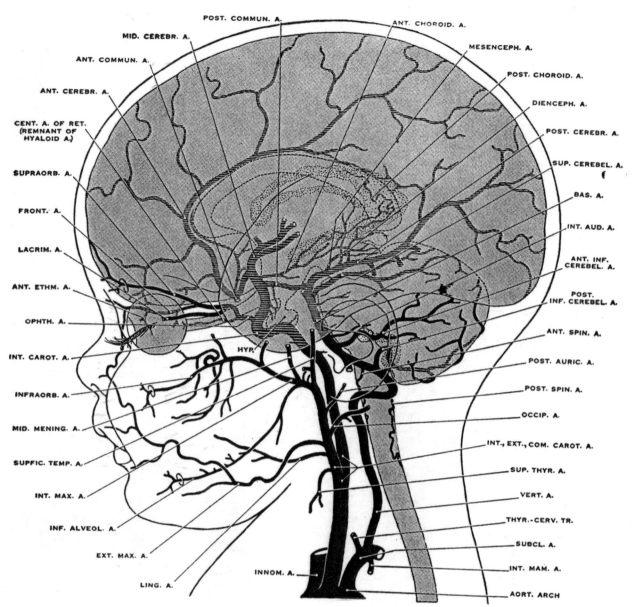

POST. COMMUN. A.
MID. CEREBR. A.
ANT. COMMUN. A.
ANT. CEREBR. A.
CENT. A. OF RET. (REMNANT OF HYALOID A.)
SUPRAORB. A.
FRONT. A.
LACRIM. A.
ANT. ETHM. A.
OPHTH. A.
INT. CAROT. A.
INFRAORB. A.
MID. MENING. A.
SUPFIC. TEMP. A.
INT. MAX. A.
INF. ALVEOL. A.
EXT. MAX. A.
LING. A.
HYP.
INNOM. A.

ANT. CHOROID. A.
MESENCEPH. A.
POST. CHOROID. A.
DIENCEPH. A.
POST. CEREBR. A.
SUP. CEREBEL. A.
BAS. A.
INT. AUD. A.
ANT. INF. CEREBEL. A.
POST. INF. CEREBEL. A.
ANT. SPIN. A.
POST. AURIC. A.
POST. SPIN. A.
OCCIP. A.
INT., EXT., COM. CAROT. A.
SUP. THYR. A.
VERT. A.
THYR.-CERV. TR.
SUBCL. A.
INT. MAM. A.
AORT. ARCH

H   Arterial System of Newborn

FIGURE 1–8 *(Continued)*

■ The Cerebral Venous System

Dorcas Padget similarly classified the developing venous system into eight stages (designated 1 to 7 and 7a).[4] Overall, venous development lags behind arterial development and shows a greater range of variation (**Fig. 1–9**).[4] The pial venous system lies deep to the cerebral arterial system.

Venous Stage 1

In stage 1 (CRL 4 mm, EGA 28 days), an endothelial meshwork extends upward from the paired first aortic arches and passes over the forebrain and midbrain in the midline to become the primary head-plexus. Longitudinal channels connect the head-plexus to the anterior cardinal veins, the future internal jugular veins. The primary head-plexus and the longitudinal channels constitute a primitive system of proliferating endothelium that gives rise to the veins of the brain.[1]

Venous Stage 2

In stage 2 (CRL 5 to 8 mm, EGA 32 days), the midline primary head-plexus disappears and is replaced by paired paramedian primary head-sinuses that provide the first true venous drainage for the developing brain. The primary head-sinuses course medial to the trigeminal ganglia and lateral to the otic capsules and the glossopharyngeal nerves en route to the internal jugular veins. Via superficial anastamosing loops, the paired primary head-sinuses connect with the capillary network investing the neural tube. These superficial anastamosing

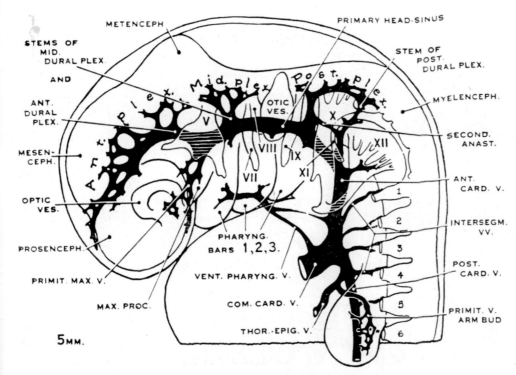

A Venous Stage 1

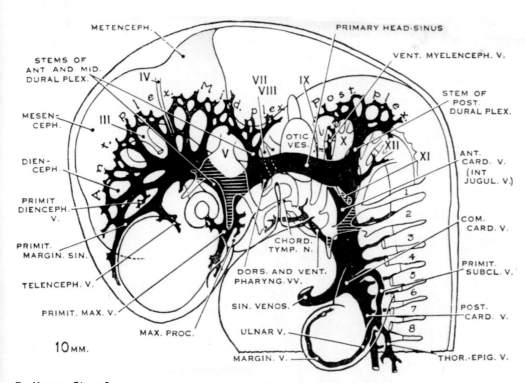

B Venous Stage 2

FIGURE 1–9 The cerebral venous system. **(A–H)** The eight sequential stages of venous formation detailed in the text. (Reprinted with permission from Padget DH. The cranial venous system in man in reference to development, adult configuration, and relation to the arteries. Am J Anat 1956;98:307–356, Plates 1 and 2, pp. 343 and 345.)

loops lie dorsally and are arranged into three major groups: the anterior, middle, and posterior dural plexi. The anterior dural plexi drain the forebrain and midbrain into the pre-trigeminal segments of the primary head-sinuses. The middle dural plexi drain the cerebellum into the otic segments of the primary head veins. The posterior dural plexi join the primary head-sinuses near to the vagus nerves.

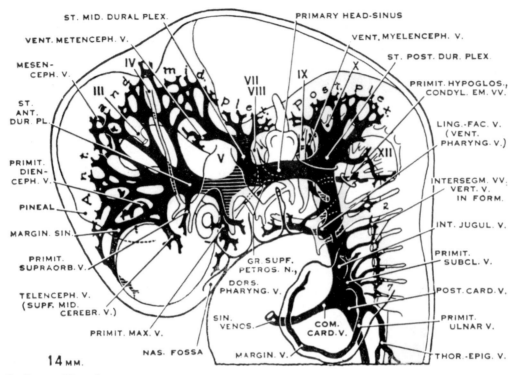

C   Venous Stage 3

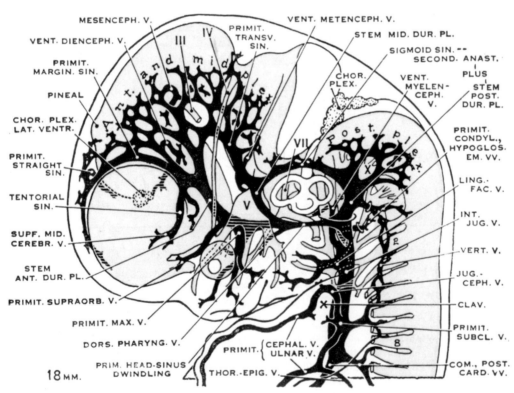

D   Venous Stage 4

FIGURE 1–9 *(Continued)*

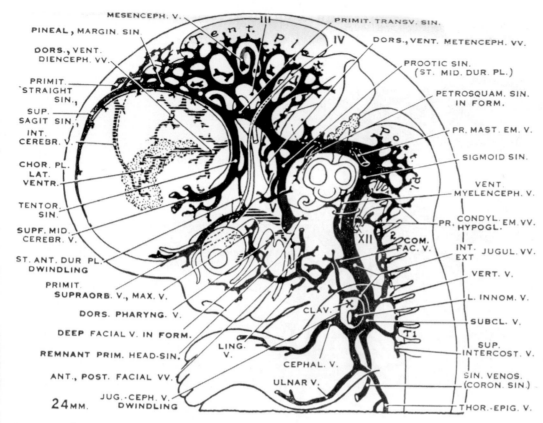

MESENCEPH. V.
PINEAL, MARGIN. SIN.
DORS., VENT. DIENCEPH. VV.
PRIMIT. STRAIGHT SIN.
SUP. SAGIT SIN.
INT. CEREBR. V.
CHOR. PL. LAT. VENTR.
TENTOR. SIN.
SUPF. MID. CEREBR. V.
ST. ANT. DUR PL. DWINDLING
PRIMIT. SUPRAORB. V., MAX. V.
DORS. PHARYNG. V.
DEEP FACIAL V. IN FORM.
REMNANT PRIM. HEAD-SIN.
ANT., POST. FACIAL VV.
JUG.-CEPH. V. DWINDLING

III
IV

Vent. Plex.
Post. Pl.

V
XII
CLAV.
LING. V.
CEPHAL. V.
ULNAR V.
X
T1
COM. FAC. V.

PRIMIT. TRANSV. SIN.
DORS., VENT. METENCEPH. VV.
PROOTIC SIN. (ST. MID. DUR. PL.)
PETROSQUAM. SIN. IN FORM.
PR. MAST. EM. V.
SIGMOID SIN.
VENT. MYELENCEPH. V.
PR. CONDYL. EM. VV. HYPOGL.
INT. JUGUL. VV. EXT
VERT. V.
L. INNOM. V.
SUBCL. V.
SUP. INTERCOST. V.
SIN. VENOS. (CORON. SIN.)
THOR.-EPIG. V.

24 MM.

E   Venous Stage 5

FIGURE 1–9 *(Continued)*

Ventrally, the paired ventral pharyngeal veins drain the mandibular and hyoid pharyngeal bars. The maxillary veins drain the developing maxillary processes.

Venous Stage 3

In stage 3 (CRL 8 to 11 mm, EGA 37 days), the marginal sinuses develop along the mesial borders of the anterior dural plexi. The marginal sinuses contribute to the developing transverse and superior sagittal sinuses. The stems of the posterior dural plexi change configuration to become the caudal ends of the sigmoid sinuses. The maxillary veins now drain both the optic and the olfactory regions. Paired primitive telencephalic and diencephalic veins arise in conjunction with the developing telencephalon and diencephalon.

> **PEARL** Arteriovenous malformations may arise in the few areas where the veins and arteries course parallel to each other, not at right angles, as in the choroid plexi.

Venous Stage 4

Stage 4 (CRL 11 to 16 mm, EGA 41 days) is significant for the separation of the meninges into the pia-arachnoid and the overlying dura.[28] In stage 4, pia-arachnoidal veins traverse the subarachnoid space to connect the dural plexi with the developing pial veins. The pial veins then form multiple interconnecting anastamoses that envelop the entire neural tube. Pial veins characteristically run at right angles to the overlying arteries. Arteriovenous malformations may arise in the few areas where the veins and arteries course parallel to each other, not at right angles, as in the choroid plexi.

The supraorbital veins develop and drain the optic vesicles into the stems of the anterior dural plexi between the fourth and fifth cranial nerves. The diencephalic veins give rise to ventral and dorsal branches. Mesencephalic veins now arise from the anterior dural plexi to drain the developing mesencephalon.

Venous Stage 5

In stage 5 (CRL 17 to 20 mm, EGA 44 to 48 days), the middle and posterior dural plexi anastamose to form the sigmoid sinuses. As the otic capsules enlarge, they compress the adjacent primary head-sinuses, so the primary head-sinuses largely regress. Therefore, flow reverses in the middle dural plexi so they begin to drain into the sigmoid sinuses. The residual stems of the middle dural plexi persist as the pro-otic sinuses.[4]

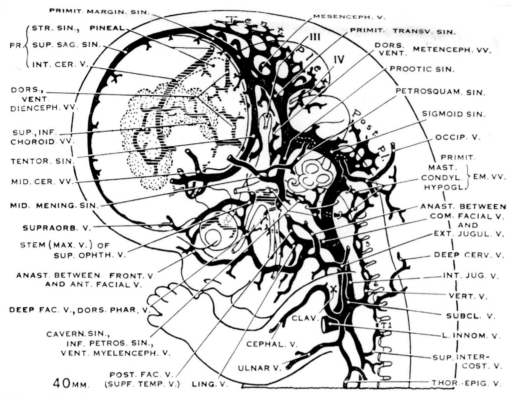

F Venous Stage 6

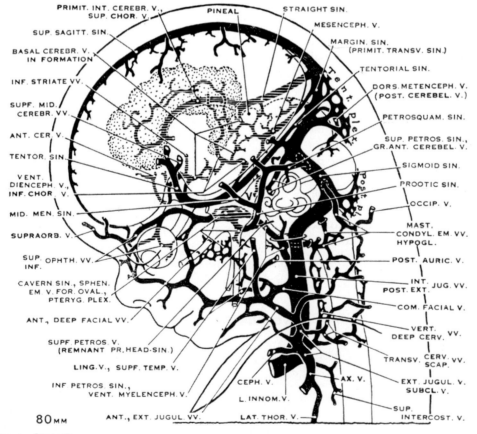

G Venous Stage 7

FIGURE 1–9 *(Continued)*

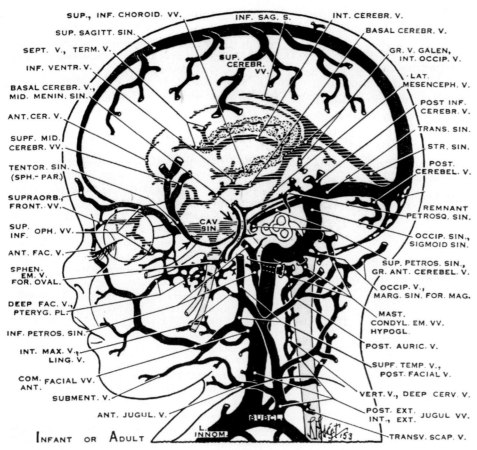

H   Venous System Newborn

FIGURE 1–9 *(Continued)*

Venous Stage 6

In stage 6 (CRL 20 to 24 mm, EGA 51 days) the anterior and middle dural plexi have joined to form the tentorial plexi. The marginal sinuses form the medial portions of the transverse sinuses. The supraorbital veins now drain through the remnants of the primitive head-sinuses to the pro-otic sinuses (the former stems of the middle dural plexi).

Venous Stage 7

In stage 7 (CRL 40 mm, EGA ~9 wks), the venous system begins to take final form. The medial aspects of the marginal sinuses join together, and through a series of anastamoses, form the superior sagittal sinus. The supraorbital and maxillary veins join to form the superior ophthalmic veins. Plexiform extensions from the pro-otic sinuses form the cavernous sinuses. The inferior petrosal sinuses form and connect the cavernous sinuses with the internal jugular veins. The choroid plexi drain through the ventral diencephalic veins to the transient median prosencephalic vein.[8]

Venous Stage 7a

In stage 7a (CRL 60 to 80 mm, EGA 10 to 12 wks), continued growth of the cerebrum and cerebellum shift the transverse sinuses laterally toward their adult position. The superior petrosal sinuses develop, completing the network of basal dural venous sinuses. The paired internal cerebral veins now arise in response to increased venous drainage from the developing basal ganglia. The internal cerebral veins join the posterior end of the median prosencephalic vein to form the vein of Galen. The internal cerebral veins gradually annex the drainage of the choroid plexus, so the median prosencephalic vein regresses. The basal cerebral veins form from highly variable anastamoses among the telencephalic veins, the ventral and dorsal diencephalic veins, and the mesencephalic veins.[29] Arteriovenous malformations and fistulae in the drainage of the median prosencephalic vein may cause increased flow through the system, persistence of the median prosencephalic vein, marked enlargement of the vein of Galen, persistence of a falcine sinus, and enlargement (or absence) of the straight sinus: key components of the vein of Galen malformation.[8]

■ Conclusion

Embryology provides the framework for deeper understanding of the normal model of the arteriovenous system of the brain, and its numerous variations. It is hoped that this summary will orient the reader to the major stages of embryogenesis and provide the vocabulary needed for further reading. Familiarity with this embryology will help to elucidate the origins of "anomalous vessels," origins of collateral feeders to arteriovenous malformations, patterns of collateral supply to ischemic regions, and potential routes of access for endovascular therapy.

ACKNOWLEDGMENTS

The authors thank Dr. Kenneth Faulder, Sydney, Australia for his help with reviewing the literature for this chapter.

REFERENCES

1. Streeter GL. The developmental alterations in the vascular system of the brain of the human embryo. Contrib Embryol 1918;8:5–38
2. Padget DH. The development of the cranial arteries in the human embryo. Contrib Embryol 1948;32:205–261
3. Padget DH. Designation of the embryonic intersegmental arteries in reference to the vertebral arteries and subclavian stem. Anat Rec 1954;119:349–356
4. Padget DH. The cranial venous system in man in reference to development, adult configuration, and relation to the arteries. Am J Anat 1956;98:307–356
5. Congdon ED. Transformation of the aortic arch system during the development of the human embryo. Contrib Embryol 1922;14: 47–110
6. Kier EL. Development of cerebral vessels. In: Newton TH, Potts DG, eds. Radiology of the Skull and Brain. Saint Louis, CV Mosby; 1974:1089–1141
7. Lasjaunias P, Berenstein A. Functional Anatomy of Craniofacial Arteries. Berlin, Hiedelberg: Springer-Verlag; 1987:1–143. Surgical Neuroangiography; vol 1
8. Raybaud CA, Strother CM, Hald JK. Aneurysms of the vein of Galen: embryonic considerations and anatomical features relating to the pathogenesis of the malformation. Neuroradiology 1989; 31:109–128
9. Naidich TP, Blaser SI, Delman BN, et al. Congenital anomalies of the spine and spinal cord: embryology and malformations. In: Atlas SW, ed. Magnetic Resonance Imaging of the Brain and Spine. Philadelphia: Lippincott Williams and Wilkins; 2002: 1527–1537
10. Osborn AG. Diagnostic Neuroradiology. St. Louis: Mosby; 1999
11. Truwit CL. Embryology of the cerebral vasculature. Neuroimaging Clin N Am 1994;4:663–689
12. McLone DG, Naidich TP. Embryology of the cerebral vascular system. In: Edwards MSB and Hoffman HJ, eds. Cerebral Vascular Disease in Children and Adolescents. Baltimore: Williams and Wilkins; 1989:1–16
13. Langman J. Medical Embryology. Baltimore: Williams and Wilkins; 1975
14. Larsen WJ. Differentiation of the somites and the nervous system: segmental development and integration. In: Larsen WJ, Sherman LS, Potter SS, Scott WJ, eds. Human Embryology. Philadelphia: Churchill Livingstone; 2001:79–98
15. Bär T. The vascular system of the cerebral cortex. Adv Anat Embryol Cell Biol 1980;59:1–62
16. Duckett S. The establishment of the internal vascularization in the human telencephalon. Acta Anat (Basel) 1971;80:107–113
17. Plate KH. Mechanisms of angiogenesis in the brain. J Neuropathol Exp Neurol 1999;58:313–320
18. Risau W. Mechanisms of angiogenesis. Nature 1997;386:671–674
19. Breier G, Risau W. The role of VEGF in blood vessel formation. Trends Cell Biol 1996;6:454–456
20. Gilbert SF. Lateral plate mesoderm and endoderm. In: Developmental Biology. Sunderland, MA: Sinauer Associates; 2000: 471–498
21. Kirks DR. Practical Pediatric Radiology: Diagnostic Imaging of Infants and Children. Philadelphia: Lippincott-Raven; 1998:581
22. Brismar J. Persistent hypoglossal artery, diagnostic criteria. Acta Radiol Diagn (Stockh) 1976;17:160–166
23. Reynolds AF Jr, Stovring J, Turner PT. Persistent otic artery. Surg Neurol 1980;13:115–117
24. Caldemeyer KS, Carrico JB, Mathews VB. The radiology and embryology of anomalous arteries of the head and neck. AJR Am J Roentgenol 1998;170:197–203
25. Salas E, Zkiyal IM, Sekhar LN, Wright DC. Persistent trigeminal artery: an anatomic study. Neurosurgery 1998;43:557–562
26. Andrews BT, Brant-Zawadzki M, Wilson CB. Variant aneurysms of the fenestrated basilar artery. Neurosurgery 1986;18:204–207
27. Sanders WP, Sorek PA, Menta BA. Fenestration of intracranial arteries with special attention to associated aneurysms and other anomalies. AJNR Am J Neuroradiol 1993;14:675–678
28. McLone DG, Naidich TP. Developmental morphology of the subarachnoid space, brain vasculature, and contiguous structures, and the cause of the Chiari II malformation. AJNR Am J Neuroradiol 1992;13:463–482
29. Suzuki Y, Ikeda H, Shimadu M, Ikeda Y, Matsumoto K. Variations of the basal vein: identification using three-dimensional CT angiography. AJNR Am J Neuroradiol 2001;22:670–676

2

Neurovascular Disorders and Syndromes in Children

E. STEVE ROACH AND CESAR C. SANTOS

Several congenital or hereditary disorders cause cerebrovascular dysfunction. This chapter reviews the major hereditary conditions with frequent cerebrovascular complications, such as hereditary hemorrhagic telangiectasia (HHT), Ehlers-Danlos syndrome (EDS), and pseudoxanthoma elasticum (PXE). Other conditions like Sturge-Weber syndrome (SWS) and progeria, where cerebrovascular dysfunction occur sporadically, are also reviewed.

■ Sturge-Weber Syndrome

SWS is a rare neurocutaneous syndrome characterized by a facial cutaneous angioma (port-wine nevus) and a leptomeningeal angiomatosis, which often occur ipsilaterally to the facial lesion. Classic neurological findings include epileptic seizures, mental retardation, contralateral hemiparesis and hemiatrophy, and homonymous hemianopia.[1–3] However, the clinical features vary widely, and many patients who have the typical skin lesion and seizures have normal intelligence and no focal neurological deficit. The syndrome occurs sporadically and in all races.[2,4]

Cutaneous Features of Sturge-Weber Syndrome

The nevus classically involves the forehead and upper eyelid, but it commonly affects both sides of the face and may extend onto the trunk and extremities (**Fig. 2–1**). The facial angioma is usually evident at birth. Patients whose nevus involves only the trunk, or the maxillary

or mandibular area, but not the upper face, do not develop neurological complications from an intracranial angioma.[5–7] The leptomeningeal angioma is typically ipsilateral to a unilateral facial nevus. However, bilateral brain lesions occur in at least 15% of patients, including those with unilateral facial nevi. Only 10 to 20% of children with a port-wine nevus of the forehead also have a leptomeningeal angioma.[6] The occurrence of the characteristic neurological and radiographic features of SWS without a skin lesion is quite rare.

Ophthalmologic Features of Sturge-Weber Syndrome

Glaucoma is the main ophthalmologic problem of patients with SWS.[8,9] The risk of developing glaucoma is highest in the first decade, although young adults occasionally develop glaucoma. In one study, 36 of 51 patients (71%) had glaucoma; 26 of these developed glaucoma by age 2 years.[8] Buphthalmos and amblyopia are present in some newborns, evidently due to an anomalous anterior chamber angle.[10,11] In other individuals, glaucoma becomes symptomatic later in life, and if not treated, causes progressive blindness. Thus periodic measurement of the intraocular pressure is essential, especially when the nevus is near the eye.

Diffuse choroidal hemangioma is another characteristic ophthalmologic finding in patients with SWS. It can be seen in up to 71% of cases.[12] It is characterized as a red, flat to moderately elevated lesion that produces a classic "tomato ketchup" appearance on funduscopic examination. It is almost always associated with leptomeningeal angiomatosis; therefore, when found, magnetic resonance imaging (MRI) of the brain should be obtained.

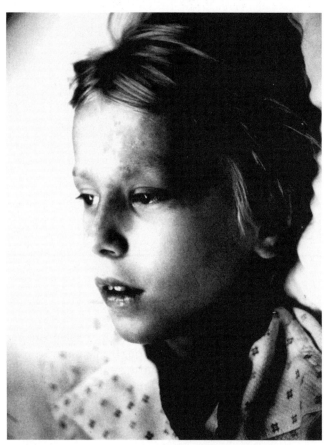

FIGURE 2–1 A patient with the classic distribution of the port-wine nevus of Sturge-Weber syndrome on the upper face and eyelid. (Reprinted with permission from Roach ES. Congenital cutaneovascular syndromes. In: Vinken PV, Bruyn GW, Klawans HL, eds. Vascular Diseases. Amsterdam: Elsevier; 1989:443–462. Handbook of Clinical Neurology; vol 11.)

Neurological Features of Sturge-Weber Syndrome

Epileptic seizures, mental retardation, and focal neurological deficits are the principal neurological abnormalities of SWS. Intracranial hemorrhage due to SWS is rare. Seizures usually start acutely in conjunction with hemiparesis. The age when symptoms begin and the overall clinical severity can both vary, but onset of seizures prior to age 2 increases the likelihood of mental retardation and refractory epilepsy. Patients with refractory seizures are more likely to be mentally retarded, whereas patients who have never had seizures are typically normal. Rarely would a patient develop severe intellectual impairment if normal past age 3.

Seizures eventually develop in 72 to 80% of SWS patients with unilateral lesions and in 93% of patients with bihemispheric involvement.[13,14] Seizures can begin at any time from birth to adulthood, but 75% of those with seizures begin during the first year, 86% by age 2, and 95% prior to age 5.[9] Thus the risk of a child developing seizures is highest in the first 2 years. Focal motor seizures or generalized tonic clonic seizures are characteristic of SWS initially, but infantile spasms, myoclonic seizures, and atonic seizures have been reported.[15,16] The first few seizures are often focal, even in patients who later develop generalized tonicoclonic seizures or infantile spasms.[15] Older children and adults are more likely to have complex partial seizures or focal motor seizures. Some patients continue to have daily seizures after the initial deterioration in spite of various daily anticonvulsant medications, whereas others have long seizure-free intervals, sometimes even without medication, punctuated by clusters of seizures.[16]

Many patients do not develop permanent focal neurological signs. In those who do, the specific deficit varies with the location of the intracranial vascular lesion. The occipital region is often affected, so visual field deficits are common.[17] Hemiparesis often develops acutely, in conjunction with the initial flurry of seizures. Although often attributed to postictal weakness, hemiparesis may be permanent or it can persist much longer than the few hours typical of a postictal deficit. Some children suddenly develop weakness without seizures, either as repeated episodes of weakness similar to transient ischemic attacks or as a single strokelike episode with persistent deficit.[18] In patients with both hemiparesis and seizures, it is difficult to establish which came first.

Early developmental milestones are usually normal, but mild to profound mental deficiency eventually develops in at least half of SWS patients.[19] Only 8% of the patients with bilateral brain involvement are intellectually normal.[13] Behavioral abnormalities are often problematic, even in patients who are not mentally retarded. The clinical condition eventually stabilizes after a few years without further deterioration.

Diagnostic Studies in SWS

Most of the children with facial port-wine nevi do not have an intracranial angioma, and neuroimaging studies and other tests help to distinguish the children with SWS from those with an isolated cutaneous lesion. Although gyral calcification is a classic feature of SWS, the "trolley track" appearance first described on standard radiographs is uncommon, especially in neonates. Intracranial calcification is best demonstrated with computed tomography (**Fig. 2–2**). Extensive cerebral atrophy is apparent even with computed tomography, but subtle atrophy is more readily demonstrated by MRI.[20,21]

MRI with gadolinium contrast (**Fig. 2–3**) effectively demonstrates the abnormal intracranial vessels in individuals with SWS.[20,22,23] It is currently the best test to determine intracranial involvement. Magnetic resonance

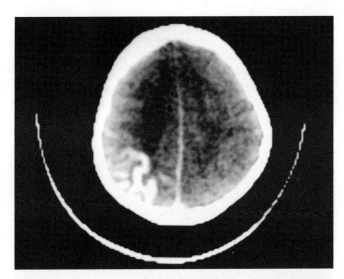

FIGURE 2–2 Computed cranial tomography demonstrates an occipital gyriform calcification typical of Sturge-Weber syndrome. (Reprinted with permission from Garcia JC, Roach ES, McLean WT. Recurrent thrombotic deterioration in the Sturge-Weber syndrome. Child's Brain 1981;8:427–433.)

angiography has recently been used to directly image the larger abnormal vessels.[24]

Cerebral angiography is not necessary for most patients with SWS, but it is sometimes useful in atypical patients or prior to epilepsy surgery. The veins are more abnormal than the arteries.[25] The subependymal and medullary veins are enlarged and tortuous, and the superficial cortical veins tend to be sparse.[26] Failure of the sagittal sinus to opacify after ipsilateral carotid injection may be secondary to obliteration of the superficial cortical veins by thrombosis.[27] The abnormal deep venous channels act as collaterals from the cerebral cortex to the deep veins.[25,27]

Positron emission tomography (PET) demonstrates reduced metabolism of the brain adjacent to the leptomeningeal lesion.[28] However, patients with recent-onset seizures may have increased cerebral metabolism near the lesion. Single photon emission tomography (SPECT) shows reduced perfusion of the affected brain.[29] Both PET and SPECT often indicate vascular alterations more extensive than those shown by computed cranial tomography.[28,30] Although functional imaging is not necessary

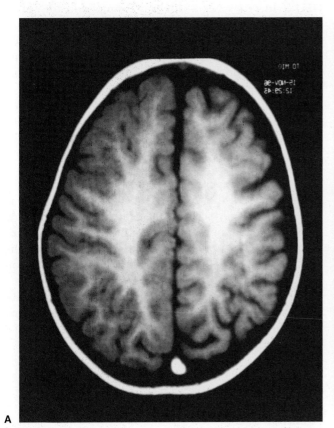

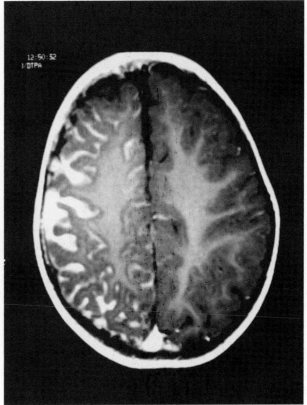

A   B

FIGURE 2–3 (A) Normal T1-weighted magnetic resonance scan without contrast infusion from a child with Sturge-Weber syndrome. **(B)** On the coronal view with gadolinium, his scan reveals a left-sided leptomeningeal and intraparenchymal angioma. (Reprinted with permission from Roach ES, Bodensteiner JB. Neurologic complications. In: Bodensteiner JB, Roach ES, eds. The Sturge-Weber Syndrome. New York: Sturge-Weber Foundation; 1999.)

for all patients, these tests may help to establish a diagnosis and localize the lesion prior to surgery.

> **PEARL** Resection of the brain containing the vascular abnormality sometimes improves seizure control and promotes intellectual development.

Treatment of Sturge-Weber Syndrome

Resection of the brain containing the vascular abnormality sometimes improves seizure control and promotes intellectual development.[31,32] Despite the general agreement that surgical resection is effective, there is debate about patient selection and timing of surgery. Almost one patient in five has bilateral cerebral lesions, limiting the surgical options unless one hemisphere is clearly causing most of the seizures. There is also reluctance to resect a still functional portion of the brain and cause a new deficit.[33] Surgery is often reserved for patients with severe seizures who do not respond to medication and who already have clinical dysfunction of the area to be removed (e.g., hemiparesis or hemianopia), similar to the approach in children with refractory epilepsy from other causes.[34] Outcome following hemispherectomy is encouraging with 81% of patients becoming seizure-free, with over half of the patients off of antiepileptic medications.[35]

Prophylactic daily aspirin has been suggested for SWS because of the frequent occurrence of transient neurological deficits without seizures and the idea that thromboses of the abnormal veins initiate episodes of clinical deterioration in patients with SWS.[18] This recommendation is difficult to study because of the variability of the clinical manifestation of SWS.

■ Hereditary Hemorrhagic Telangiectasia

HHT (Osler-Weber-Rendu disease) is an autosomal dominant disorder that features telangiectasias of the skin, mucous membranes, and various internal organs.[36–39] Clinical diagnostic criteria have been published.[39] However, both the clinical manifestations and the age of presentation are variable, and diagnosis may be difficult in younger patients without the full array of signs.[39,40]

Cutaneous Features of Hereditary Hemorrhagic Telangiectasia

Cutaneous telangiectasias occur more often on the face, lips, and hands than on the trunk or legs.[37,41] Epistaxis due to telangiectasias of the nasal mucosa is often the first indication of HHT.[37,42,43] About a third of patients have conjunctival telangiectasias and 10% have retinal vascular malformations, but visual loss from these lesions is uncommon.[44] Although telangiectasias are not often conspicuous during the first decade, thereafter they tend to enlarge and multiply.[43]

Arterial Lesions of Hereditary Hemorrhagic Telangiectasia

In addition to the vascular lesions affecting the central nervous system, vascular malformations affect the lungs, gastrointestinal tract, or genitourinary system and can lead to hemoptysis, hematemesis, melena, or hematuria.[37,41,43,45]

Neurological Features of Hereditary Hemorrhagic Telangiectasia

Headache, dizziness, and seizures are common in individuals with HHT.[46–48] More severe but fortunately less common problems include paradoxical embolism with stroke, intraparenchymal and subarachnoid hemorrhage, meningitis, and cerebral abscess.

Paradoxical embolism through a pulmonary arteriovenous fistula can cause cerebral infarction in patients with HHT.[49] In rare cases a clot may form within the fistula itself before migrating into the arterial circulation.[50] Intermittent symptoms follow repeated small emboli with subsequent improvement. Transient deficits during hemoptysis could result from air embolism via a bleeding pulmonary arteriovenous fistula.[51–53]

An estimated 1% of HHT patients develop cerebral abscess or meningitis, probably resulting from septic microemboli that bypass the normal filtration of the pulmonary circulation via a pulmonary arteriovenous fistula.[54] Mycotic aneurysms develop the same way.

Vascular anomalies may be found anywhere in the brain, spinal cord, or meninges,[55–57] and more than one type of lesion may occur in the same individual.[55] Intracerebral vascular anomalies occur more often than once suspected. One summary of 90 HHT patients from the literature recorded 17 (19%) with arteriovenous malformations and 36 (40%) with telangiectasias or angiomas.[55] Fulbright and colleagues identified 42 patients with various types of cerebral vascular anomalies among 184 consecutive HHT patients who underwent cranial MRI studies.[58]

> **PEARL** Intracranial vascular lesions of HHT are less likely to bleed than sporadic arteriovenous malformations.

Many of these patients remained asymptomatic, and there is some evidence that the intracranial vascular lesions of HHT are less likely to bleed than sporadic arteriovenous malformations.[59] However, in patients younger than 45 years of age, male HHT patients are 20 times more likely to develop cerebral hemorrhage compared with the general population.[60] These data support a more aggressive approach to the evaluation and treatment of these patients. HHT should be considered in patients with multiple cerebrovascular malformations.[59,61–63]

Saccular aneurysms are much less common in HHT patients than arteriovenous malformations.[55,64,65] The number of individuals with both HHT and intracranial aneurysm is small enough that the association could be coincidental. The same is true of spontaneous carotid-cavernous fistula.[66]

Genetics of Hereditary Hemorrhagic Telangiectasia

HHT is an autosomal dominant disorder with age-related penetrance and variable expressivity. Its occurs in 1 in 10,000 individuals,[67] ~30% of the time via spontaneous mutation.

Genes on chromosomes 9 and 12 are responsible for HHT1 and HHT2, respectively. The HHT1 gene at 9q33–34 codes for endoglin, an accessory membrane glycoprotein expressed at high levels in vascular endothelium.[67] HHT2 results from mutation of the ALK1 activin receptor-like kinase-1 gene at 12q13. Like endoglin, ALK1 is expressed at high levels in endothelial cells.[68] Individuals with HHT1 have a greater risk of pulmonary arterial malformations than those with HHT2, whereas those with HHT2 tend to have a milder phenotype and later onset of symptoms.[67] Molecular genetic testing for HHT is currently available. It is currently indicated in individuals with symptoms strongly suggestive of the disease and in asymptomatic first-degree relatives of an affected individual.[69]

■ Ehlers-Danlos Syndrome

Several subtypes of EDS can be defined by clinical features, inheritance patterns, and distinctive molecular defects.[70–72] Collectively these syndromes are characterized by fragile or hyperelastic skin (**Fig. 2–4**), hyperextensible joints, vascular lesions, easy bruising, and excessive scarring after injuries.[71] About 80% of the patients with EDS have types I, II, or III, and the other subtypes are less common.[71] Most of the vascular complications such as aneurysm and arterial dissection occur with type IV EDS, and these complications often lead to premature death.[73] All of the familial Ehlers-Danlos patients with a documented abnormality of type III collagen have displayed autosomal dominant inheritance.[71]

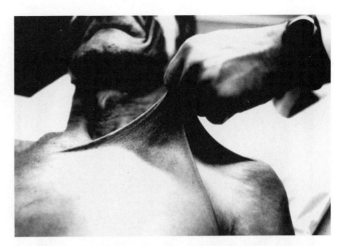

FIGURE 2–4 Hyperelasticity of the skin in a patient with EDS. (Reprinted with permission from Roach ES. Congenital cutaneovascular syndromes. In: Vinken PV, Bruyn GW, Klawans HL, eds. Vascular Diseases. Amsterdam: Elsevier; 1989:443–462. Handbook of Clinical Neurology; vol 11.)

Neurovascular Complications of Ehlers-Danlos Syndrome

Rubinstein and Cohen[74] first reported a woman with EDS and aneurysms of both the internal carotid and vertebral arteries. Many other individuals with extracranial and intracranial aneurysms have since been reported, including several people with multiple intracranial aneurysms.[75–77] Most patients became symptomatic in early adulthood, but children and adolescents are occasionally affected.

The internal carotid artery is the most likely intracranial vessel to develop an aneurysm due to EDS type IV (**Fig. 2–5**). Typically, the aneurysm develops in the cavernous sinus or just as the carotid emerges from the sinus.[74,77,78] Rupture of an aneurysm in this location creates a cavernous-carotid fistula. Aneurysms also affect various other intracranial arteries,[79] and these are more likely to present with subarachnoid hemorrhage. In one EDS family, members of three different generations suffered subarachnoid hemorrhage.[77]

Surgery is difficult because the arteries are friable and difficult to suture.[76,80] The arteries fail to hold sutures, and handling the tissue leads to tears of the artery or separation of the arterial layers.[81]

> **PEARL** The vascular fragility of type IV EDS makes both standard angiography and intravascular occlusion of the fistula more difficult.

Carotid-cavernous fistula has been documented in several individuals with EDS, sometimes following minor

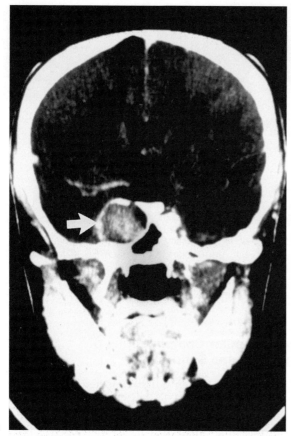

FIGURE 2–5 (A) Coronal computed tomography with contrast (from an 18-year-old with headaches and a family history of Ehlers-Danlos syndrome type IV) reveals a large aneurysm (arrow) of the intracavernous carotid artery. **(B)** Internal carotid angiogram confirms the giant aneurysm of the intracavernous carotid artery. (Reproduced with permission from Roach ES and Zimmerman CF. Ehlers-Danlos syndrome. In: Bogousslavsky J, Caplan LR, eds. Stroke Syndromes. London: Cambridge University Press; 1995:491–496.)

head trauma but for the most part spontaneously.[76] Intracranial aneurysms and carotid-cavernous fistulae often occur together.[84,85] Rupture of an internal carotid artery aneurysm within the cavernous sinus probably causes many of the fistulae.[83,86,87] However, spontaneous fistula formation without an aneurysm does occur.[88,89] Fragmentation of the internal elastic membrane and fibrosis of portions of the carotid wall are typically found at autopsy.[76,90]

The vascular fragility of type IV EDS makes both standard angiography and intravascular occlusion of the fistula very difficult.[85,86,91,92] Nevertheless, intravascular occlusion is sometimes successful.[93,94]

Arterial dissection due to EDS has been documented in most of the intracranial and extracranial arteries, and the clinical presentation depends primarily on which artery is affected.[95] Dissection of an intrathoracic artery can secondarily occlude cervical vessels,[96] and distal embolism from a dissection can cause cerebral infarction, sometimes weeks or months after the dissection occurs.

Genetics of Ehlers-Danlos Syndrome Type IV

EDS type IV is an autosomal dominant disorder with frequent spontaneous mutations. It results from a mutation of the COLA3A1 gene on chromosome 2, a gene that codes for the α 1 chain of type III collagen, which is expressed in high levels in blood vessels.[97] Various COLA3A1 mutations have been identified, but there is no consistent genotype–phenotype correlation.[97–102] Unsuspected mutations of the COLA3A1 gene that cause EDS type IV were not found in a cohort of 58 patients with an intracranial aneurysm or cervical dissection but no other signs of EDS.[82]

■ Pseudoxanthoma Elasticum

PXE is a hereditary connective tissue disorder with skin, ophthalmic, and vascular manifestations.[103,104] The clinical presentation and rate of progression vary considerably even among affected members of the same family.[105] Both autosomal dominant and autosomal recessive forms of PXE exist.[106]

Cutaneous Lesions of Pseudoxanthoma Elasticum

Cutaneous signs consist of yellowish plaques or papules of the neck, axilla, and abdomen, and the inguinal, decubital, or popliteal areas. Similar-looking lesions have been observed in the mucous membranes or intestinal mucosa. Older patients share a facial resemblance due to the lax redundant cutaneous changes of the face and neck.[107] Pregnancy, puberty, and stressful emotional situations may increase the rate of progression of the cutaneous lesions.[108] Although the skin lesions of PXE become apparent during the first decade in about half of the patients,[108] occlusive or hemorrhagic vascular complications occur primarily in adults.

Ophthalmic Lesions of Pseudoxanthoma Elasticum

Angioid streaks of the ocular fundus, the result of ruptures of Bruch's membrane, occur in 85% of individuals with PXE. These ocular lesions are gray or red irregular lines that radiate away from the optic disk.[109,110] Gradual visual loss may develop from macular degeneration, or visual loss can develop acutely from retinal hemorrhage.[103]

Arterial Lesions of Pseudoxanthoma Elasticum

Most of the systemic complications of PXE result from arterial degeneration and occlusion, but the exact clinical presentation depends largely on which organ system is affected. Progressive occlusion of the large arteries of the limbs may lead to intermittent claudication. Large arteries are sometimes palpably rigid, and radiographs of the extremities sometimes show arterial calcification.[111] Coronary artery disease sometimes occurs in young patients with PXE.[112] Gastrointestinal hemorrhage occurs primarily in adults, but it also occurs in children.[113–115] Pregnancy may increase the frequency of gastrointestinal hemorrhage.[116,117] Epistaxis, hematuria, and hemoptysis occur but less often than gastrointestinal hemorrhage.[118]

Neurological Dysfunction with Pseudoxanthoma Elasticum

Neurological dysfunction is due to vascular compromise. Brain dysfunction can result either directly from arterial occlusion or rupture or indirectly from systemic hypertension or cardiovascular disease.[119] Cerebrovascular lesions due to PXE do not usually manifest until adulthood, when single or multiple cerebrovascular occlusions result from progressive narrowing and then occlusion of an artery.[120,121] The angiographic pattern resembles that of severe atherosclerosis,[122] but gradual vessel occlusion sometimes allows sufficient collateral flow to avert a stroke.[121]

Aneurysms of the intracranial carotid artery are common,[119] and aneurysms of the other intracranial arteries also occur.[123,124]

Genetics of Pseudoxanthoma Elasticum

PXE results from a mutation of an ABC transporter gene at 16p13.1.[125–128] Both the autosomal dominant and autosomal recessive forms of PXE have been linked to 16p13.1, suggesting that allelic heterogeneity of a single gene accounts for all of the cases.[129,130]

■ Progeria

Hutchinson-Gilford syndrome or progeria (derived from *pro*, before, and *geras*, old age) is a rare condition characterized by premature aging (**Fig. 2–6A**) and the early occurrence of age-related complications. DeBusk estimates that one person in 8 million develops progeria.[131]

Clinical Features of Progeria

The signs of progeria usually become apparent during the first 2 years of life. Some features may be subtle or absent initially, then worsen over time. Alopecia, for example, may not be present at first, but is almost universal by adolescence (**Fig. 2–6B**). The most common early features are short stature, decreased subcutaneous fat stores, joint restriction, and alopecia.[131,132] Skeletal changes include thinning of the bones, coxa valga, and small clavicles. Some children have repeated poorly healing fractures.[133] The characteristic physical appearance of progeria results from a combination of postural changes, decreased subcutaneous fat, alopecia, and facial hypoplasia and micrognathia.

Children with progeria eventually develop premature atherosclerosis, leading to coronary artery disease or stroke (**Fig. 2–6C**).[134,135] Heart disease is the chief cause of death in patients with progeria.[135] Survival into middle age has been described, but death during the second decade is typical.[135]

Several other syndromes also cause signs of premature aging or carotid occlusion with stroke, and these disorders constitute the differential diagnosis of progeria. Werner's syndrome is an autosomal recessive disorder characterized by cataracts, scleroderma with subcutaneous calcium deposition, a beaklike nose, and the premature appearance usually associated with aging, such as graying of the

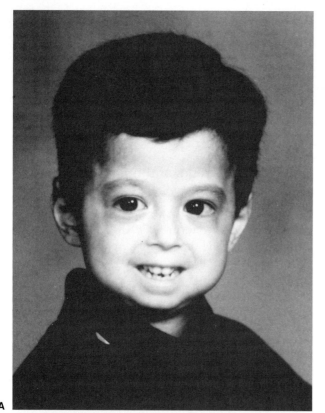

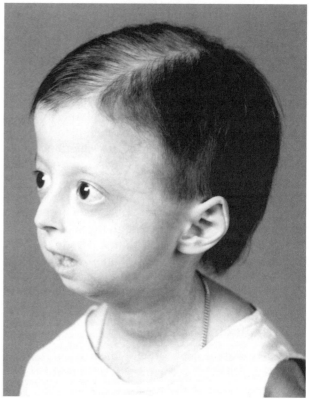

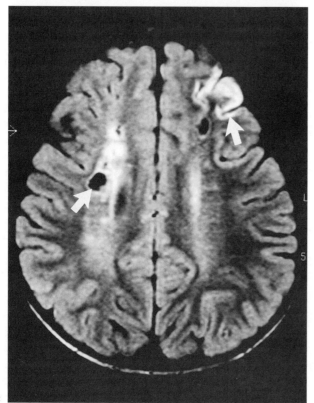

FIGURE 2–6 Premature aging in a young boy with multiple ischemic infarctions. **(A)** School portrait prior to the onset of symptoms. **(B)** Later photograph reveals hair loss, stooped posture, and loss of subcutaneous fat. **(C)** Magnetic resonance image shows multiple ischemic infarctions of different ages (arrows). (Reprinted with permission from Miller VS, Roach ES. Neurocutaneous syndromes. In: Bradley W, Daroff RB, Fenichel GM, Marsden CD, eds. Neurology in Clinical Practice. 3rd ed. Boston: Butterworth-Heinemann; 2000.)

hair, senile macular degeneration, osteoporosis, diabetes, malignancies, and atherosclerosis.[132,136,137] Werner's syndrome has been described as adult progeria.[138] Affected individuals often live well into adulthood, and, even so, death from cardiac disease and stroke seem to be less common than in patients with progeria. Mandibuloacral dysplasia is another autosomal recessive disorder characterized by alopecia and short stature, along with clavicular and mandibular hypoplasia, stiff joints, and persistently open cranial sutures. Whether this is an entirely distinct condition is still in question.

Pathophysiology of Progeria

Patients with progeria do not reproduce and most do not have affected family members. Some of the children who do have affected siblings have had atypical features,[139,140] leading to debate about the genetic nature of progeria. Both autosomal dominant and recessive traits have been proposed, but the clinical pattern is perhaps best explained by a dominant trait, usually arising via spontaneous mutation, with occasional instances of germline mosaicism in the families with affected siblings.

The pathogenesis of progeria is not well understood. In one study, cultured fibroblasts derived from an individual with progeria became senescent earlier than control cells, and the patient's fibroblasts had reduced levels of messenger ribonucleic acid coding for the macromolecules of the extracellular matrix.[141] Progeria could be explained by an abnormality of telomerase, shown recently to determine the number of cell replications before cellular senescence, but this remains speculative. A more recent article showed that cellular aging of the patient's fibroblasts is characterized by a period of hyperproliferation terminating in a large increase in the rate of apoptosis.[142]

Genetics of Progeria

Laminopathies are a group of genetic conditions that result from mutations of the LMNA gene that encodes nuclear lamin A/C. Hutchinson-Gilford progeria syndrome belongs to this group of diseases, the autosomal recessive form of which has been found to be due to homozygous missense mutation in the LMNA gene.[143] The autosomal dominant form of the disease on the other hand has been attributed to heterozygous, recurrent de novo mutation in the lamin A/C gene.[144,145]

REFERENCES

1. Alexander GL, Norman RM. Sturge-Weber Syndrome. Bristol: John Wright & Sons Ltd; 1960
2. Roach ES. Neurocutaneous syndromes. Pediatr Clin North Am 1992;39:591–620
3. Bodensteiner JB, Roach ES, eds. Sturge-Weber Syndrome. Mt. Freedom, NJ: Sturge-Weber Foundation; 1999
4. Peterman AF, Hayles AB, Dockerty MB, Love JG. Encephalotrigeminal angiomatosis (Sturge-Weber disease): clinical study of thirty-five cases. JAMA 1958;167:2169–2176
5. Uram M, Zubillaga C. The cutaneous manifestations of Sturge-Weber syndrome. J Clin Neuroophthalmol 1982;2:245–248
6. Enjolras O, Riche MC, Merland JJ. Facial port-wine stains and Sturge-Weber syndrome. Pediatrics 1985;76:48–51
7. Tallman B, Tan OT, Morelli JG, et al. Location of port-wine stains and the likelihood of ophthalmic and/or central nervous system complications. Pediatrics 1991;87:323–327
8. Sullivan TJ, Clarke MP, Morin JD. The ocular manifestations of the Sturge-Weber syndrome. J Pediatr Ophthalmol Strabismus 1992;29:349–356
9. Sujansky E, Conradi S. Sturge-Weber syndrome: age of onset of seizures and glaucoma and the prognosis for affected children. J Child Neurol 1995;10:49–58
10. Wagner RS, Caputo AR, Del Negro RG, Neigel J. Trabeculectomy with cyclocryotherapy for infantile glaucoma in the Sturge-Weber syndrome. Ann Ophthalmol 1988;20:289–291
11. Cibis GW, Tripathi RC, Tripathi BJ. Glaucoma in Sturge-Weber syndrome. Ophthalmology 1984;91:1061–1071
12. Sullivan TJ, Clarke MP, Morin JD. The ocular manifestations of Sturge-Weber syndrome. J Pediatr Ophthalmol Strabismus 1992;29:349–356
13. Bebin EM, Gomez MR. Prognosis in Sturge-Weber disease: comparison of unihemispheric and bihemispheric involvement. J Child Neurol 1988;3:181–184
14. Oakes WJ. The natural history of patients with the Sturge-Weber syndrome. Pediatr Neurosurg 1992;18:287–290
15. Fukuyama Y, Tsuchiya S. A study on Sturge-Weber syndrome. Eur Neurol 1979;18:194–204
16. Chevrie JJ, Specola N, Aicardi J. Secondary bilateral synchrony in unilateral pial angiomatosis: successful surgical management. J Neurol Neurosurg Psychiatry 1988;51:663–670
17. Aicardi J, Arzimanoglou A. Sturge-Weber syndrome. Int Pediatr 1991;6:129–134
18. Garcia JC, Roach ES, McLean WT. Recurrent thrombotic deterioration in the Sturge-Weber syndrome. Childs Brain 1981;8:427–433
19. Sujansky E, Conradi S. Outcome of Sturge-Weber syndrome in 52 adults. Am J Med Genet 1995;57:35–45
20. Elster AD, Chen MY. Magnetic resonance imaging of Sturge-Weber syndrome: role of gadopentetate dimeglumine and gradient-echo techniques. AJNR Am J Neuroradiol 1990;11:685–689
21. Chamberlain MC, Press GA, Hesselink JR. MR imaging and CT in three cases of Sturge-Weber syndrome: prospective comparison. AJNR Am J Roentgenol 1989;10:491–496
22. Lipski S, Brunelle F, Aicardi J, Hirsch JF, Lallemand D. Gd-DOTA-enhanced MR imaging in two cases of Sturge-Weber syndrome. AJNR Am J Neuroradiol 1990;11:690–692
23. Benedikt RA, Brown DC, Walker R, Ghaed VN, Mitchell M, Geyer CA. Sturge-Weber syndrome: cranial MR imaging with Gd-DTPA. AJNR Am J Neuroradiol 1993;14:409–415
24. Vogl TJ, Stemmler J, Bergman C, Pfluger T, Egger E, Lissner J. MR and MR angiography of Sturge-Weber syndrome. AJNR Am J Neuroradiol 1993;14:417–425
25. Probst FP. Vascular morphology and angiographic flow patterns in Sturge-Weber angiomatosis. Neuroradiology 1980;20:73–78
26. Farrell MA, DeRosa MJ, Curran JG, et al. Neuropathologic findings in cortical resections (including hemispherectomies) performed for the treatment of intractable childhood epilepsy. Acta Neuropathol (Berl) 1992;83:246–259
27. Bentson JR, Wilson GH, Newton TH. Cerebral venous drainage pattern of the Sturge-Weber syndrome. Radiology 1971;101:111–118

28. Chugani HT, Mazziotta JC, Phelps ME. Sturge-Weber syndrome: a study of cerebral glucose utilization with positron emission tomography. J Pediatr 1989;114:244–253

29. Chiron C, Raynaud C, Tzourio N, et al. Regional cerebral blood flow by SPECT imaging in Sturge-Weber disease: an aid for diagnosis. J Neurol Neurosurg Psychiatry 1989;52:1402–1409

30. Maria BL, Neufeld JA, Rosainz LC, et al. Central nervous system structure and function in Sturge-Weber syndrome: evidence of neurologic and radiologic progression. J Child Neurol 1998;13: 606–618

31. Carson BS, Javedan SP, Freeman JM, et al. Hemispherectomy: a hemidecortication approach and review of 52 cases. J Neurosurg 1996;84:903–911

32. Vining EP, Freeman JM, Pillas DJ, et al. Why would you remove half a brain? The outcome of 58 children after hemispherectomy: the Johns Hopkins experience: 1968 to 1996. Pediatrics 1997;100: 163–171

33. Arzimanoglou A, Aicardi J. The epilepsy of Sturge-Weber syndrome: clinical features and treatment in 23 patients. Acta Neurol Scand Suppl 1992;140:18–22

34. Roach ES, Riela AR, Chugani HT, Shinnar S, Bodensteiner JB, Freeman J. Sturge-Weber syndrome: recommendations for surgery. J Child Neurol 1994;9:190–193

35. Kossoff EH, Buck C, Freeman JM. Outcomes of 32 hemispherectomies for Sturge-Weber syndrome worldwide. Neurology 2002;59: 1735–1738

36. Garland HG, Anning ST. Hereditary haemorrhagic telangiectasia: a genetic and bibliographical study. Brit J Dermatol Syphil 1950; 62:289–310

37. Reilly PJ, Nostrant TT. Clinical manifestations of hereditary hemorrhagic telangiectasia. Am J Gastroenterol 1984;79:363–367

38. Guillen B, Guizar J, de la Cruz J, Salamanca F. Hereditary hemorrhagic telangiectasia: report of 15 affected cases in a Mexican family. Clin Genet 1991;39:214–218

39. Shovlin CL, Guttmacher AE, Buscarini E, et al. Diagnostic criteria for hereditary hemorrhagic telangiectasia (Rendu-Osler-Weber syndrome). Am J Med Genet 2000;91:66–67

40. McCue CM, Hartenberg M, Nance WE. Pulmonary arteriovenous malformations related to Rendu-Osler-Weber syndrome. Am J Med Genet 1984;19:19–27

41. Bird RM, Hammarsten JF, Marshall RA, Robinson RR. A family reunion: a study of hereditary hemorrhagic telangiectasia. N Engl J Med 1957;257:105–109

42. Bean WB. Congenital and hereditary lesions and birthmarks. In: Vascular Spiders and Related Lesions of the Skin. Springfield, IL: Charles C Thomas; 1958:132–194

43. Plauchu H, de Chadarevian JP, Bideau A, Robert JM. Age-related clinical profile of hereditary hemorrhagic telangiectasia in an epidemiologically recruited population. Am J Med Genet 1989; 32:291–297

44. Brant AM, Schachat AP, White RI. Ocular manifestations in hereditary hemorrhagic telangiectasia (Rendu-Osler-Weber disease). Am J Ophthalmol 1989;107:642–646

45. Peery WH. Clinical spectrum of hereditary hemorrhagic telangiectasia (Osler-Weber-Rendu disease). Am J Med 1987;82:989–997

46. Reagan TJ, Bloom WH. The brain in hereditary hemorrhagic telangiectasia. Stroke 1971;2:361–368

47. Adams HP, Subbiah B, Bosch EP. Neurologic aspects of hereditary hemorrhagic telangiectasia. Arch Neurol 1977;34:101–104

48. Bloom VR, Moynahan EJ. Hereditary haemorrhagic telangiectasia. Br J Dermatol 1960;72:312–317

49. Sisel RJ, Parker BM, Bahl OP. Cerebral symptoms in pulmonary arteriovenous fistula: a result of paradoxical emboli? Circulation 1970;41:123–128

50. Hunter DD. Pulmonary arteriovenous malformation: an unusual cause of cerebral embolism. Can Med Assoc J 1965;93:662–665

51. Bergqvist N, Hesen I, Hey M. Arteriovenous pulmonary aneurysms in Osler's disease (telangiectasia hereditaria haemorrhagica). Acta Med Scand 1962;171:301–309

52. Boczko ML. Neurological implications of hereditary hemorrhagic telangiectasis. J Nerv Ment Dis 1964;139:525–536

53. Le Roux BT. Pulmonary arteriovenous fistulae. Q J Med 1959; 28:1–20

54. Press OW, Ramsey PG. Central nervous system infections associated with hereditary hemorrhagic telangiectasia. Am J Med 1984;77: 86–92

55. Roman G, Fisher M, Perl DP, Poser CM. Neurological manifestations of hereditary hemorrhagic telangiectasia (Rendu-Osler-Weber disease): report of 2 cases and review of the literature. Ann Neurol 1978;4:130–144

56. Heffner RR, Solitare GB. Hereditary haemorrhagic telangiectasia: neuropathological observations. J Neurol Neurosurg Psychiatry 1969;32:604–608

57. Courville CB. Encephalic lesions in hereditary hemorrhagic telangiectasis (Rendu-Osler-Weber disease). Bull Los Angeles Neurol Soc 1957;22:28–35

58. Fulbright RK, Chaloupka JC, Putman CM, et al. MR of hereditary hemorrhagic telangiectasia: prevalence and spectrum of cerebrovascular malformations. AJNR Am J Neuroradiol 1998;19: 477–484

59. Willemse RB, Mager JJ, Westermann CJJ, Overtoom TT, Mauser H, Wolbers JG. Bleeding risk of cerebrovascular malformations in hereditary hemorrhagic telangiectasia. J Neurosurg 2000;92: 779–780

60. Easey AJ, Wallace GMF, Hughes JMB, Jackson JE, Taylor WJ, Shovlin CL. Should asymptomatic patients with hereditary haemorrhagic telangiectasia (HHT) be screened for cerebral vascular malformations? Data from 22,061 years of HHT patient life. J Neurol Neurosurg Psychiatry 2003;74:743–748

61. Aesch B, Lioret E, De Toffol B, Jan M. Multiple cerebral angiomas and Rendu-Osler-Weber disease: case report. Neurosurgery 1991; 29:599–602

62. Willinsky RA, Lasjaunias P, Terbrugge K, Burrows P. Multiple cerebral arteriovenous malformations (AVMs): review of our experience from 203 patients with cerebral vascular lesions. Neuroradiology 1990;32:207–210

63. Sobel D, Norman D. CNS manifestations of hereditary hemorrhagic telangiectasia. AJNR Am J Neuroradiol 1984;5:569–573

64. Grollmus J, Hoff J. Multiple aneurysms associated with Osler-Weber-Rendu disease. Surg Neurol 1973;1:91–93

65. Fisher M, Zito JL. Focal cerebral ischemia distal to a cerebral aneurysm in hereditary hemorrhagic telangiectasia. Stroke 1983; 14:419–421

66. Von Rad M, Tornow K. Spontane carotis-cavernosus-fistel bei morbus Osler-Rendu. J Neurol 1975;209:237–242

67. Pece-Barbara N, Cymerman U, Vera S, Marchuk DA, Letarte M. Expression analysis of four endoglin missence mutations suggests that haploinsufficiency is the predominant mechanism for hereditary hemorrhagic telangiectasia type 1. Hum Mol Genet 1999;8:2171–2181

68. Abdalla SA, Pece-Barbara N, Vera S, et al. Analysis of ALK-1 and endoglin in newborns from families with hereditary hemorrhagic telangiectasia type 2. Hum Mol Genet 2000;9: 1227–1237

69. Bayrak-Toydemir P, Mao R, Lewin S, McDonald J. Hereditary hemorrhagic telangiectasia: an overview of diagnosis and management in the molecular era for clinicians. Genet Med 2004; 6:175–191

70. Roach ES, Zimmerman CF. Ehlers-Danlos syndrome. In: Bogousslavsky J, Caplan LR, eds. Cerebrovascular Syndromes. London: Oxford University Press; 1995:491–496

71. Beighton P. The Ehlers-Danlos syndromes. In: Beighton P, ed. Heritable Disorders of Connective Tissue. St Louis: Mosby-Year Book; 1993:189–251

72. Byers PH, Holbrook KA, McGillivray B, MacLeod PM, Lowry RB. Clinical and ultrastructural heterogeneity of type IV Ehlers-Danlos syndrome. Hum Genet 1979;47:141–150

73. Pepin M, Schwartze U, Superti-Furga A, Byers PH. Clinical and genetic features of Ehlers-Danlos syndrome type IV, the vascular type. N Engl J Med 2000;342:673–680

74. Rubinstein MK, Cohen NH. Ehlers-Danlos syndrome associated with multiple intracranial aneurysms. Neurology 1964;14: 125–132

75. Mirza FH, Smith PL, Lim WN. Multiple aneurysms in a patient with Ehlers-Danlos syndrome: angiography without sequelae. AJR Am J Roentgenol 1979;132:993–995

76. Krog M, Almgren B, Eriksson I, Nordstrom S. Vascular complications in the Ehlers-Danlos syndrome. Acta Chir Scand 1983;149: 279–282

77. Schievink WI, Limburg M, Oorthuys JW, Fleury P, Pope FM. Cerebrovascular disease in Ehlers-Danlos syndrome type IV. Stroke 1990;21:626–632

78. McKusick VA. Heritable Disorders of Connective Tissue. St. Louis: CV Mosby; 1972

79. Imahori S, Bannerman RM, Graf CJ, Brennan JC. Ehlers-Danlos syndrome with multiple arterial lesions. Am J Med 1969;47:967–977

80. Edwards A, Taylor GW. Ehlers-Danlos syndrome with vertebral artery aneurysm. Proc R Soc Med 1969;62:734–735

81. Sheiner NM, Miller N, Lachance C. Arterial complications of Ehlers-Danlos syndrome. J Cardiovasc Surg (Torino) 1985;26: 291–296

82. Kuivaniemi H, Prokop DJ, Wu Y, et al. Exclusion of mutations in the gene for type III collagen (COL3A1) as a common cause of intracranial aneurysms or cervical artery dissections: results from sequence analysis of the coding sequences of type III collagen from 55 unrelated patients. Neurology 1993;43:2652–2658

83. Graf CJ. Spontaneous carotid-cavernous fistula. Arch Neurol 1965; 13:662–672

84. Farley MK, Clark RD, Fallor MK, Geggel HS, Heckenlively JR. Spontaneous carotid-cavernous fistula and the Ehlers-Danlos syndromes. Ophthalmology 1983;90:1337–1342

85. Lach B, Nair SG, Russell NA, Benoit BG. Spontaneous carotid-cavernous fistula and multiple arterial dissections in type IV Ehlers-Danlos syndrome. J Neurosurg 1987;66:462–467

86. Cikrit DF, Miles JH, Silver D. Spontaneous arterial perforation: the Ehlers-Danlos specter. J Vasc Surg 1987;5:248–255

87. Fox R, Pope FM, Narcisi P, et al. Spontaneous carotid cavernous fistula in Ehlers-Danlos syndrome. J Neurol Neurosurg Psychiatry 1988;51:984–986

88. Schievink WI, Piepgras DG, Earnest F IV, Gordon H. Spontaneous carotid-cavernous fistulae in Ehlers-Danlos syndrome type IV. J Neurosurg 1991;74:991–998

89. Halbach VV, Higashida RT, Dowd CF, Barnwell SL, Hieshima GB. Treatment of carotid-cavernous fistulas associated with Ehlers-Danlos syndrome. Neurosurgery 1990;26:1021–1027

90. Schoolman A, Kepes JJ. Bilateral spontaneous carotid-cavernous fistulae in Ehlers-Danlos syndrome. J Neurosurg 1967;26:82–86

91. Beighton P, Thomas ML. The radiology of the Ehlers-Danlos syndrome. Clin Radiol 1969;20:354–361

92. Driscoll SHM, Gomes AS, Machleder HI. Perforation of the superior vena cava: a complication of digital angiography in Ehlers-Danlos syndrome. AJR Am J Roentgenol 1984;142: 1021–1022

93. Kashiwagi S, Tsuchida E, Goto K, et al. Balloon occlusion of a spontaneous carotid-cavernous fistula in Ehlers-Danlos syndrome type IV. Surg Neurol 1993;39:187–190

94. Kanner AA, Maimin S, Rappaport ZH. Treatment of spontaneous carotid-cavernous fistula in Ehlers-Danlos syndrome by transvenous occlusion with Guglielmi detachable coils: case report and review of the literature. J Neurosurg 2000;93:689–692

95. Pope FM, Kendall BE, Slapak GI, et al. Type III collagen mutations cause fragile cerebral arteries. Br J Neurosurg 1991;5:551–574

96. Hunter GC, Malone JM, Moore WS, Misiorowski DL, Chvapil M. Vascular manifestations in patients with Ehlers-Danlos syndrome. Arch Surg 1982;117:495–498

97. Gilchrist D, Schwarze U, Shields K, MacLaren L, Bridge PJ, Byers PH. Large kindred with Ehlers-Danlos syndrome type IV due to a point mutation (G571S) in the COLA1 gene of type III procollagen: low risk of pregnancy complications and unexpected longevity in some affected relatives. Am J Med Genet 1999; 82:305–311

98. Kontusaari S, Tromp G, Kuivaniemi H, Stolle C, Pope FM, Prockop DJ. Substitution of aspartate for glycine 1018 in the type III procollagen (COL3A1) gene causes type IV Ehlers-Danlos syndrome: the mutated allele is present in most blood leukocytes of the asymptomatic and mosaic mother. Am J Hum Genet 1992;51:497–507

99. Sillence DO, Chiodo AA, Campbell PE, Cole WG. Ehlers-Danlos syndrome type IV: phenotypic consequences of a splicing mutation in one COL3A1 allele. J Med Genet 1991;28:840–845

100. Tsipouras P, Byers PH, Schwartz RC, et al. Ehlers-Danlos syndrome type IV: cosegregation of the phenotype to a COL3A1 allele of type III procollagen. Hum Genet 1986;74:41–46

101. Richards AJ, Lloyd JC, Narcisi P, et al. A 27-bp deletion from one allele of the type III collagen gene (COL3A1) in a large family with Ehlers-Danlos syndrome type IV. Hum Genet 1992;88: 325–330

102. Schwarze U, Goldstein JA, Byers PH. Splicing defects in the COL3A1 gene: marked preference for 5′ (donor) splice-site mutations in patients with exon-skipping mutations and Ehlers-Danlos syndrome type IV. Am J Hum Genet 1997;61:1276–1286

103. Carlborg U, Ejrup B, Gronblad E, Lund F. Vascular studies in pseudoxanthoma elasticum and angioid streaks. Acta Med Scand 1959;166(Suppl 350):1–84

104. Viljoen D. Pseudoxanthoma elasticum. In: Beighton P, ed. McKusick's Heritable Disorders of Connective Tissue. St. Louis: Mosby-Year Book; 1993:335–365

105. Altman LK, Fialkow PJ, Parker F, Sagebiel RW. Pseudoxanthoma elasticum: an underdiagnosed genetically heterogeneous disorder with protean manifestations. Arch Intern Med 1974;134:1048–1054

106. Pope FM. Historical evidence for the genetic heterogeneity of pseudoxanthoma elasticum. Br J Dermatol 1975;92:493–509

107. Goodman RM, Smith EW, Paton D, et al. Pseudoxanthoma elasticum: a clinical and histopathological study. Medicine 1963; 42:297–334

108. Reeve EB, Neldner KH, Subryan V, Gordon SG. Development and calcification of skin lesions in thirty-nine patients with pseudoxanthoma elasticum. Clin Exp Dermatol 1979;4:291–301

109. Connor PJ, Juergens JL, Perry HO, Hollenhorst RW, Edwards JE. Pseudoxanthoma elasticum and angioid streaks. Am J Med 1961; 30:537–543

110. Secretan M, Zografos L, Guggisberg D, Piguet B. Chorioretinal vascular abnormalities associated with angioid streaks and pseudoxanthoma elasticum. Arch Ophthalmol 1998;116:1333–1336

111. Wahlqvist ML, Fox RM, Beech AM, Favilla I. Peripheral vascular disease as a mode of presentation of pseudoxanthoma elasticum. Aust N Z J Med 1977;7:523–525

112. Kevorkian JP, Masquet C, Kural-Menasche S, Le Dref O, Beaufils P. New report of severe coronary artery disease in an eighteen-year-old girl with pseudoxanthoma elasticum. Angiology 1997; 48:735–741

113. Wolff HH, Stokes JF, Schlesinger BE. Vascular abnormalities associated with pseudoxanthoma elasticum. Arch Dis Child 1952; 27:82–88

114. Schachner L, Young D. Pseudoxanthoma elasticum with severe cardiovascular disease in a child. Am J Dis Child 1974;127:571–575

115. Spinzi G, Strocchi E, Imperiali G, Sangiovanni A, Terruzzi V, Minoli G. Pseudoxanthoma elasticum: a rare cause of gastrointestinal bleeding. Am J Gastroenterol 1996;91:1631–1634

116. Berde C, Willis DC, Sandberg EC. Pregnancy in women with pseudoxanthoma elasticum. Obstet Gynecol Surv 1983;38:339–344

117. Yoles A, Phelps R, Lebwohl M. Pseudoxanthoma elasticum and pregnancy. Cutis 1996;58:161–164

118. Tay CH. Pseudoxanthoma elasticum. Postgrad Med J 1970; 46:97–108

119. Munyer TP, Margulis AR. Pseudoxanthoma elasticum with internal carotid artery aneurysm. AJR Am J Roentgenol 1981;136: 1023–1029

120. Messimy R, Metzger J, Schaison G, Pfister A, Laccourreye H. Elastopathie cutanee et anomalies vasculaires associees avec troubles neurologiques. Rev Neurol 1975;131:419–431

121. Rios-Montenegro EN, Behrens MM, Hoyt WF. Pseudoxanthoma elasticum. Arch Neurol 1972;26:151–155

122. Prick JJG, Thijssen HOM. Radiodiagnostic signs in pseudoxanthoma elasticum generalisatum (dysgenesis elastofibrillaris mineralisans). Clin Radiol 1977;28:549–554

123. Goto K. Involvement of central nervous system in pseudoxanthoma elasticum. Folia Psychiatr Neurol Jpn 1975;29:263–277

124. Scheie HG, Hogan TF Jr. Angioid streaks and generalized arterial disease. AMA Arch Ophthalmol 1957;57:855–868

125. Le Saux O, Urban Z, Tschuch C, et al. Mutations in a gene encoding an ABC transporter cause pseudoxanthoma elasticum. Nat Genet 2000;25:223–227

126. Bergen AA, Plomp AS, Schuurman EJ, et al. Mutations in ABCC6 cause pseudoxanthoma elasticum. Nat Genet 2000;25:228–231

127. Cai L, Struk B, Adams MD, et al. A 500-kb region on chromosome 16p.13.1 contains the pseudoxanthoma elasticum locus: high-resolution mapping and genomic structure. J Mol Med 2000;78: 36–46

128. Le Saux O, Urban Z, Goring HH, et al. Pseudoxanthoma elasticum maps to an 820-kb region of the p13.1 region of chromosome 16. Genomics 1999;62:1–10

129. Struk B, Neldner KH, Rao VS, St Jean P, Lindpaintner K. Mapping of both autosomal recessive and dominant variants of pseudoxanthoma elasticum to chromosome 16p.13.1. Hum Mol Genet 1997;6:1823–1828

130. van Soest S, Swart J, Tijmes N, Sandkuiji LA, Rommers J, Bergen AA. A locus for autosomal recessive pseudoxanthoma elasticum, with penetrance of vascular symptoms in carriers, maps to chromosome 16p.13.1. Genome Res 1997;7:830–834

131. DeBusk FL. The Hutchinson-Gilford progeria syndrome. J Pediatr 1972;80:697–724

132. Gilkes JJH, Sharvill DE, Wells RS. The premature aging syndromes: report of eight cases and description of a new entity named metageria. Br J Dermatol 1974;91:243–262

133. Gabr M, Hashem N, Hashem M, Fahmi A, Safouh M. Progeria, a pathologic study. J Pediatr 1960;57:70–77

134. Matsuo S, Takeuchi Y, Hayashi S, Kinugasa A, Sawada T. Patient with unusual Hutchinson-Gilford syndrome (progeria). Pediatr Neurol 1994;10:237–240

135. Dyck JD, David TE, Burke B, Webb GD, Henderson MA, Fowler RS. Management of coronary artery disease in Hutchinson-Gilford syndrome. J Pediatr 1987;111:407–410

136. Goto M, Tanimoto K, Horiuchi Y, Sasazuki T. Family analysis of Werner's syndrome: a survey of 42 Japanese families with a review of the literature. Clin Genet 1981;19:8–15

137. Epstein CJ, Martin GM, Schultz AL, Motulsky AG. Werner syndrome: a review of its symptomatology, pathologic features, genetics and relationship to the natural aging process. Medicine 1966;45:177–221

138. Thannhauser SJ. Werner's syndrome (progeria of the adult) and Rothmund's syndrome: two types of closely related heredofamilial atrophic dermatoses with juvenile cataracts and endocrine features: a critical study with five new cases. Ann Intern Med 1945;23: 559–626

139. Viegas J, Souza LR, Salzano FM. Progeria in twins. J Med Genet 1974;11:384–386

140. Parkash H, Sidhu SS, Raghavan R, Deshmukh RN. Hutchinson-Gilford progeria: familial occurrence. Am J Med Genet 1990; 36:431–433

141. Colige A, Roujeau JC, De la Rocque F, Lapiere CM. Abnormal gene expression in skin fibroblasts from a Hutchinson-Gilford patient. Lab Invest 1991;64:799–806

142. Bridger JM, Kill IR. Aging of Hutchinson-Gilford progeria syndrome fibroblasts is characterized by hyperproliferation and increased apoptosis. Exp Gerontol 2004;39:717–724

143. Plasilova M, Chattopadhyay C, Pal P, et al. Homozygous missense mutation in the lamin A/C causes autosomal recessive Hutchinson-Gilford progeria syndrome. J Med Genet 2004;41:609–614

144. Eriksson M, Brown WT, Gordon LB, et al. Recurrent de novo point mutations in lamin A cause Hutchinson-Gilford progeria syndrome. Nature 2003;423:293–298

145. De Sandre-Giovannoli A, Bernard R, Cau P, et al. Lamin A truncation in Hutchinson-Gilford progeria. Science 2003; 300:2055

3
...

Etiology and Management of Stroke in Children

DAVID S. LIEBESKIND AND JEFFREY L. SAVER

Approximately half of the children with a first stroke have an identifiable predisposing cause, with the absence of a clear etiology in the remainder.[1] The term *cryptogenic* is often used to describe this subset of patients, despite the frequently limited diagnostic evaluation pursued in these cases. Genetic and metabolic causes of stroke are more prominent in the pediatric age group, with ramifications on counseling and disease prevention in family members.[2] Hemorrhagic strokes are more common than ischemic events,[3,4] and prompt diagnosis may facilitate requisite endovascular or surgical treatment of an underlying vascular lesion.

Few population-based reports or large cohort studies have delineated the occurrence of stroke subtypes in infants and children.[5,6] Primary stroke prevention is feasible in selected populations, such as sickle cell disease patients, employing transcranial Doppler ultrasonography and directed administration of periodic transfusions. Large case-control studies will be required for evaluation of treatment strategies in rare diseases associated with stroke, and evidence-based approaches will need to incorporate novel standardized outcome measures tailored to the pediatric population.

■ Epidemiology

The incidence of pediatric stroke worldwide varies due to genetic heterogeneity, geographical variation, and differential impact of infectious etiologies. Reported incidence ranges from 2.5 to 2.7 cases per 100,000 per year.[7] The incidence rate of 2.5 cases per 100,000 children stems from a population-based study observing only four incident cases of stroke accrued during a 10-year period prior to the advent of contemporary imaging modalities.[3]

A more recent estimate based on 16 cases yielded an incidence of 2.7 per 100,000 children. In this study, ischemic stroke incidence was 1.2 per 100,000 children per year, with a combined intracerebral and subarachnoid hemorrhage incidence rate of 1.5 per 100,000 children per year.[4] Approximately 20 to 30% of infants of less than 35 weeks gestational age sustain germinal matrix hemorrhage (**Fig. 3–1**).[8] A proportionately higher rate of intracranial hemorrhage afflicts children, even after exclusion of germinal matrix hemorrhage. The Canadian Pediatric Ischemic Stroke Registry, an ongoing project including more than 620 neonates and children less than 18 years of age with stroke, provides substantial data concerning pediatric stroke incidence. This registry estimated the incidence of arterial ischemic stroke at over 2.6 per 100,000 children per year,[9] compared with previous estimates ranging from 0.6 to 1.2 per 100,000 children per year.[3,4]

> **PEARL** Pediatric stroke is not as rare as previously estimated.

■ Etiology

Although traditional adult stroke risk factors account for a proportion of pediatric stroke, a much wider array of causes are involved in children.[10] Cardiac, hematologic, infectious, inflammatory, metabolic, and genetic causes of stroke may afflict children. In the neonatal population, neurological sequelae may be due to intrauterine or perinatal injury. Perinatal complications, accounting for 47% of neonatal strokes,[9] may involve asphyxia, trauma, or premature delivery. Neonatal causes typically include

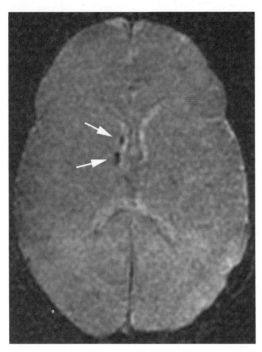

FIGURE 3–1 Germinal matrix hemorrhage (arrows) demonstrated by gradient echo magnetic resonance imaging.

congenital heart disease, respiratory distress syndrome, infection, and disseminated intravascular coagulation.

Because most strokes occur in previously healthy children, ascribing a causative risk factor is a difficult clinical task. Although cryptogenic stroke accounts for a sizable fraction of pediatric stroke, systematic efforts such as the Canadian Pediatric Stroke Registry have demonstrated that these unexplained strokes are more infrequent than once believed. Attributable risk factors were identified in 72% of registry cases. The extensive list of possible stroke etiologies (**Table 3–1**) cannot be exhaustively addressed in each patient. Identification of certain risk factors does not necessarily establish a causative relationship. Furthermore, synergistic relationships may involve multiple risk factors, such as dehydration and hypercoagulable states.

Cardiac etiologies encompass numerous common causes of pediatric ischemic stroke, accounting for 24% of cases.[9] Congenital heart disease such as ventricular septal defect or tetralogy of Fallot, rheumatic heart disease, prosthetic valves, bacterial endocarditis, atrial myxomas, and myocarditis may result in stroke. Paradoxical embolization may also occur in association with patent foramen ovale (PFO). Cardiac abnormalities may exhibit synergistic pathological relationships that precipitate stroke, such as the combination of PFO and an atrial septal aneurysm, or congenital heart disease and resultant polycythemia. The treatment of congenital heart disorders or associated pulmonary complications may also elevate stroke risk because neonates on extracorporeal

TABLE 3–1 Etiology of Pediatric Stroke

Atherosclerotic	Diabetes mellitus, hyperhomocysteinemia, hyperlipidemia, hypertension, radiation exposure
Cardiogenic	Arrhythmia, atrial myxoma, atrial septal aneurysm
	Bacterial endocarditis, basal cell nevus syndrome
	Cardiac catheterization, cardiomyopathy
	Cyanotic congenital defects, mitral valve prolapse
	Myocarditis, papillary fibroelastoma
	Patent foramen ovale, prosthetic heart valve
	Rhabdomyoma, rheumatic heart disease
Cervicocephalic arterial dissection	α1-antitrypsin deficiency
	Autosomal dominant polycystic kidney disease
	Collagen mutation, cystic medial necrosis
	Ehlers-Danlos syndrome types IV and VI
	Fibromuscular dysplasia, homocystinuria
	Hypertension, Marfan's syndrome, migraine
	Mucopolysaccharide accumulation
	Neural crest disorders, oral contraceptive use
	Osteogenesis imperfecta, pseudoxanthoma elasticum
	Recent infection, redundancy of vessels
	Reticular fiber deficiency, smoking
	Williams syndrome
Genetic/metabolic	Cytochrome-*c* oxidase deficiency, Fabry's disease
	Hyperhomocysteinemia, isovaleric academia
	Kearns-Sayre syndrome, Leigh disease
	Methylmalonic acidemia
	Mitochondrial encephalopathy, lactic acidosis, and strokelike episodes (MELAS)
	Myoclonic epilepsy and ragged red fiber (MERRF) syndrome
	Propionicacidemia, urea cycle defects
Hematologic	Antiphospholipid antibodies
	Antithrombin III deficiency, cobalamin deficiency
	Disorders of fibrinolysis
	Disseminated intravascular coagulation
	Drug-induced coagulopathy
	Dysfibrinogenemia
	Essential thrombocytosis
	Factor V, VII–XIII deficiency
	Factor V Leiden mutation
	Heparin cofactor deficiency, hepatic dysfunction
	Malignancy (e.g., leukemia, lymphoma)
	Nephrotic syndrome, plasminogen deficiency
	Platelet dysfunction, polycythemia
	Prekallikrein deficiency, protein C deficiency
	Protein S deficiency
	Prothrombin 20210 gene mutation
	Sickle cell anemia, thrombocytopenia
	Thrombotic thrombocytopenic purpura
	Vitamin K deficiency, Von Willebrand disease
Infectious	Bacterial meningoencephalitis
	Basilar meningitis (e.g., tuberculous)
	Herpes simplex virus (HSV)
	Human immunodeficiency virus (HIV)

TABLE 3–1 *(Continued)*

Inflammatory	Lyme disease, *Mycoplasma*, protozoal
	Rickettsial, syphilis, varicella-zoster
	  virus
	Viral (e.g., coxsackie A)
	Ankylosing spondylitis, Behçet's disease
	Churg-Strauss syndrome, Cogan's
	  syndrome, Eales' disease
	Henoch-Schönlein purpura
	Hypersensitivity vasculitis, isolated
	  angiitis
	Kawasaki syndrome, microscopic
	  polyangiitis
	Mixed connective tissue disease
	Mixed essential cryoglobinuria
	Polyarteritis nodosa, Reiter's
	  syndrome
	Rheumatoid arthritis, scleroderma
	Sjögren's syndrome, systemic lupus
	  erythematosus
	Takayasu's arteritis, Wegener's
	  granulomatosis

Other	Alternating hemiplegia of childhood Dehydration, hypotension, Iatrogenic injury Iron deficiency, migraine Pregnancy and postpartum period
Structural or cerebrovascular lesions	Aneurysm, aortic coarctation Arteriovenous malformation Fibromuscular dysplasia Hereditary hemorrhagic telangiectasia (Osler-Weber-Rendu disease) Neoplasm, Sturge-Weber syndrome Von Hippel-Lindau disease
Toxic	Allopurinol, amphetamines, cocaine Ephedrine Ergotamine, heroin Lysergic acid dyethylamide (LSD) Pentazocine and tripelennamine Phencyclidine (PCP) Phenylpropanolamine
Trauma	Arterial dissection, blunt trauma Chiropractic manipulation, intraoral trauma Intrauterine injury, perinatal injury

Vasculopathy	Acute posterior multifocal placoid pigment
	  epitheliopathy
	Down syndrome, homocystinuria
	Inflammatory bowel disease, moyamoya
	  disease
	Neurofibromatosis, neurosarcoidosis
	Sneddon syndrome

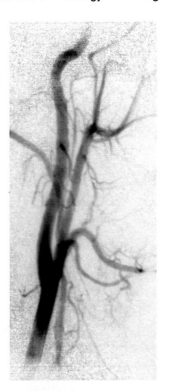

FIGURE 3–2 Segmental constriction and ectasia of the cervical internal carotid artery in fibromuscular dysplasia.

membrane oxygenation are at increased risk of ischemic and hemorrhagic stroke.

Cervicocephalic arterial dissection is a frequent cause of pediatric ischemic stroke, particularly between ages of 15 to 18 years. Traumatic and spontaneous dissections account for 8 to 20% of strokes in children.[11] Spontaneous cervicocephalic arterial dissections may be related to underlying vasculopathies including fibromuscular dysplasia (**Fig. 3–2**),[12] Marfan's syndrome,[13,14] Ehlers-Danlos syndrome types IV[15] and VI, osteogenesis imperfecta,[13] cystic medial necrosis,[16] reticular fiber deficiency,[17] accumulation of mucopolysaccharides,[18] pseudoxanthoma elasticum,[13] homocystinuria,[13] autosomal domi-

nant polycystic kidney disease,[13] α_1-antitrypsin deficiency,[19] and various collagen disorders. Neural crest disorders affecting the muscular arteries of the head and neck are suggested by an association of cervicocephalic dissections with congenital heart disease and lentiginosis.[20,21] Familial aggregations of dissection of presumed genetic origin and an association with intracranial aneurysms have also been described.[22–24] Additional dissection-associated risk factors include oral contraceptive use,[25] hypertension,[26] migraine,[27–29] recent infection,[30] smoking,[12] and redundancy of vessels.[31] Increased use of noninvasive studies is revealing dissections in several cases that may previously have been considered cryptogenic strokes.

Intracerebral and subarachnoid hemorrhages arise from diverse causes in the pediatric population. Brain tumors accounted for up to 13% of hemorrhagic strokes in one pediatric series.[32,33] Structural vascular abnormalities, including arteriovenous malformations, capillary telangiectasias, and venous or cavernous angiomas, account for ~32% of hemorrhages and over 40% of nontraumatic hemorrhages.[32] Hemorrhagic transformation of an ischemic infarct is an additional, not uncommon cause of hemorrhage in pediatric patients. Subarachnoid hemorrhage may result from trauma, intracranial aneurysms, sickle cell disease, or arteriovenous malformations. Intracranial aneurysms account for only 6% of hemorrhagic strokes in the pediatric age group. In children, these vascular lesions have a slight male predominance

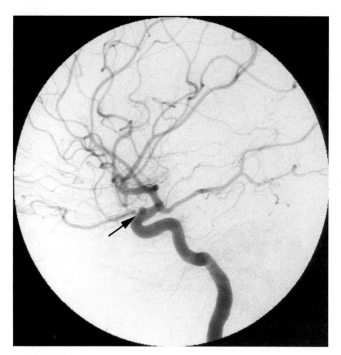

FIGURE 3–3 Saccular aneurysm (arrow) at the origin of the ophthalmic artery in polycystic kidney disease.

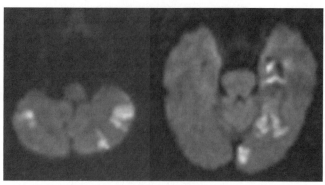

FIGURE 3–4 Multifocal posterior circulation strokes associated with sickle cell disease as illustrated by diffusion-weighted magnetic resonance imaging.

and giant aneurysms are more frequent in comparison with adults. Intracranial aneurysms may be associated with polycystic kidney disease (**Fig. 3–3**), aortic coarctation, Ehlers-Danlos syndrome, and pseudoxanthoma elasticum. Subarachnoid hemorrhage may lead to an ischemic infarct if vasospasm is present.

> **PEARL** Intracranial hemorrhage commonly presents with headache and vomiting.

Hypertensive hemorrhages are uncommon in children. Systemic hypertension may result from adrenocorticotropic hormone administration or renal insults.[32,34] Diabetes mellitus has only a minor influence, but accelerated atherosclerotic disease may be provoked by chronic elevations of insulin, proinsulin, and the development of insulin resistance.[35] Atherosclerotic-type vasculopathic changes may also be induced by radiation exposure. Minimal evidence supports moderate hypercholesterolemia as a significant stroke risk factor in children; however, genetic abnormalities producing severe dyslipidemia, such as apolipoproteinemia, may result in cerebral ischemia.[36,37]

Environmental factors account for a small proportion of stroke in children. Dehydration may contribute to cerebral venous thrombosis. Passive smoking may cause endothelial damage, but an association with stroke in children has not been proven.[38] Sleep-disordered breathing and the risk of stroke in children has yet to be elucidated. Alcohol is also unlikely to play a significant role. Illicit drug use may induce both ischemic and hemorrhagic stroke, and neonatal stroke has been associated with maternal cocaine use.[39] Inhalation of glue and abused drugs such as amphetamines, cocaine, heroin, phenylpropanolamine, combinations of pentazocine and tripelennamine, lysergic acid dyethylamide (LSD), or phencyclidine (PCP) may precipitate stroke. Stroke manifestations may present immediately or months to years following drug exposure.

Hematologic abnormalities, including prothrombotic disorders and hemorrhagic tendencies, account for ~12% of pediatric stroke cases.[9] Sickle cell disease is a well-established cause of stroke in the young. Children with sickle cell disease have an 8% incidence of stroke by age 14 years.[40,41] Sickle cell children are at risk for ischemic and hemorrhagic stroke (**Fig. 3–4**). Strokes are most commonly due to a large vessel, moyamoya-like vasculopathy related to chronic endothelial injury. If symptomatic with a transient ischemic attack, stroke risk increases substantially. Cerebral ischemia occurs in the setting of a crisis.[40,42] Transcranial Doppler (TCD) ultrasonography may be used to assess stroke risk based on blood flow velocities. Asymptomatic or silent strokes, detected on subsequent neuroimaging studies, affect 11 to 17% of children with sickle cell disease.[43,44] Although stroke has been reported in several cases of sickle cell trait,[45] this relationship awaits further clarification. Anemia severity is a risk factor for stroke in children with sickle cell disease.[46]

Antibodies directed against cell membrane phospholipids, or antiphospholipid antibodies, may precipitate arterial or venous ischemia.[47] A relationship with cerebral ischemia has been clearly established,[48–51] although clinical symptoms may manifest as migrainous episodes, chorea, amaurosis, or stroke (**Fig. 3–5**). The prevalence of these antibodies in idiopathic pediatric stroke is

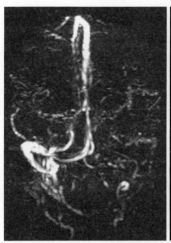 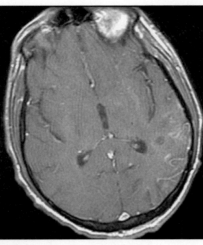

FIGURE 3–5 Cerebral venous thrombosis due to antiphospholipid antibody syndrome demonstrated by magnetic resonance venography (left) with associated temporoparietal venous infarction (right) on postgadolinium T1-weighted images.

inversely related to age.[52] These antibodies may also be detected in Sneddon syndrome, characterized by cerebral ischemia and the presence of livedo reticularis.

Numerous additional hypercoagulable states have been described that predispose to cerebral venous thrombosis in childhood. The contributions of these prothrombotic disorders to arterial ischemic stroke remain unclear. Protein C, protein S, and antithrombin III deficiencies all may precipitate childhood stroke.[53–60] Factor V Leiden mutation, the most frequent cause of activated protein C resistance, is a major cause of cerebral venous thrombosis and has also been associated with pediatric arterial ischemic stroke,[61–65] although this relationship remains contentious.[66] Similarly, the prothrombin 20210 gene mutation has been strongly associated with cerebral venous thrombosis, although its relationship with arterial stroke is loosely defined.[63,64,67–68] Additive interactions of multiple coexisting hypercoagulable states in precipitating stroke have been described, especially the combination of hyperhomocysteinemia and the factor V Leiden mutation.[67,69]

Hyperhomocysteinemia produces an elevated risk of stroke during childhood,[70–72] with increasing risk along a continuum with increasing levels of plasma homocysteine.[70,73] A combination of acquired and inherited factors influence plasma homocysteine levels.[74] Acquired causes principally involve vitamin deficiencies, although other environmental factors such as tobacco use, coffee, and alcohol consumption may cause elevations of homocysteine.[75] The antifolate effects of antiepileptic medications may also elevate plasma homocysteine.[71] These environmental factors likely underlie the reported increase of homocysteine with advancing age[76] and probably have minimal influence during childhood years. Inherited causes of hyperhomocysteinemia include enzyme deficiencies producing classic homocystinuria and the milder genetic defect of a point mutation of nucleotide

677 C → T of the N(5,10)-methylenetetrahydrofolate reductase gene.

Iron deficiency has also been proposed as a risk factor for stroke in children.[77] Cited cases have been associated with preceding viral infections. Because iron deficiency affects 20 to 25% of children worldwide, the association with stroke merits further study.

Coagulopathies may result in intracranial hemorrhage, spontaneous or triggered by major or only minimal trauma. Common coagulopathic disorders leading to hemorrhage include factor VIII deficiency, factor IX deficiency, factor XIII deficiency, hepatic dysfunction, warfarin therapy, and vitamin K deficiency. Severity of the coagulopathy, not the specific disorder, is the critical variable in propensity for intracranial hemorrhage.[78–81]

Platelet disorders, including thrombocytopenia and thrombocytosis, may lead to hemorrhagic or ischemic complications. Thrombocytopenia due to several causes may predispose individuals to hemorrhage, although spontaneous bleeding rarely occurs with platelet counts greater than 20,000.

Infectious processes are frequently associated with stroke during childhood, with estimates of recent or recurrent infection in 30 to 50% of cases.[6,82] Basal meningitides due to borreliosis, tuberculosis, and bacterial pathogens are well-recognized causes of stroke.[82,83] *Hemophilus influenza* type B and *Mycoplasma pneumoniae*[84,85] have been associated with pediatric stroke, whereas causal relationships have yet to be established for *Helicobacter* and chlamydiae. Viral infections including coxsackie A,[86] varicella-zoster virus (VZV),[87] herpes simplex virus, (HSV), and human immunodeficiency virus (HIV) may be related to stroke in children. Stroke complicates the course of chickenpox infection in one in 13,000 cases.[88,89] Ischemic manifestations usually present weeks to months after uneventful VZV infection. A transient arteriopathy, or postvaricella angiopathy, typically involves the anterior circulation, resulting in basal ganglia infarction.[90–92] Hypercoagulable states may also occur in the setting of VZV.[89] HIV may present with cerebrovascular ischemia, and therefore must be considered in the differential diagnosis of a child with abrupt, focal neurological deficits.[93,94] Both ischemic and hemorrhagic strokes may be related to HIV infection.

Nonatherosclerotic, nondissecting vasculopathies may also lead to stroke in children. A common structural vasculopathy is fibromuscular dysplasia. A variety of inflammatory vasculopathies may afflict children, although polyarteritis nodosa is perhaps the most common of the vasculitides that affect the central nervous system. Moyamoya syndrome is progressive intracranial arterial occlusions with the development of secondary telangiectasias, producing a characteristic angiographic pattern. Moyamoya syndrome may occur secondary to multiple predisposing conditions (e.g., Down syndrome, sickle cell disease) or idiopathically. Patients may present with cerebral ischemia or hemorrhage. The likelihood of recurrent neurological events diminishes about 4 years after the onset of symptoms.

Migrainous stroke is an infrequent cause of stroke in children, principally affecting the posterior circulation.[95] Migrainous infarction is usually associated with migraine with aura, rather than migraine without aura.

■ Clinical Features

Pediatric stroke typically manifests with unilateral weakness, with hemiparesis noted on examination of up to 50% of neonatal and childhood stroke patients.[9] Neonatal hemiparesis may be relatively subtle, however. Elicitation of sensory deficits, language disturbances, and visual symptoms may be difficult in the pediatric age group.[96] Basal ganglia infarction in children typically produces hemiparesis or hemisensory loss, with occasional signs of aphasia, ataxia, or mental status alterations. Speech disorders are noted in 17% of pediatric strokes.[9] Seizures frequently occur, accompanying up to 48% of childhood stroke.[9] Variable presence of additional focal neurological deficits, hypotonia, apnea, bradycardia, and hypotension may characterize neonatal stroke. Otherwise silent strokes may be clinically manifest solely as premature hand preference.

> **PEARL**   Sensory deficits, language disturbances, and visual symptoms may be difficult to assess in the pediatric age group.

Cerebral ischemia typically produces symptoms and signs reflecting the anatomical location of the lesion.

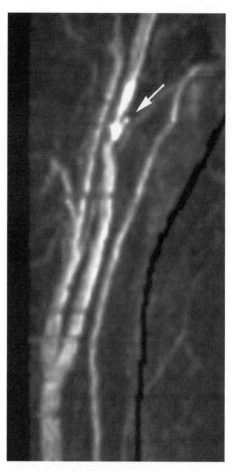

FIGURE 3–6 Magnetic resonance angiography demonstration of a distal cervical carotid dissecting aneurysm (arrow) associated with Marfan's syndrome.

The clinical presentation of cervicocephalic arterial dissection is highly variable, ranging from asymptomatic detection of the vascular abnormality to major disabling strokes in 5 to 10% of cases. Headache or neck pain is present in two thirds of cases.[12,97,98] Dissection-related expansion of the vessel wall and mechanical distortion of sympathetic fibers along the internal carotid artery may produce a Horner's syndrome (**Fig. 3–6**). Other clinical manifestations include tinnitus, an audible bruit, lower cranial neuropathies, scalp tenderness, and positive visual phenomena. Ischemic sequelae of cervicocephalic arterial dissection may affect the brain, adjacent nerves, eye, cervical roots, or spinal cord.

Extracranial carotid dissections usually produce ischemia in the middle cerebral artery territory. Border zone infarcts, retinal artery occlusion, and ischemic optic neuropathy may also occur.[99–101] Extracranial vertebral dissections typically cause lateral medullary infarcts, although other brain stem syndromes and spinal cord ischemia are possible. Intracranial dissections may present with subarachnoid hemorrhage, cerebral ischemia, or seizures. Vasculitic syndromes may produce constitutional symptoms of fever and malaise, as well as headaches and encephalopathy. Migrainous stroke may present with scintillating visual field defects, a march of symptoms over 10 to 30 minutes, headache, photophobia, and nausea. Moyamoya may cause the insidious evolution of headache, seizures, and impaired cognitive function, or present with sudden focal neurological deficits. Cerebral venous thrombosis may present with seizures, altered mental status, elevated intracranial pressure, or focal neurological deficits. Neonatal cerebral venous thrombosis may produce nonspecific findings of lethargy and seizures. Symptoms of iron deficiency include irritability, headache, and lethargy, whereas clinical signs of cognitive or motor dysfunction, papilledema, pseudotumor cerebri, and cranial neuropathies may be evident.

Although intracranial hemorrhage also produces location-dependent neurological manifestations, headache and vomiting are present in up to 59% of cases.[32] Seizures accompany the onset of symptoms in up to 37% of cases,[32] and ~3% of children present with coma. Arteriovenous malformations may present with headache or seizures; however, hemorrhage is the most common manifestation in the pediatric age group.[102] Vein of Galen malformations may lead to failure to thrive, seizures, hydrocephalus, or congestive heart failure with an audible cranial bruit in neonates and infants. Children typically suffer headaches, hydrocephalus, and subarachnoid hemorrhage. Aneurysmal subarachnoid hemorrhage may elude diagnosis in infants; children present with abrupt headache, sometimes with focal neurological deficits.

The neurological morbidity and mortality resulting from pediatric stroke are largely unknown, substantiated by only isolated reports.[103–106] Traditional stroke scales employed in adults have only limited application in the pediatric age group. The Pediatric Stroke Outcome Measure has recently been proposed as a specialized tool for evaluation of pediatric stroke outcomes.[103] Previous estimates indicate that 46% of infants and children with arterial stroke and 18% with cerebral venous thrombosis experience a poor clinical outcome, not including associated deaths. Absence of residual deficits was noted in 34%, neurological abnormalities in 56%, and death in 10% of ischemic strokes in a large Canadian study.[9] Basal ganglia strokes tend to have a favorable prognosis, characterized by survival with minimal residual deficits in the majority of cases.[83,103] Poorer outcomes have been noted in patients with cardiac or systemic disease. Although clinical outcomes in moyamoya tend to be worse, considerable variability exists. The prognosis of intracranial hemorrhage varies by size and location of the lesion. Children with arteriovenous malformations suffer a higher risk of hemorrhage and elevated mortality compared with adults. The annual hemorrhage rate is 0.5 to 3.2%. Hemorrhage associated with an arteriovenous malformation may be fatal in up to 25% of children, with complete recovery seen among 60% of children following surgical therapy. Residual neurological deficits, seizures, and intellectual dysfunction affect ~30%. The poorer prognosis in children may be due to more frequent predilection for the posterior fossa, more severe hemorrhage, and a higher rate of intraventricular extension.[107]

Vein of Galen malformations carry a mortality rate of ~30 to 40%, with even higher mortality in neonates with congestive heart failure. Neonates surviving cerebral venous thrombosis without anticoagulation experience reasonable outcomes,[7] yet mortality may be as high as 30%. Overall, outcomes appear better in the pediatric age group than in adults. Whereas physical disabilities often do not preclude regular school placement, relatively subtle intellectual and behavioral problems may necessitate special education or counseling. Seizures, headaches, and other neurological complications such as hemidystonia may have a delayed presentation and protracted course.[104]

Long-term clinical outcome may also be influenced by the rate of recurrent stroke, largely determined by stroke etiology. Recurrent stroke affects 10 to 14% of pediatric cases.[9,103] Untreated sickle cell disease carries a recurrent stroke rate of ~50%. For cervicocephalic arterial dissection, the annual rate of recurrent dissection is ~1%, affecting either the initially dissected vessel or another arterial segment.[16,22,108,109] Risk factors for recurrence include an underlying frank vasculopathy and a family history of dissection.[22,108] In one large series, the mean time to recurrence of dissection was 4.1 years, ranging from 2 days to 8.6 years.[12] The risk of recurrence with patent foramen ovale is relatively low,[2] whereas migrainous stroke carries a higher recurrence rate.[110] Moyamoya exhibits a more aggressive course in children, with protracted risk of ischemic and subsequent hemorrhagic stroke.

■ Diagnosis

Once diagnostic studies (**Table 3–2**) reveal a putative cause, evaluation of the remaining etiologies may be curtailed, although multiple causes commonly overlap. Neuroimaging modalities are indispensable for the diagnosis of pediatric stroke. In neonates and infants, ultrasonography is the primary screening modality.[111] Ultrasound and, more recently, magnetic resonance imaging (MRI), may also detect in utero vascular insults. Transfontanelle Doppler ultrasonography is useful in the detection of neonatal cerebral venous thrombosis, especially because computed tomography (CT) has a relatively high false-positive rate for this diagnosis due to elevated hematocrit during this age.

TABLE 3–2 Diagnostic Evaluation of Pediatric Stroke

Laboratory studies	Serum
	Complete blood count, platelet count
	PT, aPTT, electrolytes, glucose
	Blood urea nitrogen/creatinine
	Liver function tests, cardiac enzyme assays
	Arterial blood gas
	Pregnancy test (if of childbearing age)
	Blood cultures, lipid panel
	Sickle cell screen
	Hypercoagulable assays, including
	Functional activity and antigen levels
	Protein C, protein S
	Antithrombin III
	Factor V Leiden mutation
	Prothrombin 20210 gene mutation
	Antiphospholipid assays
	Anticardiolipin antibodies
	$\beta(2)$-glycoprotein I
	Lupus anticoagulant, DRVVT
	Homocysteine, D-dimers, fibrin split products
	Fibrinogen, erythrocyte sedimentation rate
	ANA, dsDNA, RNP, rheumatoid factor
	Cryocrit/cryoglobulins, ANCA
	C3/C4, CH-50, C-reactive protein
	Cold agglutinins, SCL70, anti-Smith antibody
	Anti-Ro and anti-LA antibodies (SS-A, SS-B)
	Immunocomplex assay, ACE, RPR, VDRL
	HIV
	Protein electrophoresis/immunoelectrophoresis
	Hepatitis serology, lyme titers, lactic acid
	Ammonia, amino acid assays
	Genetic analysis
	Cerebrospinal fluid
	Cell count, glucose, protein, cultures
	Viral titers and PCRs (HSV and VZV)
	Cytology, VDRL, ACE, IgG synthesis
	Oligoclonal bands, lactate, pyruvate
	Urine
	Urinalysis
	Culture and sensitivities
	Toxicology screen
	Organic and amino acid assays
Neuroimaging	Conventional imaging
	Noncontrast CT
	MRI with gadolinium
	Diffusion-weighted imaging
	Perfusion imaging
	CT perfusion
	MR perfusion
	Xe-CT
	SPECT
	PET
	Angiography
	CTA
	MRA
	Catheter angiography
	Ultrasonography
	Transfontanelle Doppler
	Carotid duplex
	TCD
	Functional imaging
	fMRI
	PET
	MR spectroscopy
Cardiac	Echocardiography with bubble study
	Transthoracic
	Transesophageal
	Electrocardiography
	12-lead EKG
	Continuous cardiac monitoring
Other	Pulse oximetry, chest x-ray, cervical x-rays
	Electroencephalogram, fluoroscein angiography
	Brain biopsy, muscle biopsy, skin biopsy

ACE, angiotensin-converting enzyme; ANA, antinuclear antibody; ANCA, antineutrophil cytoplasmic antibody; CT, computed tomography; CTA, computed tomographic angiography; dRVVT, dilute Russel viper venom time; dsDNA, double-stranded DNA; EKG, electrocardiogram; fMRI, functional magnetic resonance imaging; HIV, human immunodeficiency virus; HSV, herpes simplex virus; IgG, immunoglobulin G; MR, magnetic resonance; MRA, magnetic resonance angiography; PCR, polymerase chain reaction; PET, positron emission tomography; PT, prothrombin time; aPTT, partial thromboplastin time; RNP, ribonuclear protein; RPR, rapid plasma reagent; SCL70, scleroderma immunoglobulin G antibody; SPECT, single photon emission computed tomography; TCD, transcranial Doppler; VDRL, Venereal Disease Research Lab test; VZV, varicella-zoster virus; XeCT, xenon-computed tomography

Conventional parenchymal imaging modalities including CT and standard MRI sequences principally delineate regions of established infarction and hemorrhage. Noncontrast CT is most commonly acquired as the initial imaging study, yet MRI serves as the definitive technique for visualization of the parenchyma. Early after infarct onset, standard CT may be normal or reveal only subtle edematous changes within brain parenchyma and will provide minimal information with regard to vascular structures. CT helps to exclude possible diagnoses of abscess, tumor, and subdural hematoma, yet MRI usually provides further detail. Among conventional MR sequences, fluid-attenuated inversion recovery MRI sequences are particularly sensitive to cerebral ischemia (**Fig. 3–7**). MRI of metabolic disorders causing strokelike episodes may illustrate hyperintensity on T2-weighted sequences and corresponding T1 hypointensity. Gradient echo and susceptibility sequences explicitly detect regions of hemorrhage (**Fig. 3–8**).

Axial T1-weighted fat-saturation sequences enhance detection of intramural hematoma representative of dissection. An eccentric or circumferential rim of hyperintensity caused by intramural methemoglobin surrounding the arterial lumen, the crescent sign, is pathognomonic for dissection.[112,113]

Recent MRI advances pioneered in adults, such as diffusion and perfusion techniques, may play a pivotal role in the diagnostic evaluation of pediatric cerebrovascular disorders.[114] Diffusion imaging is exquisitely sensitive to ischemic edema, even during the hyperacute phase (**Fig. 3–9**). Cytotoxic edema, the incipient component of ischemic edema caused by impaired energy metabolism and ion derangements, may be detected within minutes of onset. Diffusion-weighted imaging reveals restricted diffusion of water molecules associated with intracellular swelling, and subsequent evolution of vasogenic edema due to blood–brain barrier disruption and extracellular

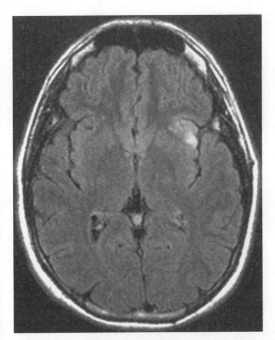

FIGURE 3–7 Left insular stroke depicted by fluid-attenuated inversion recovery in the setting of familial hyperlipidemia.

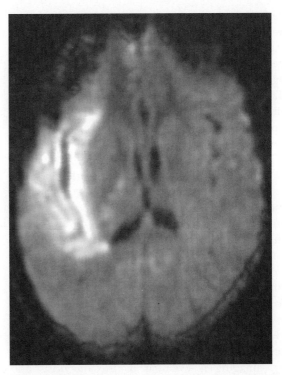

FIGURE 3–9 Diffusion-weighted magnetic resonance imaging of an embolic right middle cerebral artery stroke associated with an atrial myxoma.

fluid accumulation. Apparent diffusion coefficient maps are utilized to distinguish cytotoxic edema from vasogenic edema, apparent as hyperintensity on T2-weighted sequences, or T2 shine-through.

Perfusion MRI images may be acquired with administration of a gadolinium bolus or with an arterial spin-labeling technique. Rapid serial imaging during intravascular transit of gadolinium or a paramagnetic contrast agent or with magnetic labeling of arterial water molecules detects changes in signal intensity reflective of parenchymal perfusion. Continuous arterial spin labeling is completely noninvasive, providing quantitative measurements of

cerebral blood flow in terms of mL/100 g/min.[115] Perfusion MRI may be useful for triage of acute stroke cases and for evaluation of high-risk populations with diagnoses of moyamoya or sickle cell disease.

> **PEARL** Recent development of CT and MRI techniques may help to define regions of hypoperfusion.

Other perfusion techniques, including perfusion CT, xenon-CT, single photon emission computed tomography, and positron emission tomography (PET) may also offer critical information regarding cerebral blood flow. Assessment of cerebrovascular reserve may be achieved with simultaneous administration of acetazolamide. Fluoro-deoxyglucose PET may delineate regions of decreased glucose metabolism suggestive of mitochondrial disorders. Corresponding regions of elevated lactate may be demonstrated with magnetic resonance spectroscopy.[116]

Although perfusion techniques provide invaluable information regarding the status of cerebral blood flow, delineation of the vascular anatomy and pathophysiological blood flow patterns requires angiographic assessment. Noninvasive or conventional catheter angiographic methods may characterize a vascular stenosis or occlusion, vasculopathy, dissection, aneurysm, or arteriovenous

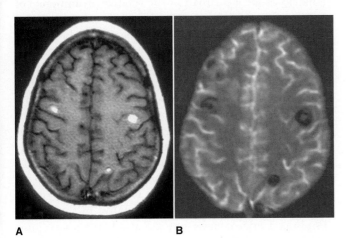

A   B

FIGURE 3–8 Multifocal intracranial hemorrhage due to thrombotic thrombocytopenic purpura depicted by **(A)** T1-weighted and **(B)** gradient echo magnetic resonance imaging.

malformation. Catheter, four-vessel angiography is the gold standard for delineation of the cerebral vasculature. Catheter angiography allows for simultaneous assessment of collateral blood flow patterns, pivotal in the pathophysiology of moyamoya and other causes of pediatric stroke. The relatively low risk of angiographic complications in a center with age-appropriate facilities and high yield of four-vessel angiography in pediatric stroke argues for routine catheter cerebral angiography in most cases of stroke in childhood. Up to 80% of children with stroke have abnormal angiographic studies, although 25 to 50% of these abnormalities subsequently resolve.[117–119] Persistent abnormalities generally encompass moyamoya and other intrinsic arteriopathies.

A transient cerebral arteriopathy characterized by segmental intracranial arterial stenoses may be demonstrated.[118] These nonspecific arterial stenoses have a similar angiographic appearance to atherosclerotic and vasculitic entities. Differential diagnoses include atherosclerosis, migraine, inflammatory vasculitides, and infections including VZV, cytomegalovirus, coxsackievirus, and cat scratch disease.[118]

Vascular imaging is essential in the diagnosis and management of the pediatric patient with cervicocephalic arterial dissection and cerebral venous thrombosis. Angiographic correlates of dissection include a string sign, gradually tapering stenosis or occlusion, intimal flap, dissecting aneurysm, distal pouch, or underlying arteriopathy. Luminal stenoses associated with dissection may appear irregular, tapered, or eccentric. Angiography may also identify structural vascular lesions in up to 41% of hemorrhagic strokes in children,[32] although the hemorrhage may obscure the underlying abnormality. The spatial distribution and relationship of structural vascular abnormalities, such as arteriovenous malformations and aneurysms, may be defined by angiography, with simultaneous assessment of vasospasm. The recent development of three-dimensional angiography promises further detail of vascular anatomical abnormalities associated with pediatric stroke. The optimal timing of angiography following hemorrhage remains controversial, however.[10]

Noninvasive angiographic modalities, including CT angiography and magnetic resonance angiography, minimize risk and provide sufficient detail for diagnostic evaluation in increasing numbers of patients. Noninvasive correlation with catheter angiography at initial diagnosis may allow serial noninvasive angiographic modalities to monitor known abnormalities and response to therapy (**Fig. 3–10**). CT angiography is an attractive imaging modality for unstable patients and those with pacemakers, implanted metal, or other MRI contraindications.

Carotid duplex and TCD ultrasonography may be used to evaluate cervical vessels and proximal segments of the intracranial vasculature. Carotid and vertebral duplex ultrasonography may confirm a diagnosis of dissection

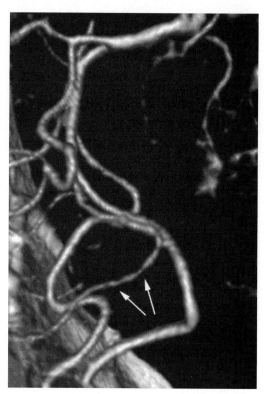

FIGURE 3–10 Computed tomographic angiography of subtle vasculitic changes (arrows) in the distal middle cerebral artery (see Color Plate 3–10).

and monitor subsequent therapy. TCD may be utilized as a screening modality to guide transfusion therapy for primary stroke prevention in sickle cell disease.[120] Proximal vascular occlusions, vasospasm, and cerebral venous thrombosis may be assessed with TCD as well. TCD may be employed for monitoring cerebral emboli, assessment of right to left cardiac shunts, and delineation of collateral blood flow patterns.

Routine evaluation of potential cardiac disorders in pediatric stroke is justified by the relative prominence of cardioembolic etiologies. A thorough cardiovascular assessment, including electrocardiography, chest x-ray, and echocardiography, may be warranted. Electrocardiograms may reveal a conduction defect or arrhythmia. Transthoracic or transesophageal echocardiography may identify structural cardiac abnormalities, including congenital anomalies, valvular disease, and right to left shunts. Transesophageal echocardiography with an intravenous contrast injection of agitated saline may be used to identify and characterize a patent foramen ovale (**Fig. 3–11**) and atrial septal aneurysms. Cardiac disorders may also be investigated with ultrafast cardiac CT and MRI.

Plain films are particularly informative in the setting of trauma. Cervical views may reveal subluxation or joint instability associated with vertebral dissection.

Histopathologic examination is infrequently involved in the diagnosis of pediatric stroke. Leptomeningeal and

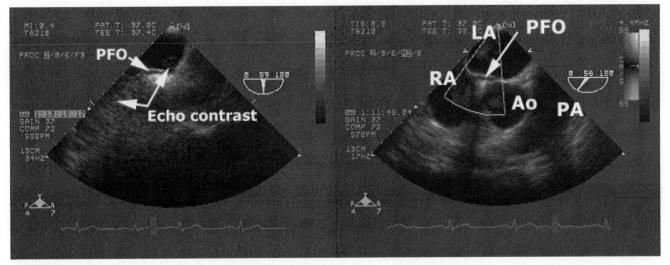

FIGURE 3–11 Transesophageal echocardiography of a patent foramen ovale (PFO) illustrating echo contrast due to the flow of agitated saline across the interatrial septum.

brain biopsy is employed to confirm vasculitic diagnoses. Other pathological studies may include skin biopsy to discern ultrastructural defects in connective tissue associated with dissection, and muscle biopsy to establish a diagnosis of mitochondrial disease.

■ Treatment

During the acute phase of pediatric stroke, general supportive measures are paramount. Following immediate triage with emergent management of airway patency and circulatory function, patients should be rapidly evaluated with brain imaging and neurological consultation.

Aspiration precautions are critical, with continuous monitoring of oxygenation and cardiovascular status. Supportive oxygenation is particularly important in fat emboli syndrome. Intravenous fluid administration should utilize normal saline with 20 mEq per liter of potassium. The rate of intravenous fluids should be adjusted for those with known renal failure or congestive heart failure. Subsequent maintenance fluids may also require adjustment if extensive cerebral edema is present. For children with congestive heart failure, furosemide and digoxin may be used, with close observation of electrolyte status. Electrolyte disturbances are common, and hyponatremia associated with cerebral salt wasting and the syndrome of inappropriate secretion of antidiuretic hormone should be aggressively corrected. Systemic blood pressure should be carefully monitored. Mild to moderate hypertension should be judiciously corrected in intracerebral hemorrhage to reduce the risk of rebleed, but tolerated acutely in cerebral ischemia to maximize collateral flow. Aggressive control of fever, hyperglycemia, and other metabolic derangements should be pursued.

Antibiotics, antiarrhythmic agents, clotting factors, and transfusions may also be indicated. In hemorrhagic events associated with oral anticoagulation, discontinuation of the antithrombotic should be followed by administration of vitamin K and fresh frozen plasma. Intravenous protamine sulfate may be given to reverse heparin in the setting of hemorrhage. Hemophiliacs with hemorrhagic stroke should immediately receive replacement of appropriate blood factor components. Elevated intracranial pressure may be rapidly reduced with hyperventilation, but intravenous mannitol, in 20% solution at a dose of 1.5 g/kg over 20 minutes, is preferred. Steroids are generally avoided due to harmful side effects and a lack of proven efficacy. Steroids may be used, however, in the treatment of purulent meningitis or to enhance platelet counts in the setting of immune thrombocytopenic purpura. Anticonvulsants may be employed for the treatment of seizures. Phenytoin is routinely employed, although phenobarbital is preferred during the neonatal period.

Thrombolytic therapy in pediatric stroke is predominantly extrapolated from clinical experience in the adult population. Although thrombolytic agents are likely effective in children as in adults, several age-related factors require further investigation. Thrombolytic pharmacodynamics may vary with age, with relatively decreased plasminogen levels and downregulation of fibrinolysis in children.[121] The vast majority of thrombolytic use in children has been associated with congenital heart disease complicated by cardiac catheterization, central venous access, and umbilical catheters.[121] Previous reports detail thrombolysis with several agents, yet tissue plasminogen activator (t-PA) is the only currently available thrombolytic approved for use in the cerebral circulation in adults. A review of thrombolysis with t-PA in the systemic circulation in 39 pediatric patients revealed successful recanalization rates, with minor bleeding in 54% and one intracranial hemorrhage. The dosage of intravenous t-PA for pediatric ischemic stroke generally recommended is that approved for adults: 0.9 mg/kg over an hour with 10% administered as a bolus over 1 to 2 minutes. Contraindications include any form of hemorrhage, clinical presentation more than 3 hours after symptom onset, radiographic findings of extensive hypodensity on CT, recent surgical procedures, or abnormal coagulation parameters. Intracranial hemorrhage is a feared complication of thrombolysis, yet only very limited data have addressed this complication in children.[121] Intra-arterial thrombolysis offers potential advantages compared with intravenous administration. Intra-arterial administration allows for selective catheterization of the occluded vessel, and direct contact with the thrombus allows mechanical interventions, with smaller thrombolytic doses and diminished systemic exposure of lytic agents.

In the absence of adequate early reperfusion, massive cerebral edema may complicate ischemic stroke leading to death. Early CT hypodensity encompassing more than half of the middle cerebral artery distribution has been correlated with up to an 80% mortality rate.[122–124] Massive cerebral edema may elevate intracranial pressure, causing ischemia in adjacent parenchyma, compressing neighboring vessels, diminishing cerebral perfusion pressure, and ultimately precipitating transtentorial herniation. Medical management of massive cerebral edema with mannitol, hyperventilation, and barbiturates has minimal, if any, effectiveness. Early decompressive surgery may improve the outcome of this catastrophic condition. Preliminary reports of decompressive surgery for middle cerebral artery ischemic stroke have demonstrated encouraging results,[125–128] with a prospective study of hemicraniectomy and duraplasty under way.[125] Decompressive hemicraniectomy requires a large craniectomy skull defect, durotomy, and potential insertion of cadaveric dura.[125] Edematous brain parenchyma is allowed to expand outward, and retrograde perfusion via leptomeningeal collaterals may be augmented. Resection of necrotic parenchyma or lobectomy is usually deferred.[125] Because early intervention is essential for the success of surgical decompression in malignant middle cerebral artery infarction, timing is critical. If pupillary dilatation consistent with transtentorial herniation is evident, decompressive surgery may be ineffective.[127] Clinical selection criteria for hemicraniectomy may be enhanced with diffusion and perfusion MRI elucidation of tissue at risk.[126] Potential disadvantages of surgical therapy for cerebral edema include trading fatal outcomes for severe disability. Refinements in surgical technique may also improve clinical outcomes. Younger patients are theoretically more likely to benefit from this procedure,[129] in part due to their greater potential for neuroplasticity and neurorepair, although very few cases have been reported

in the pediatric age group.[128] Future clinical trials may benefit from comparison with age-matched controls.[129]

> **PEARL** Decompressive hemicraniectomy requires a very large craniectomy and duraplasty to allow the edematous brain to expand outward.

In contrast to the predominantly cytotoxic cerebral edema seen in malignant ischemic infarcts, the predominantly vasogenic edema associated with cerebral venous thrombosis is more amenable to medical therapy. The management of cerebral venous thrombosis principally targets reduction of thrombus burden with subsequent resolution of venous hypertension and associated edema. Clinical trial data are conflicting, but overall suggest that anticoagulation may improve survival without considerable hemorrhagic complications.[130] In cases of progressive neurological deterioration despite anticoagulation, potential endovascular approaches may include dural sinus thrombolysis and rheolytic thrombectomy. Acetazolamide may be useful in diminishing complications of elevated intracranial pressure. Serial funduscopic examination to monitor papilledema and visual field testing may identify impending visual loss. Optic nerve sheath fenestration may avert catastrophic visual loss associated with this condition. Cerebrospinal fluid shunts may diminish the detrimental effects of hydrocephalus; however, anticoagulation or thrombolysis may be precluded by such interventions. Anticoagulation is empirically employed for 3 to 12 months. Determination of an underlying etiology is crucial because lifelong anticoagulation may be necessary for some hypercoagulable disorders.

Antithrombotic therapy is commonly employed in pediatric ischemic stroke, although therapeutic decisions must consider the risks and benefits specific to this age group. Recently published guidelines clarify the role of these agents in children.[131] Common uses of anticoagulation include treatment of arterial dissection, cerebral venous thrombosis, a high-risk embolic source, and hypercoagulable disorders. The selection of an anticoagulant and timing with regard to initiation of therapy depend on the estimated risk of recurrent ischemia. Unfractionated intravenous heparin is initially administered without a loading dose at 20 U/kg/h, although in children less than a year old the dose is 28 U/kg/h.[131] Subsequent dose titrations should aim for a target-activated partial thromboplastin time of 45 to 60 seconds. Low molecular weight heparin may also be used in children (e.g., enoxaparin given subcutaneously as 1 mg/kg, or 1.5 mg/kg in neonates every 12 hours). Warfarin is the standard oral anticoagulant used in children. The initial dose of warfarin is 0.2 mg/kg, followed by a maintenance daily dose at ~25 to 50% of the initial dose and titrated to the international normalized ratio (INR). Lower doses may be necessary in patients with hepatic dysfunction. The INR is usually maintained at 2 to 3, although an elevated therapeutic range is used for antiphospholipid antibody syndrome[132] and mechanical heart valves. Heparinization prior to initiation of warfarin is advised for protein C deficiency. Adverse side effects of anticoagulation principally encompass hemorrhagic complications, including hemorrhagic transformation of an ischemic infarct, gastrointestinal or genitourinary bleeding, and spinal epidural hematoma associated with thrombocytopenia or recent lumbar puncture. Contraindications to anticoagulation may include active bleeding, extensive cerebral infarction, thrombocytopenia, recent or pending neurosurgical procedures, concurrent medications, pregnancy, or high risk of trauma. During pregnancy, unfractionated and low molecular weight heparin is the only anticoagulant or antithrombotic agent available free of teratogenic effects. Evidence of drug hypersensitivity may also limit therapeutic options. Dietary changes and interactions with other medications that influence the INR should be carefully monitored. Treatment with anticoagulation is generally pursued when the benefit of stroke prevention exceeds the likelihood of adverse effects. Anticoagulation in cerebral venous thrombosis appears beneficial, even when intracranial hemorrhage is present. Reasonable safety without substantial hemorrhagic complications has been demonstrated in more than 100 children treated with low molecular weight heparin for systemic thromboses.[133] In children, relatively frequent trauma may elevate the risk of anticoagulation. Children on anticoagulation may need to limit exposure to contact sports, but overall clinical experience suggests reasonable safety of anticoagulation in children.

Alternative antithrombotic agents include aspirin and other antiplatelet medications. Because sparse data are available for the use of other antiplatelet medications in children, aspirin is most commonly prescribed. A dosage of 2 to 3 mg/kg effectively inhibits platelet aggregation, although clinical efficacy has yet to be established. Aspirin is routinely employed for children with stroke or transient ischemic attacks, particularly in those without obvious risk factors, isolated small to medium patent foramen ovale, contraindications to anticoagulation, or financial limitations. Ongoing aspirin therapy may be used in older children but is generally avoided in the neonatal population. Contraindications to aspirin include active bleeding, hypersensitivity, urticaria, and bronchospasm. Other considerations include the risk of Reye's syndrome and hemorrhagic complications promoted by concurrent medication use.

Specific therapies may be of benefit for select causes of pediatric stroke. Folate supplementation with vitamins or fortification of flour may counter elevations in serum homocysteine.[134] When hyperlipidemia is present, statin medications may decrease cholesterol and triglyceride levels. Alternating hemiplegia may be treated with flunarizine.[135–137] Prophylactic treatment with propanolol or verapamil may diminish migrainous complications.[110] Prophylactic therapy of hypercoagulable disorders may include long-term anticoagulation with adjusted-dose warfarin.[52,132]

Unlike other causes of pediatric stroke, considerable data are available regarding primary prevention and treatment of stroke associated with sickle cell disease. Red blood cell transfusions may prevent most strokes due to this disorder. The management of sickle cell disease has been revolutionized by Stroke Prevention Trial in Sickle Cell Anemia (STOP), demonstrating primary stroke prevention with periodic transfusions in a high-risk population identified by TCD. Children with mean blood flow velocities exceeding 200 cm/s were randomized to periodic transfusions or standard care. The clinical trial was terminated due to a 10-fold reduction in stroke in those receiving transfusions.[120] Exchange transfusions are continued on a chronic basis to reduce the level of hemoglobin S to less than 15 to 30%.[137,138] These red blood cell transfusions are typically administered every 3 to 4 weeks, although the optimal frequency is unclear. Optimal duration of therapy is also unknown, although transfusions are usually continued for 2 years. Prolonged transfusion therapy benefits in stroke risk reduction must be balanced by the possibility of secondary complications, including iron overload, sensitization to blood products, and hepatitis. Iron overload and hemosiderosis may require administration of deferoxamine, or iron chelation.[40,138,139] Elevations in serum ferritin usually prompt institution of iron chelation. Stroke risk may return following discontinuation of transfusions; optimal end points for transfusion therapy have yet to be established. Alternative approaches include bone marrow transplantation and the use of hydroxyurea.[141,142] Preliminary results of allogeneic bone marrow transplantation in selected individuals reveal beneficial effects, with decreased hemolysis and resolution of vaso-occlusive crises.[141] Financial analyses suggest that transfusions cost less than recurrent stroke, yet the added costs of chronic chelation encourage the development of cost-effective alternatives, possibly including bone marrow transplantation.[143] Finally, cardiac surgery may be indicated for the treatment of congenital heart disease and high-risk cardioembolic sources including atrial myxomas.

Rehabilitation is an important element in the management of pediatric stroke because early recognition of functional limitations and aggressive therapy may have long-term benefits. Physical, occupational, and speech therapy should be individualized based on early assessment of rehabilitative consultations. Age-appropriate facilities should be utilized and functional recovery assessed with an objective tool, such as the Pediatric

Stroke Outcome Measure.[103] Cognitive deficits may be relatively subtle but considerably disabling in school activities. Special education may be required for children with frank visual, motor, or perceptual deficits, or more subtle attentional or learning disabilities. Social work and neuropsychology referrals may be particularly helpful in the convalescent phase of pediatric stroke. Education regarding the hazards of drugs, alcohol, and tobacco are important components of stroke prevention in this younger population.

REFERENCES

1. Roach ES, Riela A. Pediatric Cerebrovascular Disorders. 2nd ed. Armonk, NY: Futura;1995
2. Natowicz M, Kelley RI. Mendelian etiologies of stroke. Ann Neurol 1987;22:175–192
3. Schoenberg BS, Mellinger JF, Schoenberg DG. Cerebrovascular disease in infants and children: a study of incidence, clinical features, and survival. Neurology 1978;28:763–768
4. Broderick J, Talbot GT, Prenger E, Leach A, Brott T. Stroke in children within a major metropolitan area: the surprising importance of intracerebral hemorrhage. J Child Neurol 1993;8:250–255
5. Williams LS, Garg BP, Cohen M, Fleck JD, Biller J. Subtypes of ischemic stroke in children and young adults. Neurology 1997;49:1541–1545
6. Kerr LM, Anderson DM, Thompson JA, Lyver SM, Call GK. Ischemic stroke in the young: evaluation and age comparison of patients six months to thirty-nine years. J Child Neurol 1993;8:266–270
7. Roach ES. Cerebrovascular disorders and trauma in children. Curr Opin Pediatr 1993;5:660–668
8. Allan WC. The IVH complex of lesions: cerebrovascular injury in the preterm infant. Neurol Clin 1990;8:529–551
9. deVeber G, Group CPISS. Canadian Pediatric Ischemic Stroke Registry: analysis of children with arterial ischemic stroke [abstract]. Ann Neurol 2000;48:514
10. Roach ES. Stroke in children. Curr Treat Options Neurol 2000;2:295–304
11. Chabrier S, Husson B, Lasjaunias P, Landrieu P, Tardieu M. Stroke in childhood: outcome and recurrence risk by mechanism in 59 patients. J Child Neurol 2000;15:290–294
12. Saver JL, Easton JD. Dissections and trauma of cervicocerebral arteries. In: Barnett HJM, Mohr JP, Stein BM, Yatsu FM, eds. Stroke: Pathophysiology, Diagnosis, and Management. Vol 1. 3rd ed. Philadelphia: Churchill Livingstone; 1998:769–786
13. Schievink WI, Michels VV, Piepgras DG. Neurovascular manifestations of heritable connective tissue disorders: a review. Stroke 1994;25:889–903
14. Youl BD, Coutellier A, Dubois B, Leger JM, Bousser MG. Three cases of spontaneous extracranial vertebral artery dissection. Stroke 1990;21:618–625
15. Schievink WI, Limburg M, Oorthuys JW, Fleury P, Pope FM. Cerebrovascular disease in Ehlers-Danlos syndrome type IV. Stroke 1990;21:626–632
16. Schievink WI, Mokri B, O'Fallon WM. Recurrent spontaneous cervical-artery dissection. N Engl J Med 1994;330:393–397
17. Hegedus K. Reticular fiber deficiency in the intracranial arteries of patients with dissecting aneurysm and review of the possible pathogenesis of previously reported cases. Eur Arch Psychiatry Neurol Sci 1985;235:102–106
18. Mokri B, Houser OW, Sandok BA, Piepgras DG. Spontaneous dissections of the vertebral arteries. Neurology 1988;38:880–885
19. Schievink WI, Prakash UB, Piepgras DG, Mokri B. Alpha 1-antitrypsin deficiency in intracranial aneurysms and cervical artery dissection. Lancet 1994;343:452–453
20. Schievink WI, Mokri B. Familial aorto-cervicocephalic arterial dissections and congenitally bicuspid aortic valve. Stroke 1995;26:1935–1940
21. Schievink WI, Michels VV, Mokri B, Piepgras DG, Perry HO. Brief report: a familial syndrome of arterial dissections with lentiginosis. N Engl J Med 1995;332:576–579
22. Schievink WI, Mokri B, Piepgras DG, Kuiper JD. Recurrent spontaneous arterial dissections: risk in familial versus nonfamilial disease. Stroke 1996;27:622–624
23. Majamaa K, Portimojarvi H, Sotaniemi KA, Myllyla VV. Familial aggregation of cervical artery dissection and cerebral aneurysm. Stroke 1994;25:1704–1705
24. Schievink WI, Mokri B, Piepgras DG, Gittenberger-de Groot AC. Intracranial aneurysms and cervicocephalic arterial dissections associated with congenital heart disease. Neurosurgery 1996;39:685–689 discussion 689–690
25. Mokri B, Sundt TM Jr, Houser OW, Piepgras DG. Spontaneous dissection of the cervical internal carotid artery. Ann Neurol 1986;19:126–138
26. Takis C, Saver JL. Cervicocephalic carotid and vertebral artery dissection: management. In: Batjer HH, Caplan LR, Friberg L, Greenlee RG Jr, Kopitnik TA Jr, Young WL, eds. Cerebrovascular Disease. Vol 1. Philadelphia: Lippincott-Raven; 1997:385–396
27. D'Anglejan-Chatillon J, Ribeiro V, Mas JL, Youl BD, Bousser MG. Migraine: a risk factor for dissection of cervical arteries. Headache 1989;29:560–561
28. Fisher CM. The headache and pain of spontaneous carotid dissection. Headache 1982;22:60–65
29. Tietjen GE. The relationship of migraine and stroke. Neuroepidemiology 2000;19:13–19
30. Grau AJ, Brandt T, Buggle F, et al. Association of cervical artery dissection with recent infection. Arch Neurol 1999;56:851–856
31. Barbour PJ, Castaldo JE, Rae-Grant AD, et al. Internal carotid artery redundancy is significantly associated with dissection. Stroke 1994;25:1201–1206
32. Al-Jarallah A, Al-Rifai MT, Riela AR, Roach ES. Nontraumatic brain hemorrhage in children: etiology and presentation. J Child Neurol 2000;15:284–289
33. McCormick WF, Rosenfield DB. Massive brain hemorrhage: a review of 144 cases and an examination of their causes. Stroke 1973;4:946–954
34. Riikonen R, Donner M. ACTH therapy in infantile spasms: side effects. Arch Dis Child 1980;55:664–672
35. Haffner SM, D'Agostino R, Mykkanen L, et al. Proinsulin and insulin concentrations in relation to carotid wall thickness: Insulin Resistance Atherosclerosis Study. Stroke 1998;29:1498–1503
36. Abram HS, Knepper LE, Warty VS, Painter MJ. Natural history, prognosis, and lipid abnormalities of idiopathic ischemic childhood stroke. J Child Neurol 1996;11:276–282
37. Saver JL, Tamburi T. Genetics of cerebrovascular disease. In: Pulst S-M, ed. Neurogenetics. New York: Oxford University Press; 2000:403–432
38. Celermajer DS, Adams MR, Clarkson P, et al. Passive smoking and impaired endothelium-dependent arterial dilatation in healthy young adults. N Engl J Med 1996;334:150–154
39. Heier LA, Carpanzano CR, Mast J, Brill PW, Winchester P, Deck MD. Maternal cocaine abuse: the spectrum of radiologic abnormalities in the neonatal CNS. AJNR Am J Neuroradiol 1991;12:951–956
40. Powars D, Wilson B, Imbus C, Pegelow C, Allen J. The natural history of stroke in sickle cell disease. Am J Med 1978;65:461–471

41. Balkaran B, Char G, Morris JS, Thomas PW, Serjeant BE, Serjeant GR. Stroke in a cohort of patients with homozygous sickle cell disease. J Pediatr 1992;120:360–366

42. Grotta JC, Manner C, Pettigrew LC, Yatsu FM. Red blood cell disorders and stroke. Stroke 1986;17:811–817

43. Pavlakis SG, Bello J, Prohovnik I, et al. Brain infarction in sickle cell anemia: magnetic resonance imaging correlates. Ann Neurol 1988;23:125–130

44. Moser FG, Miller ST, Bello JA, et al. The spectrum of brain MR abnormalities in sickle-cell disease: a report from the Cooperative Study of Sickle Cell Disease. AJNR Am J Neuroradiol 1996;17: 965–972

45. Pavlakis SG, Kingsley PB, Bialer MG. Stroke in children: genetic and metabolic issues. J Child Neurol 2000;15:308–315

46. Ohene-Frempong K, Weiner SJ, Sleeper LA, et al. Cerebrovascular accidents in sickle cell disease: rates and risk factors. Blood 1998;91:288–294

47. Carhuapoma JR, Mitsias P, Levine SR. Cerebral venous thrombosis and anticardiolipin antibodies. Stroke 1997;28:2363–2369

48. Brey RL, Hart RG, Sherman DG, Tegeler CH. Antiphospholipid antibodies and cerebral ischemia in young people. Neurology 1990;40:1190–1196

49. Asherson RA, Khamashta MA, Gil A, et al. Cerebrovascular disease and antiphospholipid antibodies in systemic lupus erythematosus, lupus-like disease, and the primary antiphospholipid syndrome. Am J Med 1989;86:391–399

50. Hess DC, Krauss J, Adams RJ, Nichols FT, Zhang D, Rountree HA. Anticardiolipin antibodies: a study of frequency in TIA and stroke. Neurology 1991;41:525–528

51. Nencini P, Baruffi MC, Abbate R, Massai G, Amaducci L, Inzitari D. Lupus anticoagulant and anticardiolipin antibodies in young adults with cerebral ischemia. Stroke 1992;23:189–193

52. Angelini L, Ravelli A, Caporali R, Rumi V, Nardocci N, Martini A. High prevalence of antiphospholipid antibodies in children with idiopathic cerebral ischemia. Pediatrics 1994;94(4 Pt 1):500–503

53. Kato H, Shirahama M, Ohmori K, Sunaga T. Cerebral infarction in a young adult associated with protein C deficiency: a case report. Angiology 1995;46:169–173

54. Brown DC, Livingston JH, Minns RA, Eden OB. Protein C and S deficiency causing childhood stroke. Scott Med J 1993;38: 114–115

55. Israels SJ, Seshia SS. Childhood stroke associated with protein C or S deficiency. J Pediatr 1987;111:562–564

56. Kohler J, Kasper J, Witt I, von Reutern GM. Ischemic stroke due to protein C deficiency. Stroke 1990;21:1077–1080

57. Koller H, Stoll G, Sitzer M, Burk M, Schottler B, Freund HJ. Deficiency of both protein C and protein S in a family with ischemic strokes in young adults. Neurology 1994;44:1238–1240

58. Uysal S, Anlar B, Altay C, Kirazli S. Role of protein C in childhood cerebrovascular occlusive accidents. Eur J Pediatr 1989;149: 216–218

59. van Kuijck MA, Rotteveel JJ, van Oostrom CG, Novakova I. Neurological complications in children with protein C deficiency. Neuropediatrics 1994;25:16–19

60. Simioni P, Battistella PA, Drigo P, Carollo C, Girolami A. Childhood stroke associated with familial protein S deficiency. Brain Dev 1994;16:241–245

61. Thorarensen O, Ryan S, Hunter J, Younkin DP. Factor V Leiden mutation: an unrecognized cause of hemiplegic cerebral palsy, neonatal stroke, and placental thrombosis. Ann Neurol 1997;42: 372–375

62. Ganesan V, Kelsey H, Cookson J, Osborn A, Kirkham FJ. Activated protein C resistance in childhood stroke. Lancet 1996;347:260

63. Zenz W, Bodo Z, Plotho J, et al. Factor V Leiden and prothrombin gene G 20210 A variant in children with ischemic stroke. Thromb Haemost 1998;80:763–766

64. McColl MD, Chalmers EA, Thomas A, et al. Factor V Leiden, prothrombin 20210G→A and the MTHFR C677T mutations in childhood stroke. Thromb Haemost 1999;81:690–694

65. Catto A, Carter A, Ireland H, et al. Factor V Leiden gene mutation and thrombin generation in relation to the development of acute stroke. Arterioscler Thromb Vasc Biol 1995;15: 783–785

66. Riikonen RS, Vahtera EM, Kekomaki RM. Physiological anticoagulants and activated protein C resistance in childhood stroke. Acta Paediatr 1996;85:242–244

67. Lalouschek W, Aull S, Serles W, et al. C677T MTHFR mutation and factor V Leiden mutation in patients with TIA/minor stroke: a case-control study. Thromb Res 1999;93:61–69

68. Gaustadnes M, Rudiger N, Ingerslev J. The 20210 A allele of the prothrombin gene is not a risk factor for juvenile stroke in the Danish population. Blood Coagul Fibrinolysis 1998;9: 663–664

69. Mandel H, Brenner B, Berant M, et al. Coexistence of hereditary homocystinuria and factor V Leiden: effect on thrombosis. N Engl J Med 1996;334:763–768

70. van Beynum IM, Smeitink JA, den Heijer M, te Poele Pothoff MT, Blom HJ. Hyperhomocysteinemia: a risk factor for ischemic stroke in children. Circulation 1999;99:2070–2072

71. Cardo E, Vilaseca MA, Campistol J, Artuch R, Colome C, Pineda M. Evaluation of hyperhomocysteinaemia in children with stroke. Eur J Paediatr Neurol 1999;3:113–117

72. Prengler M, Sturt N, Krywawych S, Surtees R, Liesner R, Kirkham F. Homozygous thermolabile variant of the methylenetetrahydrofolate reductase gene: a potential risk factor for hyperhomocysteinaemia, CVD, and stroke in childhood. Dev Med Child Neurol 2001;43:220–225

73. Clarke R, Daly L, Robinson K, et al. Hyperhomocysteinemia: an independent risk factor for vascular disease. N Engl J Med 1991; 324:1149–1155

74. Fletcher O, Kessling AM. MTHFR association with arteriosclerotic vascular disease? Hum Genet 1998;103:11–21

75. Refsum H, Ueland PM, Nygard O, Vollset SE. Homocysteine and cardiovascular disease. Annu Rev Med 1998;49:31–62

76. Nygard O, Refsum H, Ueland PM, Vollset SE. Major lifestyle determinants of plasma total homocysteine distribution: the Hordaland Homocysteine Study. Am J Clin Nutr 1998;67:263–270

77. Hartfield DS, Lowry NJ, Keene DL, Yager JY. Iron deficiency: a cause of stroke in infants and children. Pediatr Neurol 1997;16: 50–53

78. Lutschg J, Vassella F. Neurological complications in hemophilia. Acta Paediatr Scand 1981;70:235–241

79. Hoyer LW. Hemophilia A. N Engl J Med 1994;330:38–47

80. de Tezanos Pinto M, Fernandez J, Perez Bianco PR. Update of 156 episodes of central nervous system bleeding in hemophiliacs. Haemostasis 1992;22:259–267

81. Eyster ME, Gill FM, Blatt PM, Hilgartner MW, Ballard JO, Kinney TR. Central nervous system bleeding in hemophiliacs. Blood 1978; 51:1179–1188

82. Riikonen R, Santavuori P. Hereditary and acquired risk factors for childhood stroke. Neuropediatrics 1994;25:227–233

83. Brower MC, Rollins N, Roach ES. Basal ganglia and thalamic infarction in children: cause and clinical features. Arch Neurol 1996;53:1252–1256

84. Fu M, Wong KS, Lam WW, Wong GW. Middle cerebral artery occlusion after recent *Mycoplasma pneumoniae* infection. J Neurol Sci 1998;157:113–115

85. Parker P, Puck J, Fernandez F. Cerebral infarction associated with *Mycoplasma pneumoniae*. Pediatrics 1981;67:373–375

86. Roden VJ, Cantor HE, O'Connor DM, Schmidt RR, Cherry JD. Acute hemiplegia of childhood associated with coxsackie A9 viral infection. J Pediatr 1975;86:56–58

87. Askalan R, Laughlin S, Mayank S, et al. Chickenpox and stroke in childhood: a study of frequency and causation. Stroke 2001;32:1257–1262

88. Shuper A, Vining EP, Freeman JM. Central nervous system vasculitis after chickenpox: cause or coincidence? Arch Dis Child 1990;65:1245–1248

89. Ganesan V, Kirkham FJ. Mechanisms of ischaemic stroke after chickenpox. Arch Dis Child 1997;76:522–525

90. Silverstein FS, Brunberg JA. Postvaricella basal ganglia infarction in children. AJNR Am J Neuroradiol 1995;16:449–452

91. Caekebeke JF, Peters AC, Vandvik B, Brouwer OF, de Bakker HM. Cerebral vasculopathy associated with primary varicella infection. Arch Neurol 1990;47:1033–1035

92. Kovacs SO, Kuban K, Strand R. Lateral medullary syndrome following varicella infection. Am J Dis Child 1993;147:823–825

93. Park YD, Belman AL, Kim TS, et al. Stroke in pediatric acquired immunodeficiency syndrome. Ann Neurol 1990;28:303–311

94. Visudtibhan A, Visudhiphan P, Chiemchanya S. Stroke and seizures as the presenting signs of pediatric HIV infection. Pediatr Neurol 1999;20:53–56

95. Broderick JP, Swanson JW. Migraine-related strokes: clinical profile and prognosis in 20 patients. Arch Neurol 1987;44:868–871

96. Ferrera PC, Curran CB, Swanson H. Etiology of pediatric ischemic stroke. Am J Emerg Med 1997;15:671–679

97. Biousse V, D'Anglejan-Chatillon J, Massiou H, Bousser MG. Head pain in non-traumatic carotid artery dissection: a series of 65 patients. Cephalalgia 1994;14:33–36

98. Silbert PL, Mokri B, Schievink WI. Headache and neck pain in spontaneous internal carotid and vertebral artery dissections. Neurology 1995;45:1517–1522

99. Rao TH, Schneider LB, Patel M, Libman RB. Central retinal artery occlusion from carotid dissection diagnosed by cervical computed tomography. Stroke 1994;25:1271–1272

100. Biousse V, Schaison M, Touboul PJ, D'Anglejan-Chatillon J, Bousser MG. Ischemic optic neuropathy associated with internal carotid artery dissection. Arch Neurol 1998;55:715–719

101. Biousse V, Touboul PJ, D'Anglejan-Chatillon J, Levy C, Schaison M, Bousser MG. Ophthalmologic manifestations of internal carotid artery dissection. Am J Ophthalmol 1998;126:565–577

102. Kondziolka D, Humphreys RP, Hoffman HJ, Hendrick EB, Drake JM. Arteriovenous malformations of the brain in children: a forty year experience. Can J Neurol Sci 1992;19:40–45

103. deVeber GA, MacGregor D, Curtis R, Mayank S. Neurologic outcome in survivors of childhood arterial ischemic stroke and sinovenous thrombosis. J Child Neurol 2000;15:316–324

104. Lanska MJ, Lanska DJ, Horwitz SJ, Aram DM. Presentation, clinical course, and outcome of childhood stroke. Pediatr Neurol 1991;7:333–341

105. Higgins JJ, Kammerman LA, Fitz CR. Predictors of survival and characteristics of childhood stroke. Neuropediatrics 1991;22:190–193

106. Keidan I, Shahar E, Barzilay Z, Passwell J, Brand N. Predictors of outcome of stroke in infants and children based on clinical data and radiologic correlates. Acta Paediatr 1994;83:762–765

107. Celli P, Ferrante L, Palma L, Cavedon G. Cerebral arteriovenous malformations in children. Clinical features and outcome of treatment in children and in adults. Surg Neurol 1984;22:43–49

108. Leys D, Moulin T, Stojkovic T, Begey S, Chavot D, Investigators D. Follow-up of patients with history of cervical artery dissection. Cerebrovasc Dis 1995;5:43–49

109. Bassetti C, Carruzzo A, Sturzenegger M, Tuncdogan E. Recurrence of cervical artery dissection: a prospective study of 81 patients. Stroke 1996;27:1804–1807

110. Rothrock J, North J, Madden K, Lyden P, Fleck P, Dittrich H. Migraine and migrainous stroke: risk factors and prognosis. Neurology 1993;43:2473–2476

111. Barnes PD, O'Tuama L, Tzika A. Investigating the pediatric central nervous system. Curr Opin Pediatr 1993;5:643–652

112. Levy C, Laissy JP, Raveau V, et al. Carotid and vertebral artery dissections: three-dimensional time-of-flight MR angiography and MR imaging versus conventional angiography. Radiology 1994;190:97–103

113. Zuber M, Meary E, Meder JF, Mas JL. Magnetic resonance imaging and dynamic CT scan in cervical artery dissections. Stroke 1994;25:576–581

114. Gadian DG, Calamante F, Kirkham FJ, et al. Diffusion and perfusion magnetic resonance imaging in childhood stroke. J Child Neurol 2000;15:279–283

115. Detre JA, Alsop DC, Vives LR, Maccotta L, Teener JW, Raps EC. Noninvasive MRI evaluation of cerebral blood flow in cerebrovascular disease. Neurology 1998;50:633–641

116. Pavlakis SG, Kingsley PB, Kaplan GP, Stacpoole PW, O'Shea M, Lustbader D. Magnetic resonance spectroscopy: use in monitoring MELAS treatment. Arch Neurol 1998;55:849–852

117. Shirane R, Sato S, Yoshimoto T. Angiographic findings of ischemic stroke in children. Childs Nerv Syst 1992;8:432–436

118. Chabrier S, Rodesch G, Lasjaunias P, Tardieu M, Landrieu P, Sebire G. Transient cerebral arteriopathy: a disorder recognized by serial angiograms in children with stroke. J Child Neurol 1998;13:27–32

119. Ganesan V, Savvy L, Chong WK, Kirkham FJ. Conventional cerebral angiography in children with ischemic stroke. Pediatr Neurol 1999;20:38–42

120. Adams RJ, McKie VC, Hsu L, et al. Prevention of a first stroke by transfusions in children with sickle cell anemia and abnormal results on transcranial Doppler ultrasonography. N Engl J Med 1998;339:5–11

121. Leaker M, Massicotte MP, Brooker LA, Andrew M. Thrombolytic therapy in pediatric patients: a comprehensive review of the literature. Thromb Haemost 1996;76:132–134

122. Jourdan C, Convert J, Mottolese C, Bachour E, Gharbi S, Artru F. Evaluation of the clinical benefit of decompression hemicraniectomy in intracranial hypertension not controlled by medical treatment [in French]. Neurochirurgie 1993;39:304–310

123. Ropper AH, Shafran B. Brain edema after stroke: clinical syndrome and intracranial pressure. Arch Neurol 1984;41:26–29

124. von Kummer R, Meyding-Lamade U, Forsting M, et al. Sensitivity and prognostic value of early CT in occlusion of the middle cerebral artery trunk. AJNR Am J Neuroradiol 1994;15:9–15 discussion 16–18

125. Wijdicks EF. Hemicraniotomy in massive hemispheric stroke: a stark perspective on a radical procedure. Can J Neurol Sci 2000;27:271–273

126. Doerfler A, Engelhorn T, Forsting M. Decompressive craniectomy for early therapy and secondary prevention of cerebral infarction. Stroke 2001;32:813–815

127. Schwab S, Steiner T, Aschoff A, et al. Early hemicraniectomy in patients with complete middle cerebral artery infarction. Stroke 1998;29:1888–1893

128. Carter BS, Ogilvy CS, Candia GJ, Rosas HD, Buonanno F. One-year outcome after decompressive surgery for massive nondominant hemispheric infarction. Neurosurgery 1997;40:1168–1175 discussion 1175–1166

129. Wijdicks EF, Diringer MN. Middle cerebral artery territory infarction and early brain swelling: progression and effect of age on outcome. Mayo Clin Proc 1998;73:829–836

130. deVeber G, Chan A, Monagle P, et al. Anticoagulation therapy in pediatric patients with sinovenous thrombosis: a cohort study. Arch Neurol 1998;55:1533–1537

131. Monagle P, Michelson AD, Bovill E, Andrew M. Antithrombotic therapy in children. Chest 2001;119(Suppl 1):344S–370S

132. Khamashta MA, Cuadrado MJ, Mujic F, Taub NA, Hunt BJ, Hughes GR. The management of thrombosis in the antiphospholipid-antibody syndrome. N Engl J Med 1995;332:993–997

133. Massicotte P, Adams M, Marzinotto V, Brooker LA, Andrew M. Low-molecular-weight heparin in pediatric patients with thrombotic disease: a dose finding study. J Pediatr 1996;128: 313–318

134. Woodside JV, Yarnell JW, McMaster D, et al. Effect of B-group vitamins and antioxidant vitamins on hyperhomocysteinemia: a double-blind, randomized, factorial-design, controlled trial. Am J Clin Nutr 1998;67:858–866

135. Sasaki M, Sakuragawa N, Osawa M. Long-term effect of flunarizine on patients with alternating hemiplegia of childhood in Japan. Brain Dev 2001;23:303–305

136. Mikati MA, Kramer U, Zupanc ML, Shanahan RJ. Alternating hemiplegia of childhood: clinical manifestations and long-term outcome. Pediatr Neurol 2000;23:134–141

137. Casaer P, Azou M. Flunarizine in alternating hemiplegia in childhood. Lancet 1984;2:579

138. Adams RJ. Lessons from the Stroke Prevention Trial in Sickle Cell Anemia (STOP) study. J Child Neurol 2000;15:344–349

139. Cohen AR, Martin MB. Iron chelation therapy in sickle cell disease. Semin Hematol 2001;38(Suppl 1)69–72

140. Pegelow CH. Stroke in children with sickle cell anaemia: aetiology and treatment. Paediatr Drugs 2001;3:421–432

141. Hoppe CC, Walters MC. Bone marrow transplantation in sickle cell anemia. Curr Opin Oncol 2001;13:85–90

142. Vermylen C, Fernandez Robles E, Ninane J, Cornu G. Bone marrow transplantation in five children with sickle cell anaemia. Lancet 1988;1:1427–1428

143. Wayne AS, Schoenike SE, Pegelow CH. Financial analysis of chronic transfusion for stroke prevention in sickle cell disease. Blood 2000;96:2369–2372

4

Neuroangiography in Children

MANRAJ K.S. HERAN AND MICHAEL J. ALEXANDER

■ Indications

Pediatric cerebrovascular disease has been characterized by many investigators.[1-7] Advances in noninvasive imaging such as magnetic resonance imaging and magnetic resonance angiography (MRI/MRA), computed tomography and computed tomographic angiography (CT/CTA), and ultrasound, have allowed for a paradigm shift in the diagnosis of cerebrovascular conditions in the pediatric patient. However, catheter angiography continues to be the "gold standard" for many conditions (**Fig. 4–1**) and indications,[1,2,6,8-16] including the explosion of interventional neuroradiology procedures.[1,4,17-26] Some indications for pediatric cerebral angiography are listed in **Table 4–1**.

■ Radiation Protection

The patient and the personnel involved in the angiographic examination must be protected from the potentially harmful effects of ionizing radiation. The pediatric patient has been shown to be more sensitive to radiation effects than adults.[27] The concept of "as low as reasonably achievable" is extremely useful in planning and implementing methods to reduce the dose,[27,28] and principles regarding patient protection in diagnostic radiology have been reviewed elsewhere.[27]

Patient exposure can be reduced by the use of progressive pulse fluoroscopy instead of continuous fluoroscopy. Filter use, appropriate patient shielding, optimal coning, and reduction in distance between the image intensifier and the patient all allow for reduction in scattered radiation. Every attempt must also be made to reduce total fluoroscopy and angiography run times.

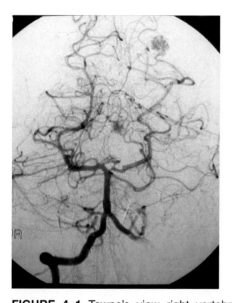

FIGURE 4–1 Towne's view right vertebral artery cerebral angiogram demonstrating two distinct small arteriovenous malformations in a 15-year-old girl with hereditary hemorrhagic telangiectasia (Osler-Weber-Rendu syndrome).

TABLE 4–1 Indications for Cerebral Angiography

Investigation and treatment of cervical, facial, and intracranial vascular abnormalities
Aneurysms
Vascular malformations
Vascular occlusive disease
Assessment/follow-up of previous therapies (e.g., clipping/coiling of aneurysm)
Workup of acute hemorrhagic/ischemic stroke, of unknown etiology, beyond neonatal period
Presurgical investigation, and possible embolization, of head and neck, and intracranial tumors
Potential vascular traumatic injury, either blunt or penetrating
Functional testing for speech and memory before planned therapeutic interventions

■ Evaluation and Preparation

Specific issues, such as allergies, antibiotic prophylaxis, serum creatinine, coagulation parameters, and bleeding tendencies must be reviewed. Clotting studies are not routinely performed unless a history of known blood dyscrasias, easy bruising, or medical conditions or medications known to affect coagulability are encountered. In most instances, elective procedures can be performed safely with an international normalized ratio (INR) <1.2. An INR <1.5 is preferred for urgent cases. Emergency cases must be evaluated on a case by case basis. Coagulopathy can be allowed to correct on its own or can be corrected emergently with oral or intravenous vitamin K or the use of fresh frozen plasma. Physical examination relevant to angiography is imperative. Cardiopulmonary and vascular assessment is mandatory, with evaluation and documentation of all peripheral pulses. The child's weight and height should be recorded. If sedation is considered, choice and route of sedation must be decided, along with desired site of vascular access. Intravenous access must be secured prior to initiation of the angiogram.

Leads and probes for routine monitoring via electrocardiogram, blood pressure, and respiratory status are placed. Because children less than 2 years of age are very susceptible to ambient temperature and temperature changes, thermal monitoring is recommended. Raising the ambient temperature of the angiography suite is often helpful, as is a warming mattress or wrapping the child. For neonates and young infants, overhead heat lamps or radiant heat warmers can be used. Urinary catheters ensure patient comfort during lengthy procedures, especially because many children are unable to void while lying supine on the angiography table. Also important is proper padding of pressure points to minimize nerve palsies,[1,28,29] and patient immobilization for optimizing image quality and minimizing angiographic runs.

> **PEARL** Thermal monitoring is recommended, particularly in children 2 years old and younger.

■ Sedation

Sedation is often necessary for angiography in children.[1,4,8,16,17,21,22,30,31] Choices for sedation/analgesia include local anesthetic alone or in combination with conscious sedation or general anesthesia. Published guidelines exist with respect to sedation of children outside the operating room or intensive care unit.[32] Whereas patients over the age of 10 years are sometimes able to tolerate cerebral angiography without conscious sedation or general anesthesia, those under 10 years almost always will require some form of sedation to ensure cooperation and adequate immobility. Lengthy procedures or planned interventions should not be done without ensuring adequate sedation or general anesthesia.[1,8,16] Newborn infants may not require sedation.[30,33] If sedation is used, their unique sensitivity to the central nervous system depressant effects of narcotics must be kept in mind.

General anesthesia is often reserved for procedures requiring complete patient cooperation, procedures that may be either painful or prolonged, or patients who have previously failed conscious sedation efforts.[22,34] Local anesthetic at the access site is still strongly recommended because it lessens postprocedure discomfort, improves cooperation, and may reduce the incidence of vasospasm.[30] Whereas lidocaine 1 to 2% is most commonly employed, combination with 0.25% bupivacaine can provide prolonged local analgesia. Lidocaine doses exceeding 6 mg/kg should be avoided because systemic neurotoxicity may occur.[30] EMLA cream applied topically at the access site is an alternative; however, its application 30 to 45 minutes prior to beginning the procedure is sometimes not possible.

Because there is no single ideal sedation drug, a working knowledge of several sedation and analgesic medications is required, as is the ability to provide emergency resuscitation. Appropriate use of reversal medications, such as naloxone (0.01 to 0.1 mg/kg IV) and flumazenil (0.01 mg/kg/dose, max dose 0.2 mg) is mandatory. Many sedation protocols exist.[28,30,35,36] Chloral hydrate (25 to 100 µg/kg, orally or rectally), a widely used agent for nonpainful and noninvasive diagnostic procedures such as CT and MRI examinations, especially in those less than 3 years of age, is not appropriate for angiography due to its lack of analgesic properties and inconsistencies of dose effectiveness.

Choice of medications now commonly includes benzodiazepines, barbiturates, and opioid narcotics. Ketamine and propofol are increasing in use.[29,30,37] Diphenhydramine (1 to 1.25 mg/kg PO/IV/IM) can be used for its sedation and antiemesis qualities. Combination of opioid analgesics and benzodiazepines provides good analgesia and anxiolysis and potential procedural amnesia.[8] Premedication using oral pentobarbital (4 mg/kg) or meperidine (3 mg/kg) is often beneficial in children over the age of 18 months. Safe sedation can be achieved using a combination of pentobarbital (3 to 6 mg/kg IV) and morphine sulfate (0.1 to 0.2 mg/kg IV), or midazolam (0.05 to 0.35 mg/kg IV) and morphine.[16] A more common conscious sedation regimen consists of short-acting IV medications such as midazolam and fentanyl. Dosing for fentanyl is higher than for adults, with children requiring 1 to 3 µg/kg. Karian et al demonstrated only a 1% sedation failure rate, with a paradoxical reaction rate of 1.2%, when modern drug combinations are administered.[38]

Before sedation, oral intake should be restricted. This decreases emesis risk, and thus the incidence and severity of aspiration, while improving absorption of medications administered orally. Although exact guidelines differ from institution to institution, general recommendations include withholding milk and solids for at least 4 hours in infants, and 6 to 8 hours in older children. Small volumes of clear liquids are permissible up to 2 hours before oral sedation medication administration, and up to 4 hours before parenteral medications.

■ Contrast

Many different choices for contrast media (CM) are commercially available. Iodine-based CM are the mainstay of pediatric cerebral angiography because carbon dioxide gas is not appropriate for use above the diaphragm.[39] Iodine-based CM can be classified as ionic or nonionic, and high-osmolar (HOCM), low-osmolar (LOCM), and iso-osmolar (IOCM). Osmotoxic effects correlate with physiological consequences such as perceived heat and discomfort.[40] Monomeric and dimeric variations of each type exist,[28] with the lowest iodine: particle ratio (3:2) seen for ionic monomers, and the highest (6:1) for nonionic dimers.[27] This translates to significant reduction in the osmolality of LOCM and IOCM compared with HOCM, which are five to eight times the normal blood osmolality (300 mOsm/kg of water). LOCM, commonly of the nonionic monomeric variety (300 to 350 mg iodine/mL), are most commonly used for pediatric cerebral angiography due to their reduced nephrotoxicity, improved patient comfort and allergy profile, and reduced osmotic load.[40–43]

Reactions to CM may be classified as idiosyncratic or nonidiosyncratic.[44] Nonidiosyncratic reactions are predictable, dose-dependent, and have a defined physicochemical basis. These include issues of contrast and osmotic-induced volume load, which can result in congestive heart failure and pulmonary edema, as well as nephrotoxicity. Many authors have evaluated these nephrotoxic effects[40,45–51] and have determined several risk factors, which are listed in **Table 4–2.**

TABLE 4–2 Risk Factors for Contrast-Induced Nephrotoxicity

Dehydration/decreased effective arterial volume
Preexisting renal insufficiency
Congestive heart failure (reduced ejection fraction)
Diabetes
Concurrent use of nephrotoxic medications (e.g., aminoglycosides)
High-contrast dose
High-osmolar contrast media
Vascular disease
Nephrotic syndrome
Cirrhosis
Short-contrast media dose interval/repeated doses

Transient renal ischemia, direct renal tubular toxicity, as well as local changes in glomerular capillary permeability have all been implicated in contrast-induced nephrotoxicity (CIN),[40,50–52] with LOCM and IOCM significantly safer than HOCM, especially in those with associated risk factors. Reducing or eliminating risk factors before beginning the angiogram is mandatory. Even when CIN occurs, serum creatinine levels usually rise transiently, and it is uncommon for CIN to become clinically significant.[51] As well, significant reduction in potential CIN is achieved via hydration alone.[40,51,53] Optimally, 0.45% normal saline hydration (1 mL/kg) should begin 12 hours before the procedure and continue for 12 hours afterward. For outpatients, oral or intravenous hydration should be given before the procedure, followed by intravenous saline for 6 hours following. Mannitol, dopamine, furosemide, and atrial natriuretic peptide have not been shown to be of benefit, and, in some cases, can worsen CIN.[48] Theophylline and acetylcysteine hold some promise in adult patients[48,51,54–56] but have not been adequately evaluated in the pediatric setting. Hemodialysis is of limited benefit and is reserved for selected patients.[52]

Idiosyncratic reactions to CM can occur with any dose and commonly present with some combination of urticaria, pruritus, angioedema or laryngeal edema, bronchospasm, and shock. They are dose-independent and unpredictable. Although less common than in adults,[33] minor and major reactions still occur, including anaphylactoid reactions. Risk of severe reaction is five times greater in those with a history of asthma.[57] Idiosyncratic reactions differ from typical allergic reactions in that they may occur on first exposure to CM, and there may be variable reactivity on subsequent exposures.[50] There is, therefore, no value in administering a "test" dose of contrast.[44,50]

> **PEARL** Adverse reactions to contrast may include urticaria, pruritis, angioedema, bronchospasm, and shock.

Neurotoxicity, although rare, is well documented.[50,58–64] Seizures occur in 0.2% of cerebral angiograms and are self-limited in almost all cases.[50,62] Transient cortical blindness occurs in 0.3 to 1% of cerebral angiograms,[58,60] occasionally accompanied by headache, nausea, vomiting, loss of coordination, aphasia, or confusion.[58] There are no definite predictive factors, and complete recovery is expected within 2 to 10 days, most resolving within 48 hours. Transient encephalopathy/global amnesia, although rare, has also been described,[50,61–63] with rapid resolution hours to days after the procedure. Characteristic imaging findings have been reported for these neurotoxic phenomena.[58,61,64]

Although the use of LOCM reduces the risk of allergic reaction substantially,[65] prophylaxis for pediatric patients undergoing cerebral angiography should be considered when there is a clear history of significant allergy. Many regimens exist,[30,33,44,65,66] with almost all including corticosteroids to target the inflammatory response, as well as histamine antagonists to counteract histamine effects. If reaction is mild, premedication with diphenhydramine (1.5 mg/kg IV) before the procedure may be satisfactory. For more severe reactions, oral prednisone (2 mg/kg/day) for 3 days prior to angiography is suggested, with diphenhydramine as already mentioned. Hydrocortisone sodium succinate (Solu-Cortef; 10 mg/kg IV) can be given as well, in the face of severe reaction, emergency medications must be readily available.

■ Vascular Access and Angiography

Often, the most challenging aspect of pediatric cerebral angiography is obtaining vascular access. Wide range in patient size, from premature infants to adults, creates many unique issues with respect to needles, wires, and catheters. Patient preparation and positioning, especially in young infants, is very important, as is deciding the preferred and backup sites for access.

Techniques for vessel cannulation in the pediatric patient are similar to those for adults, with some notable exceptions. Pediatric vasculature tends to be much straighter and has very little intrinsic vascular disease. There is an increased risk of spasm and dissection.[28] Vessels can be quite superficial, especially in the neonate or young infant. Pediatric vessels can occlude more easily due to the larger catheter:vessel ratio (**Fig. 4–2**), especially in children weighing less than 15 kg.[22,33,67]

There are many excellent articles on obtaining vascular access in the young child,[1,4,8,16,18,22,27,28,30,33,68–72] as well as the special problems encountered in low birth weight infants.[73] Although diagnostic cerebral angiography primarily requires arterial access, interventional neuroradiological procedures may require access to the venous circulation.[1,8,18,19] Many sites and approaches for vascular access are possible, from standard arterial approaches, such as common femoral arterial puncture, to uncommon approaches, such as axillary and brachial access. Venous access via nontraditional routes, such as the transhepatic approach to the inferior vena cava, has been described.[28,30] Direct carotid or vertebral arterial puncture, although rarely indicated now, is sometimes necessary.[17] Surgical access is occasionally required, especially in planned interventional procedures. Cutdown can be performed on any vessel, with certain sites, such as angular vein access to the superior ophthalmic vein, and burr-hole and puncture of the torcular

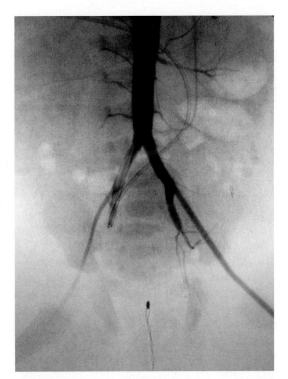

FIGURE 4–2 Anteroposterior pelvic runoff angiogram in a neonate undergoing diagnostic cerebral angiography for a complex arteriovenous fistula. Note that the 4 French sheath can be occlusive in these small vessels.

Herophili well described in the literature.[8,18,19,68,74] Direct puncture of lesions, such as low-flow or venous malformations of the face, is also sometimes indicated.[74,75]

Many different needle–wire–catheter combinations can be used. The smallest appropriate needle and catheter system should be selected, with adequate passage of the chosen wire through the needle and catheter confirmed before initiation of the procedure. Small-gauge needles are essential for access. Although standard venipuncture needles can be used for arterial puncture, dedicated vascular cannulae have a larger internal diameter than venipuncture needles of the same gauge.[72] **Table 4–3** outlines needle and wire choices for different patient weight classes. In children under 5 years of age, 22 gauge or 21 gauge argon needles are often used.

TABLE 4–3 Needle–Guide Wire–Catheter Compatibility

Patient Weight (Lb)	Needle (Gauge)	Wire Size (In.)	Catheter Size (F)
<15	21 butterfly	0.018	4
<15	21 thin-wall art	0.018	
		0.021	4
15–35	19 butterfly	0.025	5
35–60	18 thin-wall art	0.035	5

(Modified from Gerlock AJ, Mirfakhraee M. Essentials of Diagnostic and Interventional Angiographic Techniques. Philadelphia: Saunders; 1985.)

Dedicated 4 and 5 French micropuncture systems are readily available from several different manufacturers, allowing conversion from 0.018 in. compatible systems to 0.035 or 0.038 in. guide wire systems, respectively. Some angiographers prefer flexible cannulae, made from either plastic or Teflon, as opposed to rigid metal cannulae. These are inexpensive, range in size from 14 to 26 gauge, and are suitable for both venous and arterial access. The choice depends on personal experience because flexible cannula techniques, though theoretically less likely to cause intimal injury, guide wire kinking, or wire trauma, are more difficult to master.[68,72]

Puncture below the inguinal ligament is highly recommended. Local anesthetic infiltration should not obliterate the pulse. Because it is difficult to perform single-wall punctures in children, a double-wall technique can be used without significant complications unless anticoagulation is being considered. Active aspiration on the needle is not usually required for vascular access, especially of the artery. After each unsuccessful pass, the needle system should be flushed to clear the potential clot or tissue. Once good blood flow is obtained, the guide wire should advance effortlessly, its passage observed under fluoroscopy. If there is any resistance, mild manipulation of the needle may aid in guide wire passage. If difficulty is still encountered, a test injection of contrast may clarify whether the needle is truly intravascular. The wire must never be forced! Placement of a small dilator over the wire can also allow for a small test injection of contrast. Any failed attempt requires removal of all equipment and holding for at least 1 to 2 minutes for small gauge needles, and up to 5 minutes if an 18 gauge needle is used.

Once access is obtained, dilators minimize the trauma of catheter or sheath placement. Vascular sheaths are recommended, especially if several catheter exchanges, multiple manipulations, or interventional procedures are expected.[8,28,33] They allow maintenance of vascular access and precise torque of catheters.[1,8] Guide wires may be hydrophilic or nonhydrophilic and are available in variable stiffnesses. Generally speaking, angled guide wires are the mainstay of diagnostic angiography except for the Bentson wire, which, although straight, has an extremely atraumatic tip.

The smallest catheter that can accomplish the objectives of the study should be used. Most catheters come pre-shaped and are torque-controllable. Straight catheters can be shaped with steam to achieve the desired terminal curve, with slight exaggeration of the curve often necessary because there is a tendency to lose some of the curvature in the temperature of the blood circulation.[33] Braided and nonbraided catheters in several different materials exist, with several high-flow versions also available.[27] Shortening adult-length catheters is no longer required because pediatric-length catheters are now available. As a general rule of thumb, 3 to 4 French catheters should be used for children weighing less than 10 kg, 4 French for those weighing 10 to 20 kg, and 5 French for children weighing more than 20 kg.[22,76] If microcatheters are to be used, these can be advanced coaxially through catheters with an internal diameter of at least 0.038 in., or directly through 4 French arterial sheaths.[1]

The volume of contrast medium and flush injected must be carefully monitored because younger children and infants are prone to volume overload, as well as contrast nephrotoxicity. No more than 4 mL/kg of contrast should be administered to the neonate, with 6 mL/kg used as the maximum volume for pediatric patients beyond this age.[1,28,30] However, with optimal hydration and small incremental injections, larger volumes have been used during longer procedures. Guidelines for specific vessel injection rates are given in **Table 4–4**.

TABLE 4–4 Injection Rates

Vessel	Weight (kg)	Volume (mL)	Injection Time (s)
CCA	0–10	2–5	1
	10–20	5–8	1
	20–40	8–10 (max 12)	1
ICA	75% of CCA injections		
ECA	50% of CCA injections		
Vertebral	0–10	2–4	1
	10–20	4–6	1
	20–40	6–8 (max 9)	1
SCA	0–10	0.75–1 mL/kg	1–2
	10–20	0.5–0.75 mL/kg	1–2
	20–40	0.25–0.5 mL/kg (max 15)	1–2
Aortic arch	0–10	1.5 mL/kg	1–1.5
	10–20	1.5 mL/kg	1–1.5
	20–40	1.2–1.5 mL/kg (max 50)	1–1.5

CCA, common carotid artery; ECA, external carotid artery; ICA, internal carotid artery; SCA, subclavian artery.
Source: Modified from Stanley P, Miller JH, Tonkin ILD. Pediatric Angiography. Baltimore: Williams & Wilkins; 1982.

■ Special Considerations

Percutaneous vascular access has traditionally been achieved by vessel palpation. However, in the young child or infant, this can be difficult. Doppler needles have been used to expedite access.[70,77] More recently, ultrasound-guided puncture has become a safer, easier, and less traumatic option. In many instances, such as multiple previous catheterizations, known difficult access, or reduced pulses, ultrasound can be used first-line. Appropriate transducers are necessary to ensure adequate visualization.

Systemic heparinization during angiography to prevent vascular thrombosis is well accepted during pediatric angiography.[1,8,22,33,67] This is especially important for infants weighing less than 16 kg, and is administered as a bolus dose of 50 to 80 U/kg once vascular access is obtained. The activated clotting time can be monitored to ensure appropriate anticoagulation.[30] Although protamine can be administered intravenously for chemical reversal of systemic heparinization (10 mg protamine/1000 U heparin), this is often not required.[33]

Umbilical arterial/venous access is an excellent alternative to conventional access in the neonate or premature infant.[1,28,30] It allows sparing of the peripheral vasculature and can accommodate larger sheath/catheter sizes. The umbilical artery is usually patent up to at least 5 days after birth, with the vein often patent up to 1 week. A small test injection of contrast may be helpful to ensure vessel patency, especially if access beyond 1 week is considered. The artery accommodates 3 to 5 French diagnostic catheters or 4 to 5 French sheaths or delivery catheters, with larger sheath sizes possible through the vein. Hemostasis after the angiogram can be achieved by use of an umbilical tape.

Although many access closure devices exist for adult angiography, these have not been adequately evaluated for use in the pediatric setting. Suture closure devices are not recommended due to the high incidence of late stenosis; however, promising puncture-tract sealing techniques are being developed for use in selected settings.[78]

■ Complications

Although pediatric cerebral angiography is a safe procedure, especially when performed by an experienced angiographer, adverse events still occur. Differences between pediatric and adult patients result in problems unique to the child and young infant, with significant potential for serious complications.[68] It is important to recognize and treat complications quickly and appropriately.

Vascular complications continue to be the most common adverse event following angiography.[79] Iatrogenic vascular trauma is relatively common, especially in the neonate or young infant, due to the small size of their vessels.[80,81] Vitiello et al reported an overall incidence of arterial complications of 3.7%, with 7.3% incidence in those less than 1 year of age.[79] Hematoma, pseudoaneurysm formation, vessel dissection, and acute thrombosis can all occur but rarely require surgical intervention. There is at least a 0.5% incidence of local hematoma or pseudoaneurysm formation in the routine diagnostic setting, higher if therapeutic procedures or device insertion are performed.[80] Pseudoaneurysms can be observed or treated with nonoperative methods such as ultrasound-guided compression therapy or percutaneous thrombin injection.[80] Ensuring arterial access is below the inguinal ligament can prevent retroperitoneal hematomas.

> **PEARL** Iatrogenic vascular trauma is relatively common, especially in the neonate.

Vranicar et al described loss of pulses following angiography in 6% of their pediatric patients.[67] Although vasospasm is often the cause, which pediatric patients are especially prone to developing, thrombosis at the access site is not rare, especially in patients weighing less than 15 kg. This is in stark contrast to adults, where acute arterial occlusion occurs in less than 1% of diagnostic angiograms.[80] Duplex ultrasonography may allow a rapid determination of vasospasm versus thrombosis.[82] Many authors have suggested treatment regimens in this setting.[1,22,28,30,67] Most advocate keeping the patient warm, especially the affected limb, with observation for 2 to 4 hours. Before sheath/catheter removal, in the setting of diminished or absent pulses, 2 to 3 mg/kg of nitroglycerin can be instilled intra-arterially in an attempt to relieve vasospasm.[1] If distal pulses have not returned, systemic heparinization is recommended, with a bolus of 75 to 100 U/kg, and infusion to maintain a partial thromboplastin time approximately twice normal. This is continued until pulses return, or 24 hours. Almost always, pulses return. If pulses are still absent after a 24-hour period, thrombolytics have been used to restore arterial patency.[22,28,67,83]

Children have a tremendous capacity for collateral circulation development in response to arterial occlusion. Operative therapy is only performed in the rare event of impending limb loss or vascular injury proximal to the common femoral artery bifurcation.[81] Palpable pulses can be a false indicator of vessel patency. Ultrasonography can confirm if the vessel is truly patent. However, because of collaterals, even persistent femoral arterial occlusion results in fewer than 10% of pediatric patients having future claudication or limb length discrepancy.[80]

Complications related to catheter manipulation underscore the need for meticulous technique. Pettersson et al reported inadvertent embolization during pediatric cerebral angiography occurring at the same frequency as in adults, at 0.9%, with the vast majority of emboli going to the middle cerebral artery circulation.[76] However, they found the immediate and permanent clinical consequences were much milder than expected. This may be, in part, due to more readily lysable fibrin clot development, lack of intrinsic vascular disease in children, as well as rapid development of collateral circulation.

Venous access has the usual associated risks of stenosis, thrombosis, and inadvertent arterial puncture, as well as pneumothorax, hemothorax, and nerve injury when neck or arm access is performed. Chylothorax and air embolism have also been reported.[68] Arteriovenous (AV) fistulae occur when there is simultaneous puncture of both artery and vein. They occur more frequently with low groin punctures.[80] Most are asymptomatic, with ~80% closing spontaneously within 3 months. If both arterial and venous access is obtained, separate sheath/catheter removal can reduce the incidence of AV fistula formation.

Low-grade fevers can occur after angiography, lasting up to 8 hours after the procedure.[28] Cellulitis at the access site has been described. Hypothermia in the neonate or young infant can easily be prevented if the necessary precautions are taken. Hypoglycemia in premature babies and neonates can also occur, sometimes requiring bolus of 25% glucose solutions.[30] Other unique complications include those related to umbilical arterial catheterization. Partial or complete iliac artery or aortic thrombosis has been described, as have embolic complications to the visceral or peripheral vasculature.[80] Initial management is anticoagulation, with the natural history generally one of continued improvement. Thrombolytic therapy, although controversial, has been used in neonates with some success.[80]

Admission of the child may be indicated if fever is present, fluid intake is poor, or a complication requires further observation or therapy. Occasionally, parental choice is enough to warrant admission to the hospital.

■ Alternatives to Conventional Angiography

The remarkable developments in ultrasound, CT, and MRI technology, as well as marked improvements in available computing hardware and software, now afford opportunities at imaging the cerebrovascular circulation without invasive catheter angiography.[14,84–98] Many traditional indications for catheter angiography are now assessible using MRA and CTA, with reduction or elimination of radiation exposure, and, in the case of MRI,

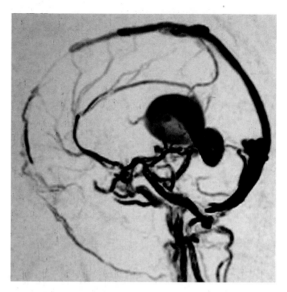

FIGURE 4–3 Sagittal magnetic resonance angiography/magnetic resonance venography (MRA/MRV) image in an infant with an arteriovenous fistula to the vein of Galen. Note the MRA is able to demonstrate pericallosal and posterior cerebral artery feeders, as well as a straight sinus venous constriction or occlusion

eliminating risks associated with conventional contrast agents.[99,100] Transcranial Doppler ultrasonography is effective in evaluating some types of vascular disease, such as vasculopathy related to sickle cell anemia, as well as following therapeutic efforts.[101–105]

MR technology has revolutionized diagnostic neuroradiology.[90] MRA can now confidently assess the arterial and venous circulation of the pediatric brain (**Fig. 4–3**). Two-dimensional or three-dimensional time-of-flight imaging can provide angiographic images without the use of gadolinium, whereas contrast-enhanced techniques have proven safe[103] and can evaluate the cerebral vasculature with amazing clarity. MRA has been used for evaluation of pediatric stroke, arteriovenous malformations, aneurysms, sickle cell anemia, dural sinus thrombosis, extracorporeal membrane oxygenation (ECMO) therapy and follow-up, as well as congenital vascular abnormalities. In combination with conventional MRI, MRA can diagnose arterial dissection.[92,106] Vascular occlusive disease, including moyamoya disease, can be characterized and followed.[107] Cryptic vascular malformations are often more readily appreciated on MRI/MRA imaging.[108]

The role of CTA is also increasing in importance.[109] Multidetector helical technology now allows for extremely rapid image acquisition, potentially decreasing the need for sedation while still producing diagnostic studies able to be rendered into three-dimensional datasets with amazing detail.[110] However, unique technical issues must be addressed to successfully perform CTA in children, such as contrast volume, injection rates, radiation dose, sedation, breath-holding factors, and timing of scan initiation.[111]

There are still some drawbacks to these technologies. Pediatric CTA and MRA studies must be customized for each case because of the variation in size of children. Small vessel size continues to challenge the resolution of these noninvasive imaging techniques.[93] MRA, especially time-of-flight imaging, is still prone to exaggerating stenosis, and to mischaracterizing high-grade stenoses as occlusions.[93] MRI/MRA is expensive and time intensive, and repeated CTA examinations can deliver high radiation doses, especially if multidetector technology is used. The dynamic nature of collateral flow has been difficult to assess with both modalities in the setting of ischemic disease. However, continued advances may allow further improvements in noninvasive diagnosis.

■ Summary

Pediatric neuroangiography remains an extremely important method of interrogating the cerebrovascular system. Technological advances have improved procedural safety, while new contrast agents reduce associated risks of allergic reaction and contrast-induced nephrotoxicity. Noninvasive modalities, such as ultrasound, CT/CTA, and MRI/MRA, complement and, in some cases, replace traditional indications for catheter angiography. Modern neuroangiographic techniques not only allow for better diagnostic abilities but have also expanded the therapeutic possibilities in the exciting world of pediatric neurointervention. Although many unique issues are raised when cerebral angiography is contemplated on the pediatric patient, a multidisciplinary approach, along with common sense and meticulous attention to detail, ensures the safety of the child while providing vital information.

REFERENCES

1. Burrows PF, Robertson RL, Barnes PD. Angiography and the evaluation of cerebrovascular disease in childhood. Neuroimaging Clin N Am 1996;6:561–588
2. Ball WS Jr. Cerebrovascular occlusive disease in childhood. Neuroimaging Clin N Am 1994;4:393–421
3. Kim SK, Wang KC, Kim DG, et al. Clinical feature and outcome of pediatric cerebrovascular disease: a neurosurgical series. Childs Nerv Syst 2000;16:421–428
4. Harwood-Nash DCE. Neuroradiology in Infants and Children. St. Louis: Mosby; 1976
5. Ventureyra EC, Higgins MJ. Traumatic intracranial aneurysms in childhood and adolescence: case reports and review of the literature. Childs Nerv Syst 1994;10:361–379
6. Proust F, Toussaint P, Garnieri J, et al. Pediatric cerebral aneurysms. J Neurosurg 2001;94:733–739
7. Puri V, Riggs G. Case report of fibromuscular dysplasia presenting as stroke in a 16-year-old boy. J Child Neurol 1999;14:233–238
8. Viñuela F, Halbach VV, Dion J. Interventional Neuroradiology: Endovascular Therapy of the Central Nervous System. New York: Raven; 1992
9. Faerber EN. Digital Subtraction Imaging in Infants and Children. Mount Kisco, NY: Futura; 1989
10. Soh G, Calvin S, Sellar R. 3D catheter angiography. Pract Neurol 2003;3:110–111
11. Ghosh S, Levy ML, Stanley P, Nelson M, Giannotta SL, McComb JG. Intraoperative angiography in the management of pediatric vascular disorders. Pediatr Neurosurg 1999;30:16–22
12. Isono M, Ishii K, Kamida T, Inoue R, Fujiki M, Kobayashi H. Long-term outcomes of pediatric moyamoya disease treated by encephalo-duro-arterio-synangiosis. Pediatr Neurosurg 2002;36:14–21
13. Lindqvist M, Karlsson B, Guo WY, Kihlstrom L, Lippitz B, Yamamoto M. Angiographic long-term follow-up data for arteriovenous malformations previously proven to be obliterated after gamma knife radiosurgery. Neurosurgery 2000;46:803–808 discussion 809–810
14. Young WF, Pattisapu JV. Ruptured cerebral aneurysm in a 39-day-old infant. Clin Neurol Neurosurg 2000;102:140–143
15. Allison JW, Davis PC, Sato Y, et al. Intracranial aneurysms in infants and children. Pediatr Radiol 1998;28:223–229
16. Hubbard AM, Fellows KE. Pediatric interventional radiology: current practice and innovations. Cardiovasc Intervent Radiol 1993;16:267–274
17. Huber P. Cerebral Angiography. New York: Thieme-Stratton; 1982
18. Holtzman RNN, Stein BM, Winston H. Endovascular Interventional Neuroradiology. New York: Springer-Verlag; 1995
19. AANS Publications Committee. Endovascular Neurological Intervention. New York: American Association of Neurological Surgeons; 1995
20. Carlson MD, Leber S, Deveikis J, Silverstein FS. Successful use of rt-PA in pediatric stroke. Neurology 2001;57:157–158
21. Christensen R. Invasive radiology for pediatric trauma. Semin Pediatr Surg 2001;10:7–11
22. Chait P. Future directions in interventional pediatric radiology. Pediatr Clin North Am 1997;44:763–782
23. Hoh BL, Ogilvy CS, Butler WE, Loeffler JS, Putman CM, Chapman PH. Multimodality treatment of nongalenic arteriovenous malformations in pediatric patients. Neurosurgery 2000;47:346–357 discussion 357–348
24. Iizuka Y, Rodesch G, Garcia-Monaco R, et al. Multiple cerebral arteriovenous shunts in children: report of 13 cases. Childs Nerv Syst 1992;8:437–444
25. Towbin RB. Pediatric interventional radiology. Curr Opin Radiol 1991;3:931–935
26. Burrows PE, LasJaunias P, TerBrugge KG. A 4-F coaxial catheter system for pediatric vascular occlusion with detachable balloons. Radiology 1989;170(3 Pt 2):1091–1094
27. Freedom RM. Congenital Heart Disease: Textbook of Angiocardiography. Armonk, NY: Futura; 1997
28. Lock JE, Keane JF, Perry SB. Diagnostic and Interventional Catheterization in Congenital Heart Disease. 2nd ed. Boston: Kluwer Academic; 2000
29. Masters LT, Perrine K, Devinsky O, Nelson PK. Wada testing in pediatric patients by use of propofol anesthesia. AJNR Am J Neuroradiol 2000;21:1302–1305
30. Garson A. The Science and Practice of Pediatric Cardiology. 2nd ed. Baltimore: Williams & Wilkins; 1998
31. Towbin RB, Ball WS Jr. Pediatric interventional radiology. Radiol Clin North Am 1988;26:419–440
32. American Academy of Pediatrics CoD. Guidelines for monitoring and management of pediatric patients during and after sedation for diagnostic and therapeutic procedures. Pediatrics 1992;89:1110–1115
33. Stanley P, Miller JH, Tonkin ILD. Pediatric Angiography. Baltimore: Williams & Wilkins; 1982

34. Handa F, Tanaka M, Shiga M, et al. Anesthetic management in pediatric interventional cardiology [in Japanese]. Masui 2000;49:509–513

35. Thompson JR, Schneider S, Ashwal S, Holden BS, Hinshaw DB Jr, Hasso AN. The choice of sedation for computed tomography in children: a prospective evaluation. Radiology 1982;143:475–479

36. Javorski JJ, Hansen DD, Laussen PC, Fox ML, Lavoie J, Burrows FA. Paediatric cardiac catheterization: innovations. Can J Anaesth 1995;42:310–329

37. Mason KP, Michna E, DiNardo JA, et al. Evolution of a protocol for ketamine-induced sedation as an alternative to general anesthesia for interventional radiologic procedures in pediatric patients. Radiology 2002;225:457–465

38. Karian VE, Burrows PE, Zurakowski D, Connor L, Mason KP. Sedation for pediatric radiological procedures: analysis of potential causes of sedation failure and paradoxical reactions. Pediatr Radiol 1999;29:869–873

39. Kriss VM, Cottrill CM, Gurley JC. Carbon dioxide (CO_2) angiography in children. Pediatr Radiol 1997;27:807–810

40. Berg KJ. Nephrotoxicity related to contrast media. Scand J Urol Nephrol 2000;34:317–322

41. Cohen MD. A review of the toxicity of nonionic contrast agents in children. Invest Radiol 1993;28(Suppl 5):S87–S93 discussion S94

42. Dawson P. Chemotoxicity of contrast media and clinical adverse effects: a review. Invest Radiol 1985;20(Suppl 1):S84–S91

43. Nossen JO, Bach-Gansmo T, Kloster Y, Jørgensen NP. Heat sensation in connection with intravenous injection of isotonic and low-osmolar x-ray contrast media and mannitol solutions. Eur Radiol 1993;3:46–48

44. Wittbrodt ET, Spinler SA. Prevention of anaphylactoid reactions in high-risk patients receiving radiographic contrast media. Ann Pharmacother 1994;28:236–241

45. Gerlach AT, Pickworth KK. Contrast medium-induced nephrotoxicity: pathophysiology and prevention. Pharmacotherapy 2000;20:540–548

46. Solomon R. Radiocontrast-induced nephropathy. Semin Nephrol 1998;18:551–557

47. Margulies K, Schirger J, Burnett J Jr. Radiocontrast-induced nephropathy: current status and future prospects. Int Angiol 1992;11:20–25

48. Briguori C, Manganelli F, Scarpato P, et al. Acetylcysteine and contrast agent-associated nephrotoxicity. J Am Coll Cardiol 2002;40:298–303

49. Barrett BJ. Contrast nephrotoxicity. J Am Soc Nephrol 1994;5:125–137

50. Junck L, Marshall WH. Neurotoxicity of radiological contrast agents. Ann Neurol 1983;13:469–484

51. Rudnick MR, Berns JS, Cohen RM, Goldfarb S. Contrast media-associated nephrotoxicity. Semin Nephrol 1997;17:15–26

52. Sterner G, Frennby B, Kurkus J, Nyman U. Does post-angiographic hemodialysis reduce the risk of contrast-medium nephropathy? Scand J Urol Nephrol 2000;34:323–326

53. Trivedi HS, Moore H, Nasr S, et al. A randomized prospective trial to assess the role of saline hydration on the development of contrast nephrotoxicity. Nephron Clin Pract 2003;93:C29–C34

54. Huber W, Jeschke B, Page M, et al. Reduced incidence of radiocontrast-induced nephropathy in ICU patients under theophylline prophylaxis: a prospective comparison to series of patients at similar risk. Intensive Care Med 2001;27:1200–1209

55. Kay J, Chow WH, Chan TM, et al. Acetylcysteine for prevention of acute deterioration of renal function following elective coronary angiography and intervention: a randomized controlled trial. JAMA 2003;289:553–558

56. Rudnick MR, Goldfarb S, Wexler L, et al. Nephrotoxicity of ionic and nonionic contrast media in 1196 patients: a randomized trial. The Iohexol Cooperative Study. Kidney Int 1995;47:254–261

57. Bensusan D, Stevenson JD, Palmer FJ. Corticosteroid prophylaxis for patients receiving intravascular contrast agents: a survey of current practice in Australia and New Zealand. Australas Radiol 1998;42:25–27

58. Zwicker JC, Sila CA. MRI findings in a case of transient cortical blindness after cardiac catheterization. Catheter Cardiovasc Interv 2002;57:47–49

59. Sabovic M, Bonac B. An unusual case of cortical blindness associated with aortography: a case report. Angiology 2000;51:151–154

60. Alsarraf R, Carey J, Sires BS, Pinczower E. Angiography contrast-induced transient cortical blindness. Am J Otolaryngol 1999;20:130–132

61. Dangas G, Monsein LH, Laureno R, et al. Transient contrast encephalopathy after carotid artery stenting. J Endovasc Ther 2001;8:111–113

62. Muruve DA, Steinman TI. Contrast-induced encephalopathy and seizures in a patient with chronic renal insufficiency. Clin Nephrol 1996;45:406–409

63. Haley EC Jr. Encephalopathy following arteriography: a possible toxic effect of contrast agents. Ann Neurol 1984;15:100–102

64. Bendszus M, Koltzenburg M, Burger R, Warmuth-Metz M, Hofmann E, Solymosi L. Silent embolism in diagnostic cerebral angiography and neurointerventional procedures: a prospective study. Lancet 1999;354:1594–1597

65. Greenberger PA, Patterson R. The prevention of immediate generalized reactions to radiocontrast media in high-risk patients. J Allergy Clin Immunol 1991;87:867–872

66. Morcos SK, Thomsen HS, Webb JA. Prevention of generalized reactions to contrast media: a consensus report and guidelines. Eur Radiol 2001;11:1720–1728

67. Vranicar M, Hirsch R, Canter CE, Balzer DT. Selective coronary angiography in pediatric patients. Pediatr Cardiol 2000;21:285–288

68. Gauderer MW. Vascular access techniques and devices in the pediatric patient. Surg Clin North Am 1992;72:1267–1284

69. Macnab AJ, Macnab M. Teaching pediatric procedures: the Vancouver model for instructing Seldinger's technique of central venous access via the femoral vein. Pediatrics 1999;103:E8

70. Cetta F, Graham LC, Eidem BW. Gaining vascular access in pediatric patients: use of the P.D. access Doppler needle. Catheter Cardiovasc Interv 2000;51:61–64

71. Rao PS. Interventional pediatric cardiology: state of the art and future directions. Pediatr Cardiol 1998;19:107–124 discussion 125

72. Gerlock AJ, Mirfakhraee M. Essentials of Diagnostic and Interventional Angiographic Techniques. Philadelphia: Saunders; 1985

73. Rocchini AP. Pediatric cardiac catheterization. Curr Opin Cardiol 2002;17:283–288

74. Doppman JL, Pevsner P. Embolization of arteriovenous malformations by direct percutaneous puncture. AJR Am J Roentgenol 1983;140:773–778

75. Dubois JM, Sebag GH, De Prost Y, Teillac D, Chretien B, Brunelle FO. Soft-tissue venous malformations in children: percutaneous sclerotherapy with Ethibloc. Radiology 1991;180:195–198

76. Pettersson H, Fitz CR, Harwood-Nash DC, Chuang S, Armstrong E. Iatrogenic embolization: complication of pediatric cerebral angiography. AJNR Am J Neuroradiol 1981;2:357–361

77. Lobe TE, Schropp KP, Rogers DA, Rao BNA. "Smart needle" to facilitate difficult vascular access in pediatric patients. J Pediatr Surg 1993;28:1401–1402

78. Illi OE, Meier B, Paravicini G. First clinical evaluation of a new concept for puncture-site occlusion in interventional cardiology and angioplasty. Eur J Pediatr Surg 1998;8:220–223

79. Vitiello R, McCrindle BW, Nykanen D, Freedom RM, Benson LN. Complications associated with pediatric cardiac catheterization. J Am Coll Cardiol 1998;32:1433–1440

80. Nehler MR, Taylor LM Jr, Porter JM. Iatrogenic vascular trauma. Semin Vasc Surg 1998;11:283–293

81. Flanigan DP, Keifer TJ, Schuler JJ, Ryan TJ, Castronuovo JJ. Experience with Iatrogenic pediatric vascular injuries. Incidence, etiology, management, and results. Ann Surg 1983;198: 430–442

82. Kocis KC, Snider AR, Vermilion RP, Beekman RH. Two-dimensional and Doppler ultrasound evaluation of femoral arteries in infants after cardiac catheterization. Am J Cardiol 1995;75:642–645

83. Strife JL, Ball WS Jr, Towbin R, Keller MS, Dillon T. Arterial occlusions in neonates: use of fibrinolytic therapy. Radiology 1988;166:395–400

84. Patsalides AD, Wood LV, Atac GK, Sandifer E, Butman JA, Patronas NJ. Cerebrovascular disease in HIV-infected pediatric patients: neuroimaging findings. AJR Am J Roentgenol 2002;179: 999–1003

85. Levy EI, Niranjan A, Thompson TP, et al. Radiosurgery for childhood intracranial arteriovenous malformations. Neurosurgery 2000;47:834–841 discussion 841–832

86. Al-Sebeih K, Karagiozov K, Jafar A. Penetrating craniofacial injury in a pediatric patient. J Craniofac Surg 2002;13:303–307

87. Seemann MD, Englmeier K, Schuhmann DR, et al. Evaluation of the carotid and vertebral arteries: comparison of 3D SCTA and IA-DSA-work in progress. Eur Radiol 1999;9:105–112

88. Moore EA, Grieve JP, Jager HR. Robust processing of intracranial CT angiograms for 3D volume rendering. Eur Radiol 2001;11: 137–141

89. Rubin GD, Dake MD, Semba CP. Current status of three-dimensional spiral CT scanning for imaging the vasculature. Radiol Clin North Am 1995;33:51–70

90. Davis WL, Boyer RS. Magnetic resonance angiography in pediatric neuroradiology. Top Magn Reson Imaging 1993;5:50–67

91. Husson B, Rodesch G, Lasjaunias P, Tardieu M, Sebire G. Magnetic resonance angiography in childhood arterial brain infarcts: a comparative study with contrast angiography. Stroke 2002;33: 1280–1285

92. Camacho A, Villarejo A, de Aragon AM, Simon R, Mateos F. Spontaneous carotid and vertebral artery dissection in children. Pediatr Neurol 2001;25:250–253

93. Lee BC, Park TS, Kaufman BA. MR angiography in pediatric neurological disorders. Pediatr Radiol 1995;25:409–419

94. Ronkainen A, Puranen MI, Hernesniemi JA, et al. Intracranial aneurysms: MR angiographic screening in 400 asymptomatic individuals with increased familial risk. Radiology 1995;195: 35–40

95. Lewin JS, Masaryk TJ, Modic MT, Ross JS, Stork EK, Wiznitzer M. Extracorporeal membrane oxygenation in infants: angiographic and parenchymal evaluation of the brain with MR imaging. Radiology 1989;173:361–365

96. Zimmerman RA, Bilaniuk LT. Pediatric brain, head and neck, and spine magnetic resonance angiography. Magn Reson Q 1992;8: 264–290

97. Zimmerman RA, Bogdan AR, Gusnard DA. Pediatric magnetic resonance angiography: assessment of stroke. Cardiovasc Intervent Radiol 1992;15:60–64

98. Sklar EM, Quencer RM, Bowen BC, Altman N, Villanueva PA. Magnetic resonance applications in cerebral injury. Radiol Clin North Am 1992;30:353–366

99. Carr JJ. Magnetic resonance contrast agents for neuroimaging: safety issues. Neuroimaging Clin N Am 1994;4:43–54

100. Rao VM, Rao AK, Steiner RM, Burka ER, Grainger RG, Ballas SK. The effect of ionic and nonionic contrast media on the sickling phenomenon. Radiology 1982;144:291–293

101. Adams RJ, McKie VC, Carl EM, et al. Long-term stroke risk in children with sickle cell disease screened with transcranial Doppler. Ann Neurol 1997;42:699–704

102. Adams RJ, McKie VC, Hsu L, et al. Prevention of a first stroke by transfusions in children with sickle cell anemia and abnormal results on transcranial Doppler ultrasonography. N Engl J Med 1998;339:5–11

103. Verlhac S, Bernaudin F, Tortrat D, et al. Detection of cerebrovascular disease in patients with sickle cell disease using transcranial Doppler sonography: correlation with MRI, MRA and conventional angiography. Pediatr Radiol 1995;25(Suppl 1):S14–S19

104. Rodriguez RA, Hosking MC, Duncan WJ, Sinclair B, Teixeira OH, Cornel G. Cerebral blood flow velocities monitored by transcranial Doppler during cardiac catheterizations in children. Cathet Cardiovasc Diagn 1998;43:282–290

105. Siegel MJ, Luker GD, Glauser TA, DeBaun MR. Cerebral infarction in sickle cell disease: transcranial Doppler US versus neurologic examination. Radiology 1995;197:191–194

106. Uchino A, Sawada A, Takase Y, Kan Y, Matsuo M, Kudo S. Supra-clinoid carotid dissection in a pediatric patient. Clin Imaging 2001;25:385–387

107. Yamada I, Nakagawa T, Matsushima Y, Shibuya H. High-resolution turbo magnetic resonance angiography for diagnosis of Moyamoya disease. Stroke 2001;32:1825–1831

108. Ciricillo SF, Cogen PH, Edwards MS. Pediatric cryptic vascular malformations: presentation, diagnosis and treatment. Pediatr Neurosurg 1994;20:137–147

109. Coleman LT, Zimmerman RA. Pediatric craniospinal spiral CT: current applications and future potential. Semin Ultrasound CT MR 1994;15:148–155

110. Denecke T, Frush DP, Li J. Eight-channel multidetector computed tomography: unique potential for pediatric chest computed tomography angiography. J Thorac Imaging 2002;17:306–309

111. Cohen RA, Frush DP, Donnelly LF. Data acquisition for pediatric CT angiography: problems and solutions. Pediatr Radiol 2000;30:813–822

■ SECTION II ■

Surgical Treatments

5

Cavernous Malformations in Children

DAVID YEH AND KERRY R. CRONE

Cavernous malformations (also known as cavernomas and cavernous angiomas) belong to a group of angiographically occult vascular malformations that also include telangiectasias, venous malformations, and low-flow arteriovenous malformations. Cavernous malformations represent 5 to 13% of all vascular malformations. Patients typically present clinically during the third through fifth decades, and in rare instances, during childhood.[1] With the increased use of imaging modalities, such as computed tomography (CT) and magnetic resonance imaging (MRI), the detection of cavernous malformations in children has increased, leading to many controversies in terms of management. This chapter describes some of the salient characteristics of childhood cavernous malformations and provides treatment options and recommendations for their management.

■ Gross, Microscopic, and Radiographic Features

A cavernous malformation can be described as a type of hamartoma that has no potential for metastasis. Macroscopically, a cavernous malformation resembles a mulberry-like structure that may contain cystic and calcified areas. Microscopically, it is composed of thin-walled sinusoidal vessels that are compact and discrete from normal brain. The distinction from normal brain is the cardinal feature that separates cavernous malformations from other low-flow venous malformations, such as telangiectasias, which do have intervening brain tissue. Cavernous malformations rarely have gross hemorrhage but usually have pathological evidence of prior microhemorrhages that cause surrounding hemosiderin-stained gliotic tissue.

Radiologically, cavernous malformations are detectable by CT or MRI. CT scans generally demonstrate a hyperdense lesion with slight enhancement and may show evidence of calcifications, edema, cysts, or hematoma (**Fig. 5–1**). In addition, CT is useful for the detection of hemorrhagic cavernous malformations. On MRI, cavernous malformations are best seen on T2-weighted images, which show high-intensity lobulated lesions surrounded by a low-intensity hemosiderin ring that resembles a popcorn kernel (**Fig. 5–2**). Angiographically, these lesions are occult because they do not have arterial feeders. Infrequently, a blush or venous drainage may be detected.[1]

■ Types Specific to Children

Several forms of childhood cavernous malformations exist that include solitary, multiple, iatrogenic, and familial lesions. Solitary forms, which are the most common, can occur in the supertentorial region (80%), posterior fossa (15%), and spine (5%). In the cerebral hemisphere, cavernous malformations are usually found in the parietal lobe (22.6%), followed by the periventricular region (18.9%), frontal lobes (17%), temporal lobes (15.1%), and occipital lobes (6.4%).[1,2] Multiple forms are less common and are associated with the familial group. Seven families, mostly of Hispanic descent, have been reported with multiple cavernous malformations.[3,4] Genetic studies have linked cavernous malformations to the CCM1 locus on the long arm of chromosome 7 in Hispanic families[5,6] and to 7q21–22 in non-Hispanic families.[7,8] These findings suggest that more than one locus is involved in the formation of cavernous malformations. Although most are presumed to be congenital or spontaneous, radiation-induced cavernous malformations in children have been described. Larson et al[8] published a series of six children who underwent radiation therapy (1800 to 5400 Gy) for various brain tumors. Follow-up

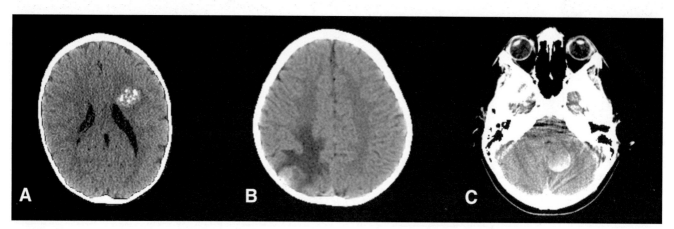

FIGURE 5–1 Axial computed tomographic images of three different patients. **(A)** Calcified areas of a left basal ganglia cavernous malformation. **(B)** Hemorrhagic and cystic components of a right parietal cavernous malformation along with evidence of cerebral edema. **(C)** A hemorrhagic cerebellar cavernous malformation with a blood-fluid level. (By permission from the Mayfield Clinic.)

imaging performed 45 to 120 months after radiation treatment showed formation of de novo cavernous malformations in the irradiated field. Furthermore, 50% of these radiation-associated cavernous malformations had hemorrhaged. The authors suggested that radiation therapy may have induced the growth of these cavernous malformations or may have stimulated their growth to a detectable size.

▪ Presentation

In a retrospective review of the literature, Fortuna et al[1] described the age distribution among children at clinical presentation (**Table 5–1**); in 56 reported cases, most presented during very young or older childhood age groups; that is, 15 (26.8%) patients presented between the ages of 0 to 2 years and 20 (35.7%) between the ages of 12 to 14 years (mean 8.3 years). Although there was no statistically significant sex predilection, more girls were more often affected.

> **PEARL** In children, cavernous malformation can present in a variety of ways, but seizures or epilepsy is the most common.

In children, cavernous malformation can present in a variety of ways (**Table 5–1**) but seizures or epilepsy (45.4%) is the most common. Some theorize that seizure is caused by one or more of the following mechanisms: cortical irritation, frequent presence of calcification and gliosis around the surround parenchyma, and

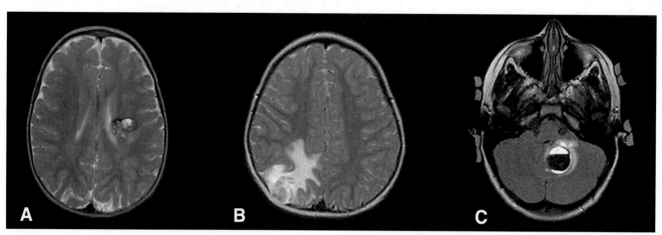

FIGURE 5–2 Axial T2-weighted magnetic resonance images of three different patients (same patients as Fig. 5–1). **(A)** "popcorn" kernel–like appearance of a left basal ganglia cavernous malformation. **(B)** Hemorrhagic and solid components of a right parietal cavernous malformation along with evidence of cerebral edema. **(C)** Hemorrhagic cerebellar cavernous malformation with a blood-fluid level in a cystic cavity. (By permission from the Mayfield Clinic.)

**TABLE 5–1 Age and Clinical Presentation for
56 Childhood Cavernous Malformations**

Age (years)	Percentage
0–2	26.8
2–4	7.1
4–6	5.4
6–8	5.4
8–10	8.9
10–12	10.7
12–16	35.7
Clinical Presentation	
Seizure/epilepsy	45.4
Hemorrhage	27.3
Headache	16.4
Focal neurological deficits	10.9

By permission from the Mayfield Clinic.

accumulation of iron-containing substances produced by silent microhemorrhages or by diffusion of pigments from the destruction of sequestered erythrocytes.[1] The second most common presentation (27.3%) is hemorrhagic syndrome, which results from increased intracranial pressures and includes symptoms of headache, nausea, vomiting, and altered mental status. Young children more often present with bleeding than older children.[2] Furthermore, hemorrhage is more frequent in cavernous malformations that have already bled.[2,9,10] Compared with adults, children less often experience headaches (16.4%) and focal neurological deficits (10.9%).

■ Natural History

Although the natural history of childhood cavernous malformations remains unclear, some information regarding hemorrhage rate, growth pattern, and de novo formation is known and is summarized in the following text.

To discuss the hemorrhage rate of childhood cavernous malformations, the hemorrhage must be precisely defined.

Although *microhemorrhage* and *overt hemorrhage* are sometimes used interchangeably in the literature, a distinction exists between these terms. The T2-hypointense hemosiderin ring around cavernous malformations is believed to be caused primarily by leakage of red blood cells or by diapedesis and is considered a microhemorrhage.[11] Although it is unusual for microhemorrhages to manifest clinically, with time, some can cause cortical irritation and seizure activity.

Unlike microhemorrhages, overt bleeding (i.e., hemorrhage) often results in sudden neurological deterioration, especially if the volume of bleeding is high or if the bleeding is located at or near eloquent areas of the brain. Robinson and Awad defined hemorrhage as the presence of acute or subacute blood outside of the hemosiderin ring or gross evidence of fresh clot outside the confines of the cavernous malformation detected during surgery.[12] Porter et al emphasized that hemorrhage must show evidence of blood inside or outside the hemosiderin ring and be accompanied by a clinical history of an apoplectic event or acute neurological deficit.[13] **Figure 5–3** illustrates a CT and gross picture of a hemorrhagic cavernous malformation. In general, hemorrhage of a cavernous malformation can usually be seen radiographically or grossly and is associated with an acute event.

> **PEARL** The ability to grow is a particular property that distinguishes cavernous malformations from other vascular malformations.

Because hemorrhage can result in catastrophic outcomes, rates and risk factors are important. In a retrospective study of 122 adult and pediatric patients with cavernous malformations, Kondziolka et al[14] analyzed

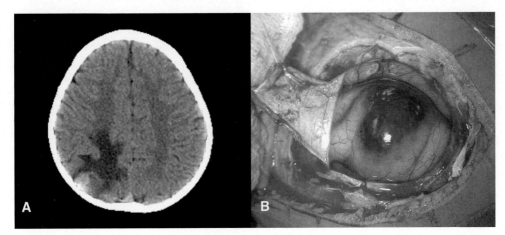

FIGURE 5–3 (A) Axial computed tomography of a right parietal cavernous malformation with evidence of acute hemorrhage. **(B)** A gross intraoperative picture shows the hemorrhagic component of the cavernous malformation (see Color Plate 5–3B). (By permission from the Mayfield Clinic.)

the risk factors and hemorrhage rates. He found that the annual risk of hemorrhage was 0.6% and that this risk increased to 4.5% for cavernous malformations with a history of hemorrhage. Furthermore, location also influenced the rate of hemorrhage: rates increased to 5.0% per year for cavernous malformations located in the brain stem region. Rebleed rates for hemorrhagic brain stem cavernous malformations have been reported to be as high as 21%.[2] Two other studies have reported a nonstatistically significant risk of bleeding between sexes and an absolute rate that appears to be higher in females.[14,15] Pregnancy appears to be an additional risk factor that may be due to hormonal substances and their fluctuations during pregnancy; these factors have been shown to increase the bleed rate and growth of other types of vascular malformations, including cavernous malformations.[16] Although others have suggested that hypertension or hypertensive events, trauma, and size[15] may also play a role, these factors were not statistically significant for cavernous malformation hemorrhage.

The ability to grow is a particular property that distinguishes cavernous malformations from other vascular malformations. The mechanism of growth is summarized by the "hemorrhagic angiogenic proliferation" theory, which suggests that recurrent microhemorrhages with ensuing occlusion of contiguous vascular channels are followed by reorganization, fibrosis, or calcification that leads to growth.[17–19] Cysts that arise are believed to originate from internal hemorrhages that rupture the septa between adjacent sinusoids.[16–18] Conversely, cavernous malformations have also been reported to regress spontaneously.[16–18]

Many biological factors also affect the growth of cavernous malformations. Estrogens are responsible for platelet-mediated thrombosis and may play a role in the growth of cavernous malformations. Cavernous malformation sizes have been shown to enlarge during pregnancy and shrink after delivery.[19] Hemangioblastoma growth is accelerated by sex hormones.[1] In females with von Hippel-Lindau disease, neurological symptoms are exacerbated with oral contraceptive use or during menses.[20] Similar to vascular tumors, cavernous malformations may also respond to hormonal changes.

De novo appearance of cavernous malformations has also been reported in children.[21] Pozzati et al[16] reported that among 145 patients with de novo–appearing cavernous malformations, three malformations developed after radiation therapy, one developed during pregnancy, and two were in patients with familial cavernous malformations; four of these six patients were children. Some authors suggested that radiation, hormones, and familial inheritance are significant factors in de novo–appearing cavernous malformations. As mentioned previously, Larson et al reported on six children who developed new cavernous malformations after radiation treatment.[8]

■ Management

In the discussion of the management options, a risk: benefit ratio for each patient should be addressed. The options that currently exist for the treatment of cavernous malformations are conservative management, surgical excision, and radiation therapy.

Conservative therapy consists of medical management (i.e., antiepileptic medications, headache drugs, or physical therapy) to control symptoms. In general, surgery is not indicated for asymptomatic lesions because these lesions are benign and typically an incidental finding during brain imaging for other reasons. Conservative therapy should also be considered for lesions associated with medically controlled seizures, lesions located in critical areas without severe symptoms, and cases of multiple cavernous malformations for which the actual symptomatic lesion is unidentified.[22]

Surgical treatment for childhood cavernous malformations should depend on several factors. In general, surgery is considered for symptomatic lesions, especially for ones located in an easily accessible area of the brain (i.e., noneloquent and superficial). As mentioned earlier, seizure is the most common presentation in children. Even when epilepsy is relatively well controlled with antiepileptic medications, a case can be made for surgical intervention because surgery can offer a cure, render the child medication free, and provide an excellent cost:benefit ratio for children with long life expectancies. In a review of 56 pediatric cavernous malformations, Fortuna et al[1] found that 41 (73.2%) patients were cured from seizures, 11 (19.6%) had improvement of their seizures, two (3.6%) remained stable, and two (3.6%) experienced worsening symptoms. In general, the literature has reported cure rates of 65 to 72% for seizures caused by cavernous malformations. Because cavernous malformations with a history of hemorrhage have a higher tendency for rebleeding, some authors advocate surgical treatment for all hemorrhagic lesions regardless of location.[2,6,17,23–25] Careful surgical techniques for noneloquent convexity cavernous malformations can be performed safely. Preoperative and intraoperative localization using image guidance and intraoperative ultrasound have allowed surgeons to minimize both craniotomy size and dissection of normal brain (**Fig. 5–4**). Any hemorrhage can supply the surgeon with an easy route to the lesion. After locating the cavernous malformation, the surgeon makes a cortical incision and dissects the margins of the lesion. The surrounding hemosiderin-stained gliotic tissue allows the development of a plane around the lesion for its complete extirpation. Generally, any associated venous

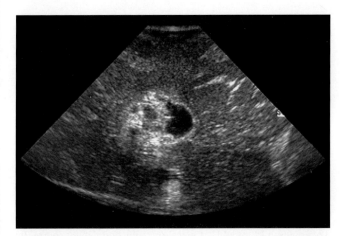

FIGURE 5–4 Intraoperative ultrasound image of a cavernous malformation demonstrating its cystic and solid components and surrounding brain edema (By permission from the Mayfield Clinic.)

angioma should be spared to minimize bleeding and the potential for venous infarction.[17,23,26] In cases of an epileptogenic cavernous malformation, Steiger et al[27] emphasized the need to remove the hemosiderin-stained capsule, which is believed to induce and contribute to the hyperexcitability of the surrounding tissue.

> **PEARL** Generally, any associated venous angioma should be spared to minimize bleeding and the potential for venous infarction.

Special surgical considerations apply to cavernous malformations located in deep or eloquent areas. Because deep lesions are associated with a higher incidence of bleeding in adults, complete excision is recommended.[28] Cavernous malformations located in eloquent cortex can become a challenge because of the risk of a significant morbidity from surgery. The potential risks versus benefits should be carefully assessed. Surgical treatment is recommended for lesions with evidence of growth, previous hemorrhage, or clinical revelations. Precise intraoperative localization is made prior to cortical incision, and piecemeal removal instead of en bloc removal is attempted.[1,2] Bleeding is usually minimal because these lesions have low arterial flow. Furthermore, the surround gliotic plane should not be violated.

Brain stem cavernous malformations present with great potentials for significant morbidities and mortalities. Those that are discovered incidentally should be treated conservatively. However, most brain stem cavernous malformations present with acute neurological deficits, particularly cranial nerve deficits. In a review of the literature, Di Rocco et al[2] found 22 reported brain stem cavernous malformations in children, including three of their own. Most (59%) were located in the pons,

followed by the pontomedullary junction (13.5%), midbrain (13.5%), medulla (9%), and pontomesencephalic junction (5%). As mentioned previously, the hemorrhage rate was 5% and, in this series, the rebleed rate was 21% per year. Therefore, early surgery is recommended for lesions that have bleeding so that reactive gliosis is not formed in the surrounding brain.[2,29] A median suboccipital approach is generally preferred for lesions located on the dorsal part of the brain stem. A retrosigmoid approach can be used for laterally situated cavernous malformations. A supracerebellar infratentorial approach can be used for midbrain lesions, and a subtemporal approach is recommended for lateral pontine lesions. Of the 22 patients reviewed by Di Rocco, all but two patients underwent surgical excision: six had excellent results, 10 had good results with neurological improvement, two had transient worsening of symptoms, and two had worsened symptoms.[2] No mortality or rebleeding was reported.

Similar to brain stem cavernous malformations, lesions located in the spine also have potential for significant morbidity and mortality. Cavernous malformations in the spinal cord are extremely rare and reported mostly in adults. The presentation varies depending on the level of the lesion. The time course consists of a rapidly developing neurological deficit followed by an evolving chronic myelopathy. Brain stem and spinal cord malformations have been associated with hydrocephalus; resolution of hydrocephalus occurs after removal.[16] Again, similar to brain stem lesions, surgical treatment should be weighed carefully for risk and potential benefits. Surgery is recommended for patients with acute or progressive neurological deficits and for patients with evidence of hemorrhage.[18,30]

Controversy continues regarding the use of radiation therapy for cavernous malformations and most studies have included only adult patients. Generally, radiation therapy should only be considered for inaccessible lesions. Several authors have advocated radiation therapy to help reduce the volume of cavernous malformations and facilitate subsequent surgical excision.[31–35] Liscak et al[11] have also reported the use of gamma knife treatment in 25 adult patients and one child who had brain stem cavernous malformations that were deemed too risky for surgical excision. At follow-up (mean 24 months), they reported a nonsignificant increase of bleed rate from 4.7% per year before radiation to 6.8% per year after radiation treatment. Liscak et al also found that 33% of patients had cavernous malformation that shrunk after treatment, 43% had improved neurological status, 28% suffered transient worsening of symptoms because of edema, 8% had permanent morbidity, and 7.7% (two patients) died due to rebleeding at 6 and 51 months after treatment. In a long-term study (mean 12.1 years) of 39 adults, Steinberg et al[35] reported the annual risk of bleed following radiation was 10.3% within 36 months and 1.1% after 36 months ($p < .001$). Complications included symptomatic edema (7%) and radiation necrosis (3%). Seven patients required subsequent surgery due to rebleeding. Clinical grade after treatment was excellent in 43%, good in 41%, poor in 3%, and dead in 13% (three of five from causes other than radiation or surgery).

Long-term effects from radiation therapy for cavernous malformation in children are unknown but its deleterious effects include edema, necrosis, tumor formation, atrophy, and cognitive deficits. In addition, radiation treatment for other central nervous system tumors has resulted in formation of de novo cavernous malformations, which have a significantly higher rebleed rate (up to 50%).[8,25] Because most patients treated with radiation for cavernous malformation were adults, definitive conclusions cannot be inferred to children. In general, radiation therapy should only be considered in children for highly inaccessible lesions for which surgery is deemed too risky.

▪ Conclusions

Although cavernous malformations are generally benign lesions, they present differently in children than in adults. Children typically present clinically with seizures or secondarily with hemorrhages. Depending on the location, hemorrhage can have devastating effects on the patient. Based on our limited experience with cavernous malformations, the knowledge gained to guide our treatment strategies includes conservative management for incidental and asymptomatic lesions and possibly more aggressive treatment for other lesions. As in all surgical endeavors, informed consent, full explanation of risks and benefits, and realistic expectations are discussed with patients and families.

REFERENCES

1. Fortuna A, Ferrante L, Mastronardi L, Acqui M, d'Addetta R. Cerebral cavernous angioma in children. Childs Nerv Syst 1989; 5:201–207
2. Di Rocco C, Iannelli A, Tamburrini G. Cavernomas of the central nervous system in children. Acta Neurochir (Wien) 1996; 138: 1267–1274
3. Bicknell JM, Carlow TJ, Kornfield M. Familial cavernous angiomas. Arch Neurol 1978;35:746–749
4. Hayman LA, Evans RA, Ferell RE, et al. Familial cavernous angiomas: natural history and genetic study over a 5-year period. Am J Med Genet 1982;11:147–160
5. Dubovsky J, Zabramski JM, Kurth J, et al. A gene responsible for cavernous malformations of the brain maps to chromosome 7q. Hum Mol Genet 1995;4:453–458
6. Gunel M, Awad IA, Anson J. Mapping of a gene causing cerebral cavernous malformation to 7q11.2–q21. Proc Natl Acad Sci U S A 1995;92:6620–6624
7. Gunel M, Awad IA, Finberg K, et al. Genetic heterogeneity of inherited cerebral cavernous malformation. Neurosurgery 1996; 38:1265–1271
8. Larson JJ, Ball WS, Bove KE, Crone KR, Tew JM Jr. Formation of intracerebral cavernous malformations after radiation treatment for central nervous system neoplasia in children. J Neurosurg 1998;88:51–56
9. Aiba T, Tanaka R, Koike T, Kameyama S, Takeda N, Komaa T. Natural history of intracranial cavernous malformations. J Neurosurg 1995;83:56–59
10. Kondziolka D, Lunsford LD, Flickinger JC, Kestle JRW. Reduction of hemorrhage risk after stereotactic radiosurgery for cavernous malformations. J Neurosurg 1995;83:820–824
11. Liscak R, Vladyka V, Simonova G, Vymazal J, Novotny J. Gamma knife radiosurgery of the brain stem cavernomas. Min Invasive Neurosurg 2000;43:210–220
12. Robinson JR, Awad IA. Clinical spectrum and natural course. In: Awad IA, Barrow DL, eds. Cavernous Malformations. Rolling Meadows, IL: AANS; 1993:25–36
13. Porter RW, Detwiler PW, Spetzler R, et al. Cavernous malformations of the brainstem: experience with 100 patients. J Neurosurg 1999; 90:50–58
14. Kondziolka D, Lunsford D, Kestle JRW. The natural history of cerebral cavernous malformations. J Neurosurg 1995;83:820–824
15. Herter T, Brandt M, Szuwart U. Cavernous hemangiomas in children. Childs Nerv Syst 1988;4:123–127
16. Pozzati E, Giuliani G, Nuzzo G, Poppi M. The growth of cerebral cavernous angiomas. Neurosurgery 1989;25:92–97
17. Giulioni M, Acciarri N, Padovai R, Frank F, Galassi E, Gaist G. Surgical management of cavernous angiomas in children. Surg Neurol 1994;42:194–199
18. Scott RM, Barnes P, Kupsky W, Adelman LS. Cavernous angiomas of the central nervous system in children. J Neurosurg 1992;76: 38–46
19. Simard JM, Garcia-Bengochea F, Ballinger WE Jr, Mickle JP, Quisling RG. Cavernous angioma: a review of 126 collected and 12 new clinical cases. Neurosurgery 1986;18:162–172
20. Ramina R, Ingunza W, Vonofakos D. Cystic cerebral cavernous angioma with dense calcifications: case report. J Neurosurg 1980; 52:259–262
21. Pozzati E, Acciarri N, Tognetti F, Marliani F, Giangaspero F. Growth, subsequent bleeding, and de novo appearance of cerebral cavernous angiomas. Neurosurgery 1996;38:662–670
22. Zeidman JM, Pressman EK, Glenn GM, Lineham WM, Oldfield EH. Hemangioblastoma of the central nervous system: hormone-induced symptomatic and radiographic progression [abstract]. J Neurosurg 1994;80:399A
23. Rigamonti D, Hadley MN, Drayer BP, et al. Cerebral cavernous malformations: incidence and familial occurrence. N Engl J Med 1988;319:343–347
24. Maggi G, Aliberti F, Ruggiero C, Pittore L. Cerebral cavernous angiomas in critical areas: reports of three cases in children. J Neurosurg Sci 1997;41:353–357
25. Rigamonti D, Spetzler RF. The association of venous and cavernous malformations: report of four cases and discussion of the pathophysiological, diagnostic, and therapeutic implications. Acta Neurochir (Wien) 1988;92:100–105
26. Sasaki O, Tanaka R, Koike T, Koide A, Koizumi T, Ogawa H. Excision of cavernous angioma with preservation of coexisting venous angioma. J Neurosurg 1991;75:461–464
27. Steiger HJ, Markwalder TM, Reulen HJ. Clinicopathological relations of cerebral cavernous angiomas: observations in eleven cases. Neurosurgery 1987;21:879–884
28. Lewis AI, Tew JM Jr. Management of thalamic-basal ganglia and brain-stem vascular malformations. Clin Neurosurg 1994; 41:83–111

29. Scott RM. Brain stem cavernous angiomas in children. Pediatr Neurosurg 1990–1991;16:281–286

30. Pagni CA, Canacero S, Forni M. Report of a cavernoma of the cauda equina and review of the literature. Surg Neurol 1990;33:124–131

31. Giombini S, Morello G. Cavernous angiomas of the brain: account of 14 personal cases and review of the literature. Acta Neurochir (Wien) 1978;40:61–82

32. Schneider RC, Liss L. Cavernous hemangiomas of the cerebral hemispheres. J Neurosurg 1958;15:392–399

33. Yamasaki T, Handa H, Yamashita J, Mortiake K, Nagasawa S. Intracranial cavernous angioma angiographically mimicking venous angioma in an infant. Surg Neurol 1984;22:461–466

34. Shibata S, Mori K. Effect of radiation therapy on extracerebral cavernous hemangioma in the middle fossa: report of three cases. J Neurosurg 1987;67:919–922

35. Steinberg G, Chang S, Marcellus M, et al. Cavernous malformation radiosurgery: long-term results (10-year minimum follow-up). Paper presented at: American Association of Neurological Surgeons; April 2003; San Diego, CA

6

Moyamoya Disease in Children

TOSHIO MATSUSHIMA, TOORU INOUE, YASUO KUWABARA, AND MASASHI FUKUI

Moyamoya disease is a cerebrovascular disorder characterized by bilateral progressive stenosis of the internal carotid arteries. It is also associated with abnormal fine collateral vessels called moyamoya vessels (**Fig. 6–1**).[1–4] However, its precise etiology is still unknown. Children with moyamoya disease often present with ischemic symptoms whereas adult patients tend to demonstrate cerebral hemorrhage.[3] Most pediatric patients first develop transient ischemic attacks (TIAs), and then demonstrate cerebral infarction later.[5] Surgical treatment for ischemic-type moyamoya disease seeks to establish an adequate and sufficient collateral circulation for the ischemic brain to prevent cerebral infarction. Multiple types of bypass procedures have proven to be effective for ischemic-type moyamoya disease, especially in pediatric patients.[3,6–8]

When children present with their first TIA, they are initially treated with aspirin. The management transitions to surgical treatment as the ischemic symptoms progress. The surgical treatment should be selected depending on the progression of ischemic events and an angiographic stage as well as impairment in the cerebral circulation and metabolism.

■ Indications for Surgery

The frequency and extent of such symptoms as TIAs, the condition of the cerebral circulation and metabolism, and the angiographic and magnetic resonance angiographic staging are useful in determining if surgery is recommended.

Transient Ischemic Attacks

Repeated TIAs strongly suggest this disease, especially when they occur after such hyperventilation as heavy crying, blowing on hot soup, or playing the harmonica.[3,5] In early stages, TIAs reflect the condition of the patient's cerebral circulation and metabolism. The frequency of such TIAs is very important, not only for the diagnosis but also to select the optimal treatment.[9,10] The side on which the TIA occurs also suggests the guilty hemisphere.[11–14] In the long-term course of the disease, the incidence of TIA diminishes but the intellectual deterioration and motor disturbance tend to increase.[5] This is due to the fact that repeated TIAs induce large infarction, usually resulting in permanent motor and mental deficits of varying degrees. The frequency and extent of the TIAs are the most reliable indicators for the surgical treatment of an affected hemisphere. Before experiencing an infarction, the patient should undergo bypass surgery. Bypass surgery is usually sufficient only on the affected hemisphere, which is responsible for the TIA or minor stroke, even when angiography demonstrates bilateral stenosis of the internal carotid arteries.

> *PEARL* The phenomenon of misery perfusion, especially with an elevation of the regional oxygen extraction fraction, and the decreased vascular response are good indicators for bypass surgery.

Regional Cerebral Circulation and Metabolism

Positron emission tomography (PET) or single photon emission tomography (SPECT) studies demonstrate the regional condition of the cerebral hemodynamics. The typical findings of the cerebral circulation and metabolism in ischemic-type pediatric patients with moyamoya disease are a reduction of the regional cerebral blood flow (rCBF), an increase of the regional oxygen extraction

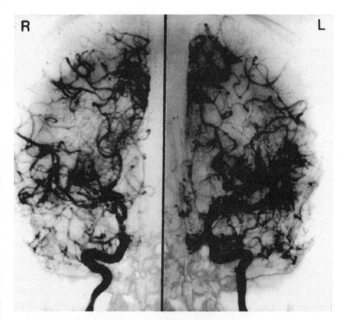

FIGURE 6–1 Internal carotid angiograms. Anteroposterior views of bilateral internal carotid angiograms show occlusion at the terminal portions of the internal carotid arteries (arrows). So-called moyamoya vessels can also be seen in the vicinity of the arterial occlusion. The posterior cerebral arteries can be seen very well, but the anterior and middle cerebral arterial groups are not well visualized.

fraction (rOEF) and the regional cerebral blood volume (rCBV) at an early stage (**Fig. 6–2**), and extensive reduction of vascular vasodilation.[8,15] At an early stage, the rCBF decreases but the regional cerebral metabolic rate of oxygen (rCMR02) does not decrease thanks to a marked elevation of the rOEF. This condition is characteristic of so-called misery perfusion. A study of the cerebral circulation and metabolism often reveals differences in the impairment between both hemispheres. In cases with a unilateral TIA, the hemisphere responsible for the symptom often shows more impairment than the other hemisphere.[9,13,14] The phenomenon of misery perfusion, especially with an elevation of the rOEF, and the decreased vascular response are good indicators for the bypass surgery.[9,15,16]

Angiographic and/or Magnetic Resonance Angiography Changes

This disease or syndrome can only be diagnosed by its characteristic radiological features on either angiograms or magnetic resonance imaging (MRI) and magnetic resonance angiography (MRA) findings.[1,17,18] The fundamental picture consists of bilateral stenosis or occlusion at the internal carotid siphon and an

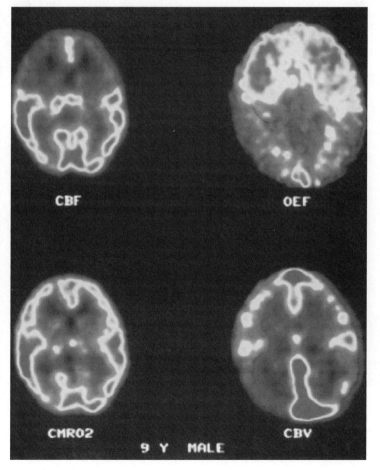

FIGURE 6–2 Preoperative positron emission tomography images reveal a decrease in regional cerebral blood flow (rCBF) bilaterally in the frontal regions. However, regional cerebral metabolic rate of oxygen (CMR02) is relatively well preserved and the regional oxygen extraction fraction (rOEF) increases in these regions. Regional cerebral blood volume (rCBV) also markedly increases in the basal ganglia (see Color Plate 6–2).

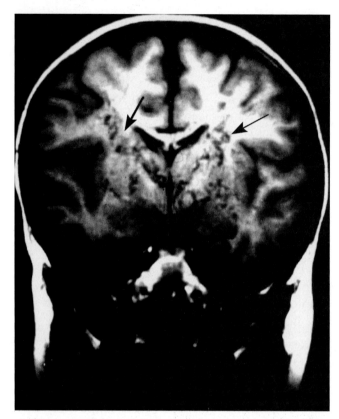

FIGURE 6–3 Magnetic resonance imaging, T1-weighted image, coronal view, demonstrates abundant moyamoya vessels in the basal ganglia and the thalamus as flow void signals (arrows).

abnormal network at the base of the brain. These findings can be seen on both sides. From the angiographic changes seen during the natural course in juveniles, Suzuki and Takaku[19] divided the disease progress into six stages as follows: stage I: narrowing of the carotid siphon; stage II: initiation of moyamoya vessels; stage III: intensification of moyamoya vessels; stage IV: minimization of moyamoya vessels; stage V: reduction of moyamoya vessels; and stage VI: disappearance of moyamoya vessels. Regarding the characteristic angiographic changes, as the narrowing of the main arteries advances, the moyamoya vessels increase in number, and thereafter, as transdural anastomoses develop, the number of moyamoya vessels decreases. In addition, the longer the time after onset, the greater the degree of transdural anastomoses tends to develop via such arteries as the middle meningeal, ethmoidal, and anterior falx arteries. After the development of MRI, MRA, and 3D-CT, angiography is not essential for a definitive diagnosis or follow-up.[1,17,18] Now we prefer MRA and 3D-CT to angiography due to safety and easiness. Patients who have TIAs often demonstrate angiographic pictures of Suzuki's stage III or IV classification, and thus the angiographic stage can also be used as a surgical indicator. A combination of a few different techniques or MRI and MRA are particularly helpful for making an accurate diagnosis (**Fig. 6–3** and **6–4**). Three-dimensional time-of-flight (3D-TOF) MRA shows the stenosis or occlusion of the internal

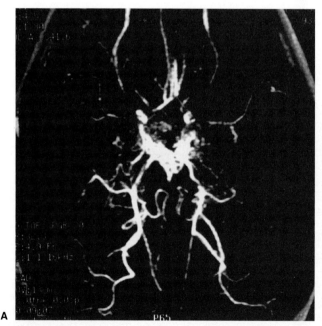

A

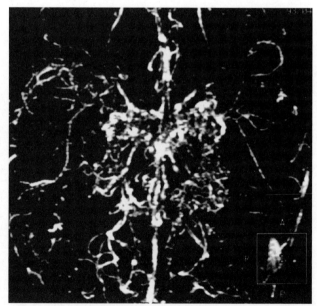

B

FIGURE 6–4 Magnetic resonance angiography (MRA), three-dimensional time-of-flight (3D-TOF) and two-dimensional (2D)-TOF. **(A)** Axial view of 3D-TOF MRA shows bilateral severe stenosis or occlusion at the terminal portions of the internal carotid arteries. A small number of moyamoya vessels

can be seen, particularly on the left side. **(B)** Axial view of 2D-TOF MRA reveals a large number of moyamoya vessels in the basal ganglia on both sides. (Reprinted with permission from Matsushima T, Ikezaki K, Mizushima A, Fukui M. MRA of moyamoya disease. Surg Cerebral Stroke 1994;22:215–219.)

carotid artery or the middle cerebral artery (MCA), and two-dimensional (2D-TOF) MRA reveals the moyamoya vessels in the basal ganglia.[18,20] In the case of MRA, however, we have to keep in mind the characteristics of MRA. MRA shows stenosis of the cerebral arteries to be more severe than angiography.[21] Moyamoya vessels also can be seen as flow voids on MRI.

■ Surgical Treatment

Up to now, various kinds of bypass procedures have been employed (**Table 6–1**). They can be divided roughly into two groups consisting of direct and indirect nonanastomotic bypass procedures. The former are represented by the superficial temporal artery to middle cerebral artery anastomosis (STA-MCA anastomosis).[22,23] On the other hand, in moyamoya disease spontaneous leptomeningeal anastomoses develop after placing donor materials supplied by the external carotid artery (ECA) directly onto the surface of the ischemic brain,[4,24–26] and this phenomenon is seen particularly often in pediatric patients. Various kinds of indirect bypass procedures have so far been developed. They include encephalo-myo-synangiosis (EMS),[24,27] encephalo-duro-arterio-synangiosis (EDAS),[25,28] the use of a split dura,[29] and omental transplantation.[30] Most of these procedures are safe and easy, but all have a few drawbacks.[9,31–33] To overcome these problems multiple indirect or combined methods have been developed.[20,34–40]

TABLE 6–1 Various Kinds of Bypass Procedures for Moyamoya Disease

A. Direct anastomosis
STA-MCA anastomosis
B. Indirect anastomosis
B1. Single indirect anastomosis
EMS
EDAS
EMAS
EAS
Transplantation of the omentum
B2. Multiple combined indirect anastomoses
Fronto-temporo-parietal combined indirect bypass procedure (frontal EMAS, frontotemporal EDAS, and temporoparietal EMS)
EDAMS
Dual EDASs using the anterior and posterior branches of the STA
Multiple (three) EDASs
B3. Additional indirect anastomosis
Frontal EMAS
Ribbon EDAMS
Use of a split dura
C. Direct and indirect combined anastomoses
STA-MCA anastomosis with EMS
STA-MCA anastomosis and EDAMS

EAS, encephalo-arterio-synangiosis; EDAS, encephalo-duro-arterio-synangiosis; EDAMS, encephalo-duro-arterio-myo-synangiosis; EMAS, encephalo-myo-arterio-synangiosis; EMS, encephalo-myo-synangiosis; STA-MCA, superficial temporal artery to middle cerebral artery.

PEARL Small pediatric patients often do not have a recipient cerebral artery large enough for direct anastomosis; such cases may require an indirect bypass.

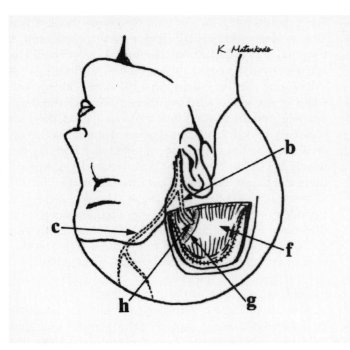

FIGURE 6–5 The operative procedure of the superficial temporal artery to middle cerebral artery anastomosis (STA-MCA anastomosis) with encephalo-myo-synangiosis as a direct anastomosis. The posterior branch of the STA is anastomosed with the cortical branch of the MCA in the bony opening through the temporoparietal craniotomy, and it is covered by the temporal muscle. b, posterior branch of the STA; c, anterior branch of the STA; f, temporal muscle; g, branch of the MCA; h, anastomosis. (Reprinted with permission from Matsushima T, Inoue TK, Ikezaki K, et al. Multiple combined indirect procedure for the surgical treatment of children with moyamoya disease: a comparison with single indirect anastomosis with direct anastomosis. Neurosurg Focus 1998;5:1–5.)

Direct Anastomosis

This anastomosis is represented by STA-MCA anastomosis. It is usually associated with the EMS (**Fig. 6–5**).[11,22,41,42] This is the most reliable method of collateral formation, but, on the other hand, it also has some technical difficulties.[42] Small pediatric patients often do not have a recipient cerebral artery large enough for direct anastomosis. In addition, the artery used in this procedure is also fragile. When the anastomosis does not remain patent, a severe stroke can occur postoperatively. As a result, only highly skilled vascular neurosurgeons should perform direct procedures in pediatric patients.

Single Indirect Anastomosis

Indirect methods started first as a single procedure such as EMS[24] and the original EDAS.[25,28] EMS[24], which is the first indirect procedure, was developed by Karasawa for cases in which the MCA was not adequate for STA-MCA anastomosis. In this method, the temporal muscle flap is used as the donor tissue, and it is placed on the exposed brain surface. The original EDAS, which was developed by Matsushima et al[25] utilizes the posterior branch of the STA together with the surrounding galea as the donor artery. The artery is exposed and freed from the scalp and a galeal strip with artery is thus formed. The edges of the galeal strip are sutured to the dural edges of the linear incision. The artery possessing the blood flow then comes in contact with the brain surface. However, these single indirect methods all have some problems. Each of the methods mentioned earlier can form collaterals but the extent of the newly formed collateral is limited. It has also been recognized that the collaterals cannot always be formed widely enough to cover the ischemic area of the brain. In our experience, 20 to 30% of the sides treated surgically by such single indirect bypass procedures as EDAS or EMS failed to produce sufficient collateral vessels.[9,31] In some cases a reoperation was required because of persistent symptoms.[12,32,33] Therefore, such single indirect methods have gradually changed into multiple combined procedures. We have therefore developed multiple indirect methods, and we believe that our fronto-temporo-parietal combined indirect bypass procedure is an ideal indirect method for pediatric patients with moyamoya disease.[35–37]

Multiple Combined Methods—Fronto-Temporo-Parietal Combined Indirect Bypass Procedure

In this procedure three indirect bypass procedures are used in combination: the encephalo-myo-arterio-synangiosis (EMAS) in the frontal region and the EDAS and the EMS in the temporoparietal region, while using the anterior and the posterior branches of the STA and the frontal and

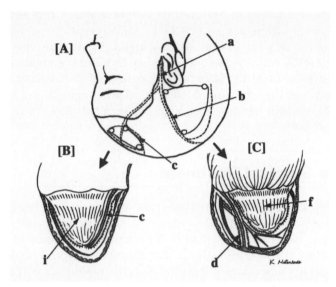

FIGURE 6–6 The operative procedures of the fronto-temporo-parietal combined procedure: the encephalo-myo-arterio-synangiosis (EMAS) in the frontal region and the encephalo-duro-arterio-synangiosis (EDAS) and encephalo-myo-synangiosis (EMS) in the temporoparietal region. **(A)** The courses of the anterior and posterior superficial temporal artery (STA) branches are shown, and the skin incisions are related to the courses of the branches. The locations of the frontal and temporoparietal craniotomies are also demonstrated. **(B)** The frontal EMAS. **(C)** The EDAS and EMS in the temporoparietal bony opening. a, main trunk of the STA; b, ; c, ; d, galeal flap; f, frontal muscle and periosteum. (Reprinted with permission from Matsushima T, Inoue TK, Ikezaki K, et al. Multiple combined indirect procedure for the surgical treatment of children with moyamoya disease: a comparison with single indirect anastomosis with direct anastomosis. Neurosurg Focus 1998;5:1–5.)

the temporal muscles (**Fig. 6–6**).[11,35–37] In the temporoparietal region, the posterior branch of the STA is first exposed using the cutdown technique. Next, a skin incision is extended posteriorly to perform a craniotomy. A temporal muscle flap is prepared for EMS. Care should be taken to avoid damaging the exposed STA with the galeal strip during the craniotomy. After the dura is incised, the edges of the galeal strip are then sutured to the dural opening, and the EDAS is thus completed. Next, the dura is partially resected and the exposed cortical surface is covered with the muscle flap to complete the EMS. In the frontal EMAS, the anterior branch of the STA is exposed using a cutdown technique, and then it is divided distally to make a muscle flap harboring it. The skin incision is extended to create a horseshoe skin flap. A craniotomy is then done and the dura is resected. The muscle flap with the arterial branch is sutured to the dural edge to make contact with the frontal cortical surface (frontal EMAS).[43] By this combined procedure, a collateral formation through at least one of the three indirect bypasses was achieved in 94% of the 16 treated sides, and the collaterals thus covered a wider area.[37,39] The clinical symptoms improved postoperatively after all operations but one.

■ Postoperative Evaluation

Observation of the Clinical Symptoms

One of the effective indicators to estimate the surgical effect is the change in frequency and the extent of such symptoms as TIA, which can easily be observed in the outpatient department. When sufficient collaterals are formed postoperatively, the TIAs markedly decrease or disappear within a few months.[9,42] In cases of indirect bypass procedures it takes longer to obtain the collateral formation and an improvement in the clinical symptoms appears even several months later. In patients whose symptoms such as TIA or headache remain, the collateral formation is neither sufficient nor precise.[12] Other matters that must be considered include the place where the procedure is done and the territory of the collaterals formed. In the surgical procedures using the posterior branch of the STA, postoperative collaterals usually cover the MCA territory, and then the TIAs of the lower limb may remain even though those of the upper limb disappear.

Magnetic Resonance Imaging–Magnetic Resonance Angiography Study

MRA can now safely demonstrate postoperative collateral formation at the outpatient department (**Fig. 6–7A**).[17,18] In most cases an MRA study is sufficient to detect postoperative collateral formation or enlargement of the size of the STA as a donor artery. However, when the collateral formation is minimal, it is very difficult to detect. Even prominent collaterals may be seen much less extensively compared with those seen on conventional angiography. It may also be difficult to visualize the collaterals in the anterior cerebral artery (ACA) territory because it usually exits in a high-convexity region of the brain. To visualize collaterals, 3D-TOF MRA with and without a saturation pulse should be used (**Fig. 6–7B,C,D**).

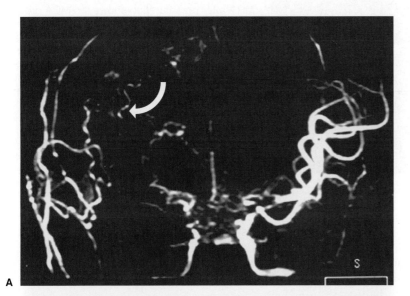

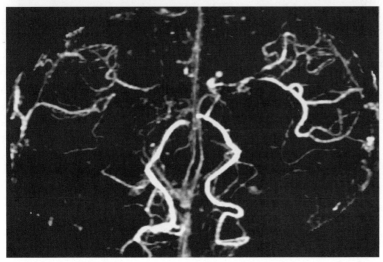

FIGURE 6–7 Postoperative magnetic resonance angiography (MRA). **(A)** Coronal view of a gadolinium (Gd)-enhanced MRA demonstrates a postoperative collateral formation on the right side. The large branches of the superficial temporal artery (STA) (arrow) supply the cortical branches of the middle cerebral artery (MCA). **(B)** Axial view of a Gd-enhanced MRA before presaturation demonstrates the MCA groups on both sides. Both posterior cerebral arteries are also well demonstrated (STA) (arrow).

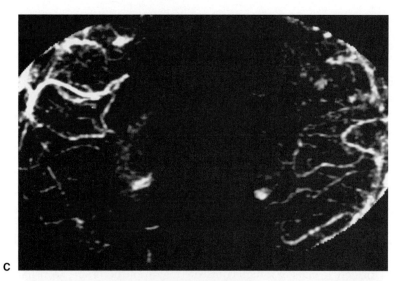

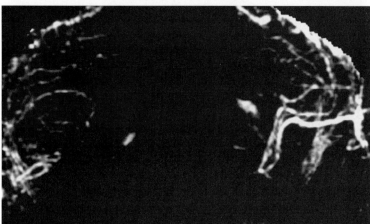

FIGURE 6–7 (*Continued*) **(C)** Axial view of an MRA after presaturation shows the MCA groups on both sides being supplied through the external carotid artery and suggesting a good postoperative collateral formation bilaterally. **(D)** Anteroposterior view of an MRA after presaturation. The MCAs are filled through the postoperative collaterals on both sides. Their shapes are very similar to those on the postoperative external carotid angiograms shown in Fig. 6–9. (**B, C,** and **D** reprinted with permission from Matsushima T, Ikezaki K, Mizushima A, Fukui M. MRA of moyamoya disease. Surg Cerebral Stroke 1994;22:215–219.)

In cases having undergone one of the indirect bypass procedures, the timing of the examination after surgery must be considered. Our previous study demonstrated the relationship between the time lapse after surgery and the visualization of postoperative collaterals using 3D-TOF MRA. MRAs can detect collaterals in most cases, especially when more than 3 months have passed since surgery.[17] However, in some cases, the collateral formation may be present 1 month after surgery, but MRA should be done 6 months after surgery to reliably detect it.

> **PEARL** A SPECT or PET study can be used not only to determine the surgical indications but also to postoperatively estimate an improvement in the cerebral hemodynamics.

Study of the Cerebral Circulation and Metabolism

A SPECT or PET study can be used not only to determine the surgical indications but also to postoperatively estimate an improvement in the cerebral hemodynamics. Collaterals that are well formed postoperatively from the ECA improve the condition of the misery perfusion (**Fig. 6–8**).[9,15,16] In this situation, the rCBF and vascular response increase, whereas the rOEF and rCBV decrease.

Angiographic Study

After development of MRI and MRA, it is not always necessary to do cerebral angiography postoperatively. Angiography is not only difficult to perform but also dangerous, particularly in small patients. Therefore, it should be confined to those with persistent symptoms

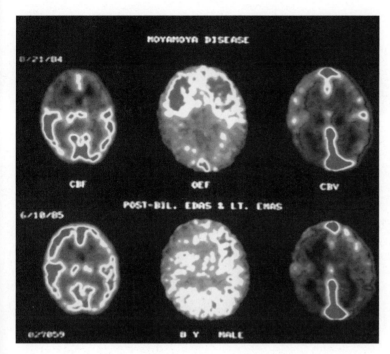

FIGURE 6–8 Pre- and postoperative positron emission tomography (PET) images. Preoperative PET (upper row) reveals decrease in the regional cerebral blood flow (rCBF) bilaterally in the frontal regions. However, the CMR02 is relatively well preserved and oxygen exraction fraction (rOEF) is observed to increase in these regions. Cerebral blood volume (rCBV) also markedly increases in the basal ganglia. Postoperative PET (lower row) demonstrates an improvement, which includes an increase in the rCBF and a decrease in the rOEF in both frontal regions (see Color Plate 6–8). (Reprinted with permission from Matsushima T. Cerebral circulation in moyamoya disease and its surgical treatment. Fukuoka Acta Medica 1994;85: 277–281.)

whose MRI and MRA findings do not precisely demonstrate postoperative collaterals. After the multiple combined indirect anastomosis consisting of three procedures to three regions, angiograms revealed collateral formation in each of the three surgical fields (**Fig. 6–9**). In our experience, the surgical effects and the improvement in the cerebral circulation and metabolism are found especially near the site of surgery.[9] The location and extent of collaterals on the angiograms may indicate the location and extent of the surgical effect.

■ Management of Treatment Failure

We first give anticoagulants such as Bufferin or aspirin to patients with persistent ischemic symptoms after surgery. During the next few months we examine changes in the symptoms and collateral formation on the MRA, and conditions of the cerebral circulation and metabolism on the SPECT or PET. A few patients need a reoperation, especially those who previously received a single indirect procedure such as EDAS.[12,32,33]

■ Indications for Reoperation

Reoperation should be considered: (1) when the patient's symptoms do not improve at all or become worse postoperatively; (2) when postoperative collaterals are only slightly found or not sufficient on cerebral angiograms; and (3) when studies on the cerebral circulation and metabolism still show misery perfusion. When it is difficult to judge or decide to perform a reoperation from the conditions already described, we continue to observe for any changes in the conditions for a few months more.

> **PEARL** When the posterior branch of the STA can be used, then STA-MCA anastomosis is the first choice for the MCA territory.

■ Methods for Reoperation

The reoperation procedure is restricted to the bypass procedures previously utilized. The area for the reoperation is limited. We have to select an appropriate procedure for each patient from the following procedures: STA-MCA anastomosis, additional EMS or EDAS, and omentum transplantation.[10,12,30,32] In selecting the procedure, we first have to know whether the posterior or anterior branch of the STA can be used. When the posterior branch of the STA can be used, then STA-MCA anastomosis is the first choice for the MCA territory. In cases completely refractory to EDAS, the posterior branch of the STA used for EDAS can be stripped and used as a donor artery for the anastomosis.[10,32] In cases

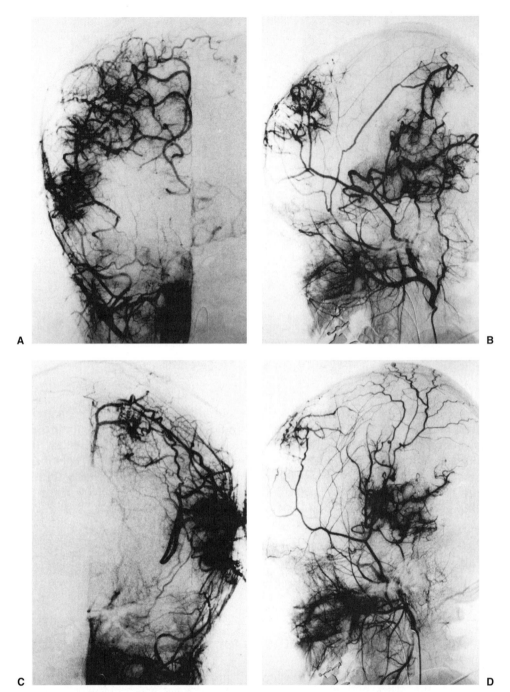

FIGURE 6–9 Postoperative external carotid angiograms. **(A)** Anteroposterior (AP) view of a right external carotid angiogram shows good collateral formation. M2 segment of the middle cerebral artery and A4 segment of the anterior cerebral artery are filled through the external carotid arteries used for bypass surgery. **(B)** Lateral view of a right external carotid angiogram demonstrates well-formed collaterals in three areas where the three bypass procedures were done. **(C)** AP view of a left external carotid angiogram shows a good collateral formation. **(D)** Lateral view of a left external carotid angiogram. (Reprinted with permission from Matsushima T, Ikezaki K, Mizushima A, Fukui M. MRA of moyamoya disease. Surg Cerebral Stroke 1994;22:215–219.)

in which the branches of the STA cannot be used, the EMS or transplantation of the omentum should be selected.[12] To improve the symptoms, the surgical field for the second bypass surgery is also very important. Collaterals should be formed in an appropriate distribution of the ACA, MCA, or posterior cerebral artery (PCA) territory responsible for the patient's symptoms.[12,40,43,44]

■ Conclusion

Collateral formation can be expected postoperatively even by indirect procedures in moyamoya disease, especially in pediatric patients. It has been proven that the average value of basic fibroblast growth factor is significantly higher in moyamoya disease patients than in the control group and this value is thus related to postoperative collateral formation.[45]

When we started our surgical treatment of moyamoya disease using the single indirect procedures, we encountered some problems.[9,12,31,42] Twenty to 30% of the operations failed to establish adequate collateral vessels. The frontal EMAS was started to obtain collateral circulation in the ACA distribution.[12,43] We therefore gradually switched our standard surgical procedure from a single one to a multiple one.[46] The symptoms improved in 94% after our procedure whereas they improved in only 76% after EDAS alone.[36,37] The combined procedure not only produced collateral formation but also improved the clinical symptoms better than the original EDAS alone. As a result, multiple combined procedures are obviously superior to any single procedure. We have not experienced any major complications after either the single or the multiple combined indirect bypass procedures.

The distribution and extension of the collateral formation through the same kind of bypass procedure vary considerably from patient to patient. Moreover, the collateral formation through the indirect bypass procedures in the three regions of the same hemisphere also tend to vary. The factors that influence the collateral formation are still not thoroughly known. A PET study has shown an increased OEF to be an important indicator for good postoperative collateral formation. It therefore seems better to design surgical fields after mapping the misery perfusion area. It is, however, difficult to do a PET study on small pediatric patients. Recently attention has been paid to surgical treatment for ischemia not only in the ACA but also in the PCA distribution, which may lead to transient visual disturbances.[40,44] Thus, at present, we believe that a combination of single indirect bypass procedures, such as ours, is the treatment of choice for pediatric patients with moyamoya disease because this procedure is safe and easy and also covers a wide area of the ischemic brain.

ACKNOWLEDGMENT

We express our thanks to Prof. Emeritus Katsutoshi Kitamura, Neurological Institute, Faculty of Medicine, Kyusu University for his continuing valuable suggestions.

REFERENCES

1. Fukui M, Members of the Research Committee on Spontaneous Occlusion of the Circle of Willis of the Ministry of Health and Welfare, Japan. Guidelines for the diagnosis and treatment of spontaneous occlusion of the circle of Willis ("moyamoya" disease). Clin Neurol Neurosurg 1997;99(Suppl 2):238–240

2. Gotoh F. Guideline to the diagnosis of occlusion of the circle of Willis. In: Goth F, ed. Annual Report (1978) of the Research Committee on Spontaneous Occlusion of the Circle of Willis ("Moyamoya" Disease) of Ministry of Health and Welfare, Japan (MHWJ). Japan: Ministry of Health and Welfare; 1978:132

3. Kitamura K, Fukui M, Oka K, Matsushima T, Kurokawa T, Hasuo K. Moyamoya disease. Handbook of Clinical Neurology 1989 (vol 11): 293–306

4. Spetzler RF, Roski RA, Kopaniky DR. Alternative superficial temporal artery to middle cerebral artery revascularization procedure. Neurosurgery 1980;7:484–485

5. Kurokawa T, Tomita S, Ueda K, et al. Prognosis of occlusive disease of the circle of Willis (moyamoya disease) in children. Pediatr Neurol 1985;1:274–277

6. Inoue TK, Matsushima T, Kuwabara Y. The effectiveness of bypass surgery for moyamoya disease: especially for ischemic type. Brain and Circulation 1997;2:223–227

7. Karasawa J, Touho H, Ohnishi H, Miyamoto S, Kikuchi H. Long-term follow-up study after extracranial-intracranial bypass surgery for anterior circulation ischemia in childhood moyamoya disease. J Neurosurg 1992;77:84–89

8. Kuwabara Y, Ichiya Y, Otsuka M, et al. Cerebral hemodynamic change in the child and the adult with moyamoya disease. Stroke 1990;21:272–277

9. Matsushima T, Fukui M, Kitamura K, Hasuo K, Kuwabara Y, Kurokawa T. Encephalo-duro-arterio-synangiosis in children with Moyamoya disease. Acta Neurochir (Wien) 1990;104:96–102

10. Matsushima T, Natori Y, Kuwabara Y, Mihara F, Fukui M. Management strategies of moyamoya disease, III: Postoperative evaluation, follow-up imaging, management of treatment failure, indication for reoperation. In: Ikezaki K, Loftus M (eds.). Moyamoya Disease. New York: Springer-Verlag; 2001:137–148

11. Matsushima T. Cerebral circulation in moyamoya disease and its surgical treatment. Fukuoka Acta Medica 1994;85:277–281

12. Matsushima T, Fujiwara S, Nagata S, Fujii M, Fukui M, Hasuo K. Reoperation for moyamoya disease refractory to encephalo-duro-arterio-synangiosis. Acta Neurochir (Wien) 1990;107: 129–132

13. Matsushima T, Inoue T, Natori Y, et al. Children with unilateral occlusion or stenosis of the ICA associated with surrounding moyamoya vessels: "unilateral" moyamoya disease. Acta Neurochir (Wien) 1994;131:196–202

14. Matsushima T, Take S. Fujii K, et al. A case of moyamoya disease with progressive involvement from unilateral to bilateral. Surg Neurol 1988;30:471–475

15. Kuwabara Y. Evaluation of CBF, OEF, CMR02 and mean transit time in moyamoya disease using positron emission computed tomography. Jpn J Nucl Med 1986;23:1381–1402

16. Ikezaki K, Matsushima T, Kuwabara Y, Suzuki SO, Nomura T, Fukui M. Cerebral circulation and oxygen metabolism in childhood moyamoya disease: perioperative PET study. J Neurosurg 1994;81: 843–850

17. Hasuo K, Mihara F, Matsushima T. MRI and MR angiography in moyamoya disease. J Magn Reson Imaging 1998;8:762–766

18. Matsushima T, Ikezaki K, Mizushima A, Fukui M. MRA of moyamoya disease. Surg Cerebral Stroke 1994;22:215–219

19. Suzuki J, Takaku A. Cerebrovascular "moyamoya" disease: disease showing abnormal net-like vessels in base of brain. Arch Neurol 1969;12:288–299

20. Sato H. Combined revascularization for moyamoya disease in children. Child Nerv Syst 1991;7:281–282

21. Mizoguchi M, Matsushima T, Ikezaki K, et al. Magnetic resonance angiography in moyamoya disease under the different magnetic field strengths. Prog Comput Imag 1995;17:165–170

22. Karasawa J, Kikuchi H, Furuse S, Kawamura J, Sasaki T. Treatment of moyamoya disease with STA-MCA anastomosis. J Neurosurg 1978;49:679–688

23. Krayenbuhl HA. The moyamoya syndrome and neurosurgeon. Surg Neurol 1975;4:353–360

24. Karasawa J, Kikuchi H, Furuse S, et al. A surgical treatment of moyamoya disease: encephalo-myo-synangiosis. Neurol Med Chir (Tokyo) 1977;17:29–37

25. Matsushima Y, Fukai N, Tanaka K, et al. A new surgical treatment of moyamoya disease in children: a preliminary report. Surg Neurol 1981;15:313–320

26. Tsubokawa T, Kikuchi M, Asano S, Ito H, Urabe M. Surgical treatment for intracranial thrombosis: case report of "durapexia." Neurol Med Chir (Tokyo) 1964;6:48–49

27. Takeuchi S, Tsuchida T, Kobayashi K, et al. Treatment of moyamoya disease by temporal muscle graft "encephalo-myo-synangiosis." Childs Brain 1983;10:1–15

28. Matsushima Y, Inaba Y. Moyamoya disease in children and its surgical treatment: introduction of a new surgical procedure and its follow-up angiograms. Childs Brain 1984;11:155–170

29. Kashiwagi S, Kato S, Yasuhara S, Wakuta Y, Yamashita T, Ito H. Use of a split dura for revascularization of ischemic hemispheres in moyamoya disease. J Neurosurg 1996;85:380–383

30. Karasawa J, Kikuchi H, Kawamura J, Sasaki T. Intracranial transplantation of the omentum for cerebrovascular moyamoya disease: a two-year follow-up study. Surg Neurol 1980;14:444–449

31. Marsushima T, Fujiwara S, Nagata S, et al. Surgical treatment for pediatric patients with moyamoya disease by indirect revascularization procedures (EDAS, EMS, EMAS). Acta Neurochir (Wien) 1989;98:135–140

32. Miyamoto S, Kikuchi H, Karasawa J, Nagata I, Yamazoe N, Akiyama Y. Pitfalls in the surgical treatment of moyamoya disease: operative techniques for refractory cases. J Neurosurg 1988;68:537–543

33. Touho H, Karasawa J, Ohnishi H, Yamada K, Shibamoto K. Surgical reconstruction of failed indirect anastomosis in childhood moyamoya disease. Neurosurgery 1993;32:935–940

34. Kinugasa K, Mandai S, Kamata I, Sugiu K, Ohmoto T. Surgical treatment of moyamoya disease: operative technique for encephalo-duro-arterio-myo-synangiosis: its follow-up, clinical results, and angiograms. Neurosurgery 1993;32:527–531

35. Matsushima T, Inoue T, Ikezaki K, Suzuki SO, Fukui M. Fronto-temporo-parietal combined indirect bypass for children with moyamoya disease, I: Surgical procedure and techniques. Nerv Sys Child 1995;20:317–321

36. Matsushima T, Inoue TK, Ikezaki K, et al. Multiple combined indirect procedure for the surgical treatment of children with moyamoya disease: a comparison with single indirect anastomosis with direct anastomosis. Neurosurg Focus 1998;5(5) 4:1–5

37. Matsushima T, Inoue TK, Suzuki SO, et al. Surgical techniques and the results of a fronto-temporo-parietal combined indirect bypass procedure for children with moyamoya disease: a comparison with results of encephalo-duro-arterio-synangiosis alone. Clin Neurol Neurosurg 1997;99(Suppl 2):S123–S127

38. Matsushima Y, Aoyagi M, Suzuki R, Nariai T, Shishido T, Hirakawa K. Dual anastomosis for pediatric moyamoya patients using the anterior and the posterior branches of the superficial temporal artery. Nerv Syst Child 1993;18:27–32

39. Suzuki SO, Matsushima T, Inoue T, Ikezaki K, Fukui M, Hasuo K. Fronto-temporo-parietal combined indirect bypass procedures for children with moyamoya disease, II: Surgical results. Nerv Sys Child 1995;20:322–326

40. Tenjin H, Ueda S. Multiple EDAS (encephalo-duro-arterio-synangiosis): additional EDAS using the frontal branch of the superficial temporal artery (STA) and the occipital artery for pediatric moyamoya patients in whom EDAS using the parietal branch of STA was insufficient. Childs Nerv Syst 1997;13:220–224

41. Houkin K, Kamiyama H, Takahashi A, Kuroda S, Abe H. Combined revascularization surgery for childhood moyamoya disease: STA-MCA and encephalo-duro-arterio-myo-synangiosis. Childs Nerv Syst 1997;13:24–29

42. Matsushima T, Inoue T, Suzuki SO, Fujii K, Fukui M, Hasuo K. Surgical treatment of moyamoya disease in pediatric patients: comparison between the results of indirect and direct revascularization procedures. Neurosurgery 1992;31:401–405

43. Inoue T, Matsushima T, Nagata S, et al. Frontal encephalo-myo-arterio-synangiosis (EMAS). Surg Cerebral Stroke 1992;20: 297–300

44. Takahashi A, Kamiyama H, Houkin K, Abe H. Surgical treatment of childhood moyamoya disease: comparison of reconstructive surgery centered on the frontal region and the parietal region. Neurol Med Chir (Tokyo) 1995;35:231–237

45. Yoshimoto T, Houkin K, Takahashi A, Abe H. Angiogenic factors in moyamoya disease. Stroke 1996;27:2160–2165

46. Matsushima T, Inoue T, Katsuta T, et al. An indirect revascularization method in the surgical treatment of moyamoya disease: various kinds of indirect procedures and a multiple combined indirect procedure. Neurol Med Chir Suppl (Tokyo) 1998;38:297–302

7

Surgical Treatment of Cerebral Aneurysms in Children

CORMAC O. MAHER AND FREDRIC B. MEYER

Intracranial aneurysms rarely present in childhood.[1] In a review of 1500 pediatric angiograms, Thompson et al found no aneurysms compared with an estimated angiographic incidence of 0.5 to 1% in adults.[2–4] Pediatric aneurysms compose only 0.6 to 2.6% of all aneurysms reported in large surgical series.[5–10] Furthermore, aneurysms are even more rare in very young children.[11] Matson's landmark series of pediatric aneurysms contained no patients younger than 16 years of age.[12] In a survey of 6368 aneurysm patients in the Cooperative Study, only one patient younger than 5 years was identified.[5] As of 1988, there were 73 reported cases of cerebral aneurysms in children younger than 5 years and 43 cases of aneurysms in infants in the world literature.[13–15] As of 1994, only 16 cases of cerebral aneurysms in neonates had been reported.[16,17] In contrast to the female predominance in adults, most pediatric cerebral aneurysms are found in males. This male preponderance varies from 1.5:1 to 2.5:1 in most series.[2,6,9,18–21] Multiple aneurysms occur less frequently in children than in adults and have been reported in 6 to 12% of cases.[8,19,22,23]

The location of aneurysms varies with age. Aneurysms at the origins of the anterior communicating and posterior communicating arteries are uncommon in children. Aneurysms involving the bifurcation of the internal carotid artery (ICA), a relatively rare location in adults, represent 29 to 54% of all pediatric aneurysms.[8,19,20,24–26] Compared with aneurysms in adults, pediatric aneurysms are more likely to be found at distal cortical branches. Although several reports suggest an apparent overrepresentation of posterior circulation aneurysms in children, this relationship has not been found in all series.[6,8,18,19,25,26] Furthermore, the frequency of specific aneurysm locations varies with age even within the pediatric population.

In very young children, the middle cerebral artery (MCA) is by far the most commonly reported origin for an aneurysm.[27,28] Posterior cerebral artery (PCA) and superior cerebellar artery (SCA) aneurysms are also thought to be more common in very young children than in adults. PCA or SCA aneurysms in these patients may result from vascular trauma as the vessel crosses the tentorial edge.[6,16]

Aneurysms in children are likely to be larger and have more complex geometry than those in adults.[6,29–31] Giant aneurysms compose 20 to 45% of all pediatric aneurysms.[6,18,22,26,32] Histological analysis demonstrates medial wall defects with injury to the internal elastic lamina in most saccular aneurysms in both children and adults. This defect, acting alone or in combination with shear stress, may lead to the formation of an aneurysm. Larger medial wall defects may play a relatively more important role in the pathogenesis of pediatric aneurysms. The complex shape and large size typical of pediatric aneurysms may be the result of larger medial wall defects.[6,33] Atherosclerosis and inflammation are not found in pediatric saccular aneurysms.[27]

Although saccular aneurysms are the most frequently encountered type of aneurysm in all age groups, mycotic or traumatic aneurysms compose a relatively greater percentage of pediatric aneurysms.[2,9,22,34] Traumatic aneurysms compose 12 to 39% of pediatric aneurysms, and nearly one quarter of all traumatic aneurysms occur in children.[2,22,30,34,35] Mycotic aneurysms are also common, composing 10 to 12% of pediatric aneurysms.[2,9,22] The relative frequency of atypical aneurysms in children may reflect the rarity of saccular aneurysms in this population. The high incidence of penetrating head injury in young adults and older adolescents is reflected in the high incidence of traumatic aneurysms in some series.[34]

83

The high frequency of these atypical aneurysms helps explain the higher incidence of aneurysms involving the distal cortical arteries in children.

Aneurysmal rupture is the most frequent cause of spontaneous subarachnoid hemorrhage in children.[25] As in adults, small aneurysms in children usually manifest with subarachnoid hemorrhage, and giant aneurysms may do so with either mass effect or subarachnoid hemorrhage.[6,8,9,13,26,36] Unruptured asymptomatic intracranial aneurysms are very rarely detected in the pediatric age group.[37] Although the presentation of subarachnoid hemorrhage in older children is indistinguishable from that in adults, the diagnosis can be challenging in neonates, infants, and younger children.[38] Infants and neonates usually become symptomatic, with irritability, seizures, vomiting, and a decline in level of consciousness. As in adults, head computed tomography (CT) should be obtained when subarachnoid hemorrhage is suspected. Although CT is usually diagnostic of subarachnoid hemorrhage, a lumbar puncture is often performed before CT because the frequency of meningitis in this age group is relatively high.

Every child with a cerebral aneurysm should undergo a general medical evaluation to screen for associated diseases or abnormalities. Connective tissue disorders have been associated with aneurysms in both children and adults.[39,40] Coarctation of the aorta occurs in 3 to 12% of children with cerebral aneurysms.[8,10,20,40–43] Children with polycystic kidney disease (PCKD) probably represent less than 5% of all pediatric aneurysms.[8,10,20,27] Aneurysms associated with PCKD, like those associated with "familial" aneurysms, usually manifest in adulthood.[20,44] Screening for the presence of unruptured aneurysms has been recommended for adults with a diagnosis of PCKD or with two first-degree relatives with intracranial aneurysms.[45–48] There is no information on the utility of specifically screening children in these families for asymptomatic aneurysms. In some cases, screening may be delayed until adulthood.

■ Perioperative Management

Although the most appropriate timing for surgical repair of a ruptured intracranial aneurysm has been the subject of considerable debate, most surgeons now advocate early surgery, especially for patients in good neurological condition.[49,50] The anesthesiologist and the intensive care unit staff must be experienced with the care of pediatric neurosurgical patients. Delays of several days are sometimes appropriate if the child is hemodynamically unstable or if an experienced group of care providers must be assembled. When required, external ventricular drains should be placed preoperatively according to standard neurosurgical protocol.

Although the incidence of vasospasm in children is not significantly different than in adults, it is probably less likely to cause ischemia.[8,10,20] Furthermore, in children, the presence of subclinical vasospasm is not predictive of outcome. Many surgeons use nimodipine after subarachnoid hemorrhage in children even though the safety and efficacy of this agent in the pediatric population have not been established. Applying the principles of intravascular volume expansion and hypertension to combat delayed ischemic deficits from vasospasm is no different in children than in adults. Catheters for monitoring central venous pressure, arterial lines, and urinary catheters should be placed in most cases.

■ Surgical Management

General Considerations

The goal of aneurysm treatment is to exclude the aneurysm from the circulation while preserving the normal vasculature, including perforating arteries. As in adults, application of a clip across the neck of an aneurysm is the standard surgical treatment of pediatric saccular aneurysms. It is important to maintain optimum body temperature during the procedure. Because of the small intravascular volume, great care should be exerted to minimize the loss of blood during the opening and exposure. Blood should be available for rapid transfusion if required. If it is necessary to occlude one or more cerebral arteries temporarily, modest hypertension should be initiated along with pharmacological agents such as barbiturates for brain protection.

> **PEARL**   Because of the smaller intravascular volume in children, great care should be taken to minimize intraoperative blood loss.

The specific surgical approach varies according to an aneurysm's location. In most cases, the child is positioned supine with the head turned. As in adults, a pterional craniotomy is advocated for the surgical treatment of most pediatric aneurysms of the anterior circulation.[49] Distal anterior cerebral artery (ACA) aneurysms are better approached interhemispherically, and posterior circulation aneurysms require subtemporal or suboccipital approaches. A single self-retaining brain retractor is usually needed. Aneurysms are exposed by sequential division of appropriate arachnoid planes using microdissectors, bipolar forceps, a microvascular suction unit, an arachnoid knife, and a microscissors. Obtaining proximal control is critical before the neck of any aneurysm is attacked.

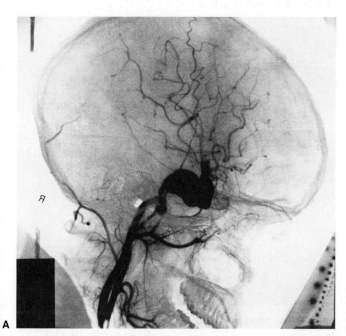
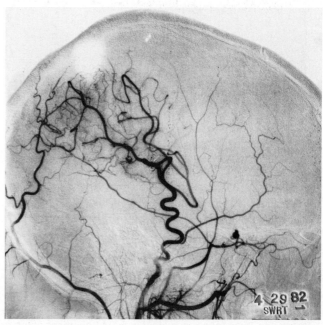

FIGURE 7–1 (A) Lateral carotid angiogram of a 12-year-old boy who presented with decreased vision in the right eye. The complex fusiform shape of this aneurysm made satisfactory clip placement impossible. This aneurysm was treated by proximal vessel ligation and a superficial temporal artery to middle cerebral artery bypass. **(B)** A postoperative lateral external carotid angiogram demonstrates excellent blood flow through the anastomosis.

Once the surgeon is satisfied that the aneurysm has been identified and exposed adequately, the aneurysm is mobilized to identify hidden perforating arteries and adjacent nerves. Temporary clipping of adjacent arteries is often helpful during the exposure of and dissection around the aneurysm. Normal vascular anatomy may be distorted by complex aneurysmal geometry.[6,51] Intraoperative angiography may assist with optimum clip placement or vessel reconstruction.[52] If adequate clip placement is impossible, vessel trapping, with or without bypass, should be considered (**Fig. 7–1**).[49,53] Although these alternative approaches have often been used in the past, they are now required less often.

Saccular Aneurysms of the Internal Carotid Artery Bifurcation

The ICA bifurcation is the most common location of saccular aneurysms in children (**Fig. 7–2**). The pterional approach is used to access aneurysms at this location. The patient is positioned supine with the head turned 15 to 20 degrees.[51] After a standard pterional craniotomy has been performed, a small scalpel is used to divide carefully the arachnoid plane above the sylvian fissure. This plane may be more difficult to identify in young people. If this proves to be the case, a subfrontal approach is used to access the proximal sylvian fissure. Consequently, it is important to ensure that the frontal craniotomy is low, just above the orbit, and extends to the inner canthus of the ipsilateral eye. Once the supraclinoid carotid artery is identified, the arachnoid of the carotid-optic cistern is incised to permit cerebrospinal fluid drainage. The arachnoid surrounding the MCA is divided to allow exposure of the proximal sylvian fissure. The arachnoid over the frontal lobe and optic apparatus is divided to facilitate retraction of the frontal brain.

> **PEARL** In cases where surgical clipping of the aneurysm neck cannot be performed, consideration should be given to trapping the vessel and performing a vascular reconstruction.

Perforating arteries rarely arise from the ICA bifurcation; however, lenticulostriate branches from the M1 segment traversing laterally to medially may adhere to the dome or back wall of the aneurysm. These arteries must be freed carefully from the aneurysm to provide safe passage for the clip. The recurrent artery of Huebner may originate from the A1 segment and may be at risk for injury as it traverses laterally. Also, the anterior choroidal artery is sometimes found along the undersurface of aneurysms in this location. The patency of these perforating arteries should be confirmed following clip placement.

Occasionally, it is impossible to obliterate the neck of the aneurysm while maintaining the integrity of the lumen of the proximal MCA. In these difficult instances,

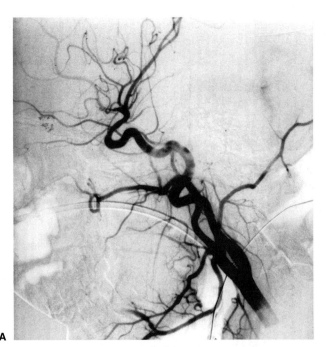
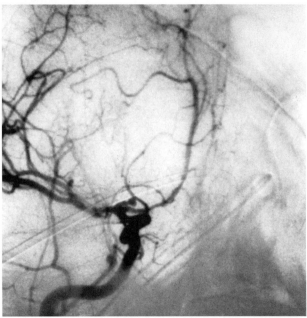

FIGURE 7–2 (A) Lateral and **(B)** oblique left internal carotid angiograms in a 16-year-old girl who presented with subarachnoid hemorrhage. Vasospasm is evident in the A1 segment of the anterior cerebral artery. The aneurysm was surgically clipped.

trapping the vessel and performing a vascular reconstruction should be considered. Most often, this strategy involves a saphenous vein bypass graft from the cervical carotid artery to the MCA distal to the aneurysm's neck (**Fig. 7–3**). This type of vascular anastomosis may fail to preserve perforators off the M1 segment. Fortunately, in our experience, fusiform aneurysms of the ICA terminus are rare. Bypass grafts are more useful in treating fusiform aneurysms of the proximal M1 segment. Bypass grafts work well in this circumstance because the perforators of this segment usually are obliterated during the initial dissection.

Saccular Aneurysms of the Basilar Apex and Proximal Posterior Cerebral Artery

The most common locations for pediatric posterior circulation aneurysms are the basilar apex, the junction of the posterior inferior cerebellar artery with the vertebral artery, and along the P1 and P2 segments of the PCA (**Fig. 7–4**). Aneurysms of the basilar apex and proximal P1 segment of the PCA are best approached through either a modified pterional (anterior temporal) or a subtemporal exposure depending on factors such as the height of the aneurysm along the clivus, the aneurysm's projection, the location of the P1 segments, and the surgeon's preference.[51] For a modified pterional approach, the patient is positioned supine with the head turned 15 degrees to the opposite side. Flexing the neck improves visualization of the aneurysm by removing the posterior clinoidal processes from the direct line of site.

After a pterional craniotomy has been performed, the anterior sylvian fissure is divided and the anterior temporal lobe is gently retracted posteriorly. Tacking the free

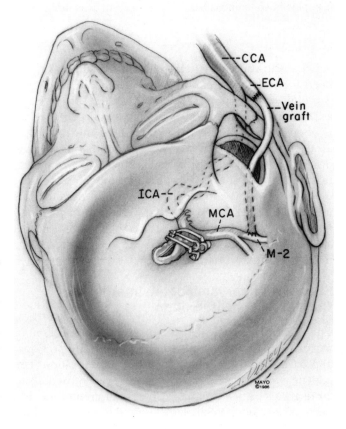

FIGURE 7–3 A vascular anastomosis should be considered when optimal clip placement is impossible without compromising the parent vessel. Illustration shows a vein graft anastomosed from the cervical carotid artery to the M-2 branch of the middle cerebral artery. CCA, common carotid artery; ECA, external carotid artery; ICA, internal carotid artery; MCA, middle cerebral artery.

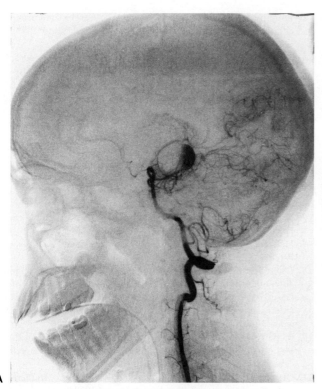

A

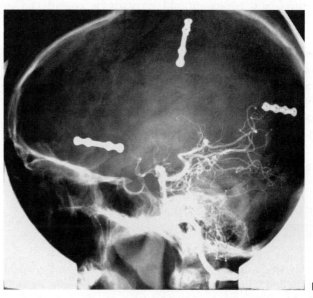

B

FIGURE 7–4 Lateral vertebral angiogram from a 13-year-old boy who presented with headaches. **(A)** Shows a giant aneurysm of the P2 segment of the posterior cerebral artery.

(B) The aneurysm was repaired surgically with a satisfactory angiographic result, and the child remains neurologically intact.

edge of the tentorium laterally to the floor of the middle fossa improves visualization of the vessels of the posterior circulation. Usually, the P2 segment of the PCA is visualized first and is followed proximally to the basilar bifurcation. If necessary, the posterior communicating artery may be ligated and divided close to its junction with the PCA. This maneuver allows the perforators to be reflected from the posterior communicating artery anteriorly and out of harm's way.

Several thalamostriate perforating arteries arise anteriorly from the posterior part of the basilar apex and proximal P1 segment. These perforating arteries may arise from the proximal aneurysm neck at its junction with the basilar artery. The success treating an aneurysm at this location largely depends on avoiding injury to these thalamostriate arteries. Before the final clip is applied, the aneurysm neck and dome should be inspected carefully for the presence of perforating arteries. Because of its location, a transient oculomotor nerve palsy is very common after this surgery.

Saccular Aneurysms of the Middle Cerebral Artery Bifurcation

MCA aneurysms are especially common in very young patients. Aneurysms of the MCA are usually found at the bifurcation of the M1 segment and usually project away from the long axis of that segment. These aneurysms are best approached by performing a standard pterional craniotomy and dividing the sylvian fissure.[51] It is often possible to follow arterial branches proximally until the MCA bifurcation is identified. Care should be taken to preserve all perforating branches arising from the M1 segment. One or two lenticulostriate branches, often originating from the distal M1 segment just below the bifurcation, are at risk during clip placement. In most cases, a clip that preserves the patency of the M1 segment and M2 branches can be placed. If complex aneurysmal geometry prohibits acceptable clip placement or compromises a branch of the MCA, reconstructing the compromised circulation with a bypass should be considered. Because it is difficult to predict the need for a bypass before surgery, it is best to preserve the superficial temporal artery during the initial exposure of broad-necked aneurysms.

Traumatic and Mycotic Aneurysms

Regardless of location, traumatic and mycotic aneurysms have certain unique features and often require different treatment strategies than saccular aneurysms. Buckingham et al have identified three common categories of traumatic aneurysms: ICA aneurysms of the petrous or cavernous segment associated with a basilar skull fracture, parafalcine ACA aneurysms, and aneurysms of distal cortical branches.[35] In general, intradural traumatic aneurysms should be explored surgically because they appear to be associated with a high risk of hemorrhage. Direct clipping may be impossible if the shape of the aneurysm is complex or a pseudoaneurysm is present (i.e., a total disruption of the vessel wall).[54–56] Surgical excision with proximal control and bypass should be strongly considered in these cases.[57] In their review of the literature, Buckingham et al found that only 17% of all pediatric traumatic aneurysms had been clipped and that 36% had been trapped or excised.[35] Balloon occlusion and aneurysmal trapping are often safe and effective procedures for traumatic aneurysms of the petrous or cavernous segments of the ICA at the skull base. A trial balloon occlusion is always indicated prior to permanent occlusion if time permits.

> **PEARL** Surgery should be considered if a mycotic aneurysm has enlarged or failed to resolve on serial angiography, or in cases where the aneurysm has ruptured.

Mycotic aneurysms most often involve distal cortical branches. They are usually fusiform with friable walls. It is often necessary to occlude the parent vessel. Medical treatment alone is indicated as the initial treatment for small, unruptured mycotic aneurysms. Surgery may be considered if the aneurysm has enlarged or failed to resolve on serial angiography or when the aneurysm has ruptured.[58,59] Stereotaxis can be a useful adjunct to locate small cortical aneurysms.

■ Conclusions

Although pediatric aneurysms are rare, they are the most frequent cause of spontaneous subarachnoid hemorrhage in children. Early diagnosis and treatment are essential. Surgical clipping and endovascular coiling provide two complementary modalities for the treatment of pediatric aneurysms. One advantage of surgical clipping in the pediatric population is its proven durability, obviously a major concern when average life expectancy is many decades.[60] Also, the complex shape and broad necks of many pediatric aneurysms may favor surgical treatment. Although older studies emphasized the frequent need for alternative treatments because of the difficulty of clip placement, excellent results are now the norm for most children with cerebral aneurysms.

REFERENCES

1. Yasargil MG. AVM of the Brain, History, Embryology, Pathological Considerations, Hemodynamics, Diagnostic Studies, Microsurgical Anatomy. New York: Thieme Stratton; 1984. Microneurosurgery; vol III A

2. Thompson JR, Harwood-Nash DC, Fitz CR. Cerebral aneurysms in children. Am J Roentgenol Radium Ther Nucl Med 1973;118: 163–175

3. Atkinson JLD, Sundt TM, Houser OW, Whisnant JP. Angiographic frequency of anterior circulation intracranial aneurysms. J Neurosurg 1989;70:551–555

4. Winn HR, Taylor J, Kaiser DL. Prevalence of asymptomatic incidental aneurysms: review of 4,568 arteriograms [abstract]. Stroke 1983;14:121

5. Locksley HB. Report on the Cooperative Study of Intracranial Aneurysms and Subarachnoid Hemorrhage, Section V, Part I: Natural history of subarachnoid hemorrhage, intracranial aneurysms and arteriovenous malformations: based on 6368 cases in the Cooperative Study. J Neurosurg 1966;25:219–239

6. Meyer FB, Sundt TM, Fode NC, Morgan MK, Forbes GS, Mellinger JF. Cerebral aneurysms in childhood and adolescence. J Neurosurg 1989;70:420–425

7. McDonald CA, Korb M. Intracranial aneurysms. Arch Neurol Psychiat, Chicago 1939;42:298–328

8. Ostergaard JR, Voldby B. Intracranial arterial aneurysms in children and adolescents. J Neurosurg 1983;58:832–837

9. Pasqualin A, Mazza C, Cavazzani P, Scienza R, DaPian R. Intracranial aneurysms and subarachnoid hemorrhage in children and adolescents. Childs Nerv Syst 1986;2:185–190

10. Richardson JC, Hyland HH. Intracranial aneurysms: clinical and pathological study of subarachnoid and intracerebral hemorrhage caused by berry aneurysms. Medicine 1941;20:1–83

11. Orozco M, Trigueros F, Quintana F, Dierssen G. Intracranial aneurysms in early childhood. Surg Neurol 1978;9:247–252

12. Matson DD. Intracranial arterial aneurysms in childhood. J Neurosurg 1965;23:578–583

13. Ferrante L, Fortuna A, Celli P, Santoro A, Fraiolo B. Intracranial arterial aneurysms in early childhood. Surg Neurol 1988;29:39–56

14. Hulsmann S, Moskopp D, Wassmann H. Management of ruptured cerebral aneurysm in infancy: report of a case of a ten-month-old boy. Neurosurg Rev 1998;21:161–166

15. Thrush AL, Marano GD. Infantile intracranial aneurysm: report of a case and review of the literature. AJNR Am J Neuroradiol 1988;9:903–906

16. Piatt JH, Clunie DA. Intracranial arterial aneurysm due to birth trauma: case report. J Neurosurg 1992;77:799–803

17. Muszynski CA, Carpenter RJ Jr, Armstrong DL. Prenatal sonographic detection of basilar aneurysm. Pediatr Neurol 1994;10:70–72

18. Amacher LA, Drake CG. Cerebral artery aneurysms in infancy, childhood and adolescence. Childs Brain 1975;1:72–80

19. Hourihan MD, Gates PC, McAllister VL. Subarachnoid hemorrhage in childhood and adolescence. J Neurosurg 1984;60:1163–1166

20. Patel AN, Richardson AE. Ruptured intracranial aneurysms in the first two decades of life: a study of 58 patients. J Neurosurg 1971; 35:571–576

21. Roche JL, Choux M, Czorny A, et al. Intracranial arterial aneurysm in children: a cooperative study. Apropos of 43 cases [in French]. Neurochirurgie 1988;34:243–251

22. Fox JL. Intracranial Aneurysms. Vol 1. New York: Springer-Verlag; 1983

23. Kassel NF, Boarini DJ. Perioperative care of the aneurysm patient. Contemp Neurosurg 1984;6:1–6

24. Almeida GM, Pindaro J, Plese P, Bianco E, Shibata MK. Intracranial arterial aneurysms in infancy and childhood. Childs Brain 1977;3: 193–199

25. Sedzimir CB, Robinson J. Intracranial hemorrhage in children and adolescents. J Neurosurg 1973;38:269–281

26. Storrs BB, Humphreys RP, Hendrick EB, Hoffman HJ. Intracranial aneurysms in the pediatric age group. Childs Brain 1982;9:358–361

27. Becker DH, Silverberg GD, Nelson DH, Hanbery JW. Saccular aneurysm of infancy and early childhood. Neurosurgery 1978;2:1–7

28. Tekkok IH, Ventureyra ECG. Spontaneous intracranial hemorrhage of structural origin during the first year of life. Childs Nerv Syst 1997;13:154–165

29. Gewirtz RJ, Broderick RW, Baumann RJ, Stevens JL. Fusiform P1 segment artery aneurysm in a pediatric patient: technical case report. Pediatr Neurosurg 1998;29:218–221

30. Herman JM, Rekate HL, Spetzler RF. Pediatric intracranial aneurysms: simple and complex cases. Pediatr Neurosurg 1991–92; 17:66–73

31. Humphreys RP, Hendrick EB, Hoffman HJ, Storrs BB. Childhood aneurysms: atypical features, atypical management. Concepts Pediatr Neurosurg 1985;6:213–229

32. Maggi G, Ruggiero C, Petrone G, Aliberti F. Giant intracavernous carotid aneurysm in a child: case report. J Neurosurg Sci. 1997; 41:349–351

33. Lipper S, Morgan D, Krigman MR, Staab EV. Congenital saccular aneurysm in a 19-day-old neonate: case report and review of the literature. Surg Neurol 1978;10:161–165

34. Yazbak PA, McComb JG, Raffel C. Pediatric traumatic intracranial aneurysms. Pediatr Neurosurg 1995;22:15–19

35. Buckingham MJ, Crone KR, Ball WS, Tomsick TA, Berger TS, Tew JM. Traumatic intracranial aneurysms in childhood: two cases and a review of the literature. Neurosurgery 1988;22:398–408

36. Baeesa SS, Dang T, Keene DL, Ventureyra EC. Unusual association of intractable temporal lobe seizures and intracranial aneurysms in an adolescent: is it a coincidence? Pediatr Neurosurg 1998;28: 198–203

37. Humphreys RP. Intracranial arterial aneurysms. In: Edwards MSB, Hoffman HJ, eds. Cerebral Vascular Disease in Children and Adolescents. Baltimore: Williams and Wilkins; 1989:247–254

38. Humphreys RP. Complications of hemorrhagic stroke in children. Pediatr Neurosurg 1991-92;17:163–168

39. Schievink WI, Mellinger JF, Atkinson JLD. Progressive intracranial aneurysmal disease in a child with progressive hemifacial atrophy (Parry-Romberg disease): case report. Neurosurgery 1996;38: 1237–1241

40. Schievink WI, Puumala, Meyer FB, Raffel C, Katzmann JA, Parisi JE. Giant intracranial aneurysm and fibromuscular dysplasia in an adolescent with alpha-1 antitrypsin deficiency. J Neurosurg 1996; 85:503–506

41. Abbot ME. Coarctation of the aorta of the adult type, II: A statistical study and historical retrospect of 200 recorded cases, with autopsy, of stenosis or obliteration of descending arch in subjects above the age of two years. Am Heart J 1928;3:392–421

42. Eppinger H. Stenosis aortae congenita seu isthmus persistens. Vjschr prakt Heilk 1871;112:31–67

43. Woltman HW, Shelden WD. Neurologic complications associated with congenital stenosis of the isthmus of the aorta: a case of cerebral aneurysm with rupture and a case of intermittent lameness presumably related to stenosis of the isthmus. Arch Neurol Psychiat, Chicago 1927;17:303–306

44. Roach ES, Riela AR. Pediatric Cerebrovascular Disorders. 2nd ed. Armonk, New York: Futura; 1995

45. Butler WE, Barker FG II, Crowell RM. Patients with polycystic kidney disease would benefit from routine magnetic resonance angiographic screening for intracerebral aneurysms: a decision analysis. Neurosurgery 1996;38:506–516

46. Ronkainen A, Puranen MI, Hernesniemi JA, et al. Intracranial aneurysms: MR angiographic screening in 400 asymptomatic individuals with increased familial risk. Radiology 1995;195:35–40

47. Schievink WI, Schaid DJ, Rogers HM, Piepgras DG, Michels VV. On the inheritance of intracranial aneurysms. Stroke 1994;25: 2028–2037

48. Wiebers DO, Torres VE. Screening for unruptured intracranial aneurysms in autosomal dominant polycystic kidney disease. N Engl J Med 1992;327:953–955

49. Meyer FB, Sundt TM, Fode NC. Cerebral aneurysms of childhood and adolescence. In: Sundt TM, ed. Surgical Techniques for Saccular and Giant Intracranial Aneurysms. Baltimore: Williams and Wilkins; 1990

50. McDonald RL. Surgical management of aneurysms in the pediatric age group. In: Welch KMA, Caplan LR, Reis DJ, Siesjo BK, Wier B, eds. Primer on Neurovascular Disease. New York: Academic; 1997

51. Meyer FB. Atlas of Neurosugery. Philadelphia: Churchill Livingstone; 1999

52. Ghosh S, Levy ML, Stanley P, Nelson M, Giannotta SL, McComb JG. Intraoperative angiography in the management of pediatric vascular disorders. Pediatr Neurosurg 1999;30:16–22

53. Lansen TA, Kasoff SS, Arguelles JH. Giant pediatric aneurysm treated with ligation of the middle cerebral artery with the Drake tourniquet and extracranial-intracranial bypass. Neurosurgery 1989;25:81–85

54. Diaz A, Taha S, Vinikoff L, Monnin L, Leriche B. Trauma-induced arterial aneurysm in childhood: report of a case and review of the literature. Neurochirurgie 1998;44:46–49

55. Gallari G, Chibbaro S, Perra G. Traumatic aneurysms of the pericallosal artery in children: case report. J Neurosurg Sci 1997;41: 189–193

56. Ventureyra EC, Higgins MJ. Traumatic intracranial aneurysms in childhood and adolescence: case reports and review of the literature. Childs Nerv Syst 1994;10:361–379

57. Regli L, Piepgras DG, Hansen K. Late patency of long saphenous vein bypass grafts to the anterior and posterior cerebral circulation. J Neurosurg 1995;83:806–811

58. Bingham WF. Treatment of mycotic intracranial aneurysms. J Neurosurg 1977;46:428–437

59. Morawetz RB, Karp RB. Evolution and resolution of intracranial bacterial (mycotic) aneurysms. Neurosurgery 1984;15:43–49

60. David CA, Vishteh AG, Spetzler RF, Lemole M, Lawton MT, Partovi S. Late angiographic follow-up review of surgically treated aneurysms. J Neurosurg 1999;91:396–401

8

Surgical Treatment of Cerebral Arteriovenous Fistulas in Children

RABIH G. TAWK, BERNARD R. BENDOK, MIR JAFER ALI, CHRISTOPHER C. GETCH, AND H. HUNT BATJER

Arteriovenous fistulas (AVFs) are defined as an abnormal connection between an artery and a vein without an intervening capillary channel.[1] They can be acquired or congenital, and in the majority of cases, drainage occurs in the transverse or sigmoid sinuses. Occasionally, they drain into the vein of Galen causing it to dilate.[1] Although frequently solitary, in the pediatric population they may be multiple with multiple feeding arteries, and are not infrequently associated with other vascular lesions such as arteriovenous malformations (AVMs), aneurysms, and venous ectasias.[1-5] Angiographically, they are characterized by an immediate arteriovenous (AV) transition, without a capillary bed or "nidus" as occurs in AVMs,[6] and typically there is rapid circulation (**Fig. 8–1**).

The occurrence of AVF, excluding the vascular malformation of the vein of Galen, is extremely rare.[1,4,7] Because it is discussed in a different chapter (see Chapter 10), this last entity was omitted from our discussion. This chapter provides an overview of the role of open surgery and endovascular options in the management of pediatric AVFs.

In the pediatric population, AVFs are uncommon vascular malformations.[8,9] They account for ~10% of all intracranial AV shunts in children, lower than the 10 to 20% estimated for adults.[10-12] The most common locations are the sigmoid–transverse, cavernous, and superior sagittal sinuses.[13] Those affecting the occipital-suboccipital region are reported to account for 50% of all dural AVFs.[9]

■ Origin and Natural History

In the pediatric population, congenital failure of involution of the primitive arterial system seems to be the likely cause.[14] The congenital basis of nontraumatic pediatric AVFs is supported by the age of these patients. The associated well-established bone defects and the abnormality of venous sinuses make a congenital etiology highly likely. Added, is the apparent association of these vascular lesions with several distinct inherited syndromes of childhood including Rendu-Osler-Weber (ROW) syndrome, Wyburn-Mason's syndrome, and Klippel-Trénaunay-Weber syndrome.[15-19] Of interest is that older children often have objective but nonsubjective cranial bruits. This suggests that the noise was always present in the natural acoustic environment of the child and thus probably present at birth.[10,20]

Not uncommonly, multiple cerebrovascular malformations coexist with these kinds of inherited disorders. ROW is a rare autosomal dominant disorder of strong penetrance but variable expression characterized by multiple mucocutaneous and visceral telangiectasias, which may result in hemorrhagic complications in adult life.[16] Associated AVMs of the nervous system are present in ~8% of these patients.[21] Because typical symptoms are unusual before puberty and the pial fistula can be the presenting manifestation, this disorder should be suspected in patients with multiple pial AVFs.[16]

Lasjaunias et al[8] have divided dural AV shunts in children into three groups: (1) dural sinus malformation with AV shunts, which typically occur in neonates, (2) infantile dural AV shunts, which occur in children, and (3) adult-type dural AV shunts, which are less frequent but also occur in children. Infantile dural sinus malformation is a developmental anomaly of the dural sinus and usually seen as a giant dural sinus lake.

The natural history of AVFs is unclear. The literature reports both gradual increase in size and symptoms and spontaneous regression.[21-27] In contrast to adults, it is

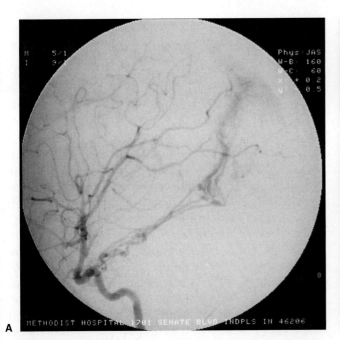 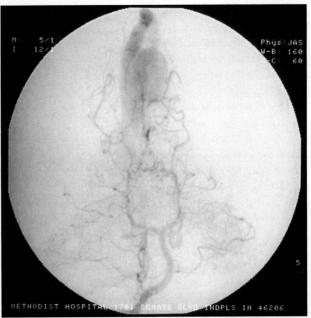

FIGURE 8–1 Arteriovenous fistula in adolescent with high output congestive heart failure. **(A)** Lateral carotid injection shows rapid fistulous connection between middle cerebral artery branches and superior sagittal sinus. **(B)** Vertebral injection illustrates posterior cerebral artery contribution to fistula.

assumed that dural AVFs in pediatric patients are congenital in origin and follow a different clinical course.[19,28,29] They tend to have more of an aggressive clinical course and a greater incidence of multifocality and complexity.[8,30,31]

■ Clinical Aspects and Presentation

Presentation is variable and is related to the age of the patient, the site and size of the fistula, and the presence of other vascular lesions.[4] Although cases have been reported at the extremes of age, AVFs typically present in childhood and early adulthood.[6]

Clinical syndromes from birth to age 15 may be categorized into three groups.[8] Group 1, representing the neonatal group, typically presents with symptoms of heart failure, cyanosis, and cranial bruits. These patients are predominantly males. This group has a poor prognosis with onset of intractable heart failure and death within days or weeks following birth. Group 2 represents predominantly children between 1 and 15 months of age and is the largest group. Patients in this category typically present with hydrocephalus and macrocrania, convulsions, and subarachnoid hemorrhage (SAH). Although short-term prognosis is better than that for group 1, these patients are frequently afflicted with neurological sequelae months to years after diagnosis. The third group typically represents patients from age 2 through 15 years or more. Clinical presentation of these patients typically includes headache, focal neurological deficits, syncope, seizures, and SAH.[32–34]

Tomlinson and colleagues[6] reported 12 cases of cerebral AVFs in an older age group. There were four children/adolescents, and one neonate. Headache and seizure were the most common presentations followed by SAH, cardiac failure, and progressive neurological dysfunction. It is interesting to note that, unlike cerebral AVMs, hemorrhage from AVFs seems relatively uncommon.

■ Diagnosis and Radiological Evaluation

Computed tomography (CT) features may suggest AVFs. They include prominent enlargement of arteries or veins, a large varix, and lack of an obvious nidus. Calcifications, either in the thrombosed portion of an associated varix or as a shell-like calcification in its wall, are seen in about half of cases. CT provides valuable information in identifying any associated alteration in ventricular size or the presence of ischemic infarction.[35] It is also important to rule out parenchymal edema related to venous hypertension, SAH, subdural hematoma, and intraparenchymal hemorrhage. On magnetic resonance imaging (MRI) studies, it is difficult to depict shunts. Only indirect manifestations, such as venous dilatations, venous infarctions, and flow voids can be seen.[36,37] However, MRI is useful for demonstrating end-organ damage to the brain, such as edema and infarction, and can help in the visualization of dilated veins.[38] Particularly in neonates, ultrasonography of the head provides a rapid and accurate demonstration of the lesion and cerebral angiography will complete the diagnosis. Because AVFs are a relatively rare cause of severe congestive heart failure in newborns, most of these infants are subjected to workups for congenital heart disease, including cardiac catheterization and angiography, before a correct diagnosis is made.[32]

At standard cerebral angiography, cerebral AVFs share some characteristics with AVMs. Nevertheless, the demonstration of an abrupt transition from artery to vein with an increase in vessel caliber and the absence of a plexiform nidus distinguish these two vascular malformations.[4,6] Adequate angiography requires selective studies of the external and internal carotid and vertebral arteries.[39–41] The role of supraselective angiography for the accurate diagnosis and location of the fistula has been emphasized.[6] Although small vessels cannot be visualized, it is essential to understand the complex architecture of these lesions. This can be accomplished with special oblique views that are essential to characterize the fistulous communications.[42]

Seldom is a malformation served by only one arterial channel. There may be only one major artery contributing to the lesion, but the surgeon should anticipate any number of minor vessels coming from pial or deep perforating sources. Distal stenosis, when present, is associated with severe episodes of recurrent hemorrhage. The most predictive angiographic finding for repeated hemorrhage is a cortically draining dural fistula with either or both high-grade stenosis and variceal enlargement of the draining vein distal to the fistula.[43] Aside from affording an accurate diagnosis and precise localization of the fistula, endovascular techniques are also valuable in successful management. They may be used for functional assessment or temporary occlusion prior to permanent surgery.[6]

■ Pathophysiology

Neonates, when shunting is severe, tend to present immediately with congestive heart failure as a result of the increased venous return and volume overload.[30] An increase in blood volume also occurs as a compensation for AV shunting. In older children, the degree of AV shunting is usually less severe. As the shunted blood is added to the systemic venous return, there is an increased volume load on all chambers of the heart as well as on the lungs and great vessels.[44] The heart failure is believed to occur as a result of the increased volume of blood passing through the shunt.[45,46] The time of its occurrence depends primarily on the size of the shunt because this determines the degree of cardiac loading and the rate at which the limit of cardiac reserve is reached.[47] It is generally accepted that the higher the flow through the malformation, the earlier the age of

presentation.[35] The largest fistulas cause congestive heart failure in infancy, whereas smaller ones cause hydrocephalus or convulsions later.[44]

Associated giant varices are uncommon.[2,4,48] Nevertheless, they have been described in several reports.[1,4,23,49–52] Presumably, the underlying pathology is high flow through a nonarterial vessel associated with distal outflow obstruction.[4]

Fortunately, in the setting of a single area of dural sinus occlusion or when a major sinus becomes occluded, the venous drainage usually reroutes without difficulties. On the other hand drainage might occur through cortical veins or deep venous sinuses. In this setting, venous drainage may prove inadequate, resulting in dangerous venous hypertension.[30] Venous hypertension has been recognized as an important cause of neurological dysfunction.[53–63] It may cause venous ischemia or infarction, hemorrhage, or problems with cerebrospinal fluid (CSF) dynamics.[30] By precluding normal absorption of the CSF, it results in hydrocephalus.[49] Hemorrhage, when it occurs, usually results from rupture of a venous aneurysm.[11,53,64] Additionally, because of the engorgement of the venous system, symptoms may result from compression by veins or may also be attributable to arterial steal.

> **PEARL** As the shunted blood is added to the systemic venous return, there is an increased volume load on all chambers of the heart as well as on the lungs and great vessels.[44] The heart failure is believed to occur as a result of the increased volume of blood passing through the shunt.

■ Carotid Cavernous Fistulas

This location of the fistula is rare in the pediatric population, and only a few cases have been reported.[65–68] As in adults, fistulous diversion of arterial blood in the cavernous sinus can produce a variety of clinical signs, including orbital or cephalic bruit, proptosis, visual failure, and chemosis. Orbital pain, facial numbness, and disrupted ocular motility have also been observed.[69]

Carotid cavernous fistulas (CCFs) can be categorized based on pathological, hemodynamic, and arteriographic criteria. These distinctions include (1) posttraumatic versus spontaneous, (2) high flow versus low flow, (3) direct versus dural [arterial flow directly from the internal carotid artery (ICA) or from dural branches of the ICA or external carotid artery (ECA)], and (4) typical versus atypical (venous drainage into the dural sinuses or through parenchymal veins).[70–73] Most often, they occur as a posttraumatic event[65] and usually consist of one or two large holes between the artery and the sinus or result from avulsion of a cavernous carotid branch.

Treatment

Although many cases may be managed conservatively, the ideal treatment should be to obliterate the fistula while maintaining patency of the carotid artery. However, in cases of clinical deterioration or radiographic evidence of retrograde leptomeningeal venous drainage, treatment is recommended. An aggressive approach is indicated in patients presenting with deterioration of vision, progressive ophthalmoplegia, or progressive and severe exophthalmos.[74]

A wide variety of techniques have been described.[75–77] Historically, CCFs have been treated surgically, after both craniotomy and exposure of the cervical ICA, with trapping of the intervening segment. The direct surgical approach to the cavernous sinus has been described by Parkinson.[78] Mullan has described the use of thrombogenic needles or bronze wire to induce thrombosis.[80] Other reported techniques include proximal ligation, direct repair, packing of the cavernous sinus, and endovascular approaches.

Presently, the first-line therapy for the majority of CCFs is an endovascular approach. Embolization represents the procedure of choice for most high-flow fistulas and for low-flow fistulas fed by the ECA.[80] However, there are situations in which endovascular approaches are inadequate. Rarely, open surgery is required, and candidates for direct obliteration procedures are those who fail endovascular therapy and continue to suffer visual loss and diplopia. Because low-flow fistulas receive blood from several sources, surgical management consists of interrupting the fistulous connections after adequate exposure of the lateral wall of the cavernous sinus. The fistula is coagulated together with the draining veins that are also coagulated and sectioned. Recurrence is not uncommon after trapping of the ICA.[68] Day and Fukushima[80] encountered a 22% incidence of complications directly attributed to overpacking the triangles, with subsequent ICA compromise. Most of the risks of this microsurgical approach were related to the difficulty of packing the cavernous sinus triangles to an optimal pressure that occludes the fistula while only minimally disturbing the ICA and cranial nerves. However, if less packing was performed, treatment might have failed and resulted in persistence of the CCF.

Ballon test occlusions may predict tolerance to sinus packing from the standpoint of carotid patency. By using intraoperative angiography, each stage of packing can be evaluated to ensure patency of the ICA and obliteration of the fistula.[80] It is of primary importance to keep the patient normotensive. Intraoperative hypotension may lead to retinal hypotension because of an inability to overcome high intraocular pressures from venous obstruction.[80]

■ Dural Arteriovenous Fistulas

Dural AVFs consist of a direct shunt located inside the dural layer, with their arterial supply from the meningeal arterial system.[53,81] Usually, they involve the walls of a dural sinus or adjacent cortical veins, and pathologically, the malformation consists of a network of AV microfistulas in the wall of a dural sinus.[12,31,82,83] A variety of cerebral venous structures can be affected, and they can present at various clinical stages ranging from simple lesions to potentially life-threatening lesions.[43] Arterial supply is similar to that in adult patients, including occipital and meningeal arteries from external carotids and the vertebral arteries, and tentorial branches from the internal carotids. These lesions are often enormous, consisting of large venous lakes, which involve the sinuses, and are irrigated by bilateral feeders. Pathologically, the dural sacs may not be connected to cerebral venous drainage.[84] Sometimes, distal cortical or dural vessels are involved, perhaps through a sump effect.[29]

Treatment

The treatment of dural AVFs is difficult and many therapeutic approaches have been proposed.[85] Although some lesions may exhibit benign courses and even heal spontaneously, others may exhibit an aggressive behavior and may be as dangerous as parenchymal AVMs.[53,64,86–88] Treatment of asymptomatic fistulas is controversial, and some groups recommend only observation.[89,90] Most authors agree on treating symptomatic patients and those with angiographic markers for a malignant course.

Because these lesions have other impacts on other systems located at a distance, management is often targeted at alleviating these secondary manifestations. Associated high output cardiac failure, whenever present, is difficult to treat prior to closure of the intracranial shunt.[35] Reportedly, it has been managed effectively by feeder ligation.[35,44,91,92] Particularly in newborns presenting at an early age with severe cardiac failure, their small vascular capacities greatly increase the surgical risk.[84,93] In these circumstance staged feeder embolization is a viable option. Morita et al[84] suggested that surgical intervention in neonates should be delayed as long as the patient can tolerate conservative management. Arterialized leptomeningeal veins or "red veins," and particularly if they are variceal, have been shown to be predictors of a malignant course.[38,94–96] When venous sinus drainage is accompanied by reflow into the leptomeningeal veins, there is a relatively high risk of intracranial bleeding, venous hypertension, high intracranial pressure, and progressive neurological deficits.[38,53,64,81,94–103] Particularly when drainage through cortical veins is associated with variceal drainage, there is a marked tendency to cause progressive neurological symptoms and hemorrhage.[64] It is now well agreed that such an angiographic appearance is a feature favoring aggressive treatment.[42] If these veins are absent, the lesions are often asymptomatic and may exhibit a benign course.[86,88,103,104]

Other factors that may enter into the decision to operate include location, depth, drainage, and associated venous restrictive disease.[38,53,64,97,99–101,105,106]

It is now accepted that arterialized leptomeningeal veins are considered indications for surgical treatment even if clinical presentation does not involve hemorrhage.

On the other hand, even adequate treatment involves risk. Occlusion of an AVF may produce significant local cerebrovascular changes with either or both edema and hemorrhage, as well as systemic hemodynamic effects and even decompensation and cardiac arrest.[107] The surgical mortality and relatively poor prognosis are closely related to the hemodynamic derangements.[4] Furthermore, surgical excision of high-risk fistulas, despite being an effective therapy, may be associated with massive intraoperative hemorrhage.[108,109]

> **PEARL** When venous sinus drainage is accompanied by reflow into the leptomeningeal veins, there is a relatively high risk of intracranial bleeding, venous hypertension, high intracranial pressure, and progressive neurological deficits.

■ Surgical Techniques

Surgical techniques vary among reports and involve one or a combination of the following:

- Skeletonization and excision of the sinus
- Packing of the sinus
- Interruption of the red veins at their connection with the sinus
- Ligation of feeding vessels
- Combination approaches with endovascular procedures
- Rerouting sinus drainage to the extracranial venous circulation

Sinus Excision

This technique has been championed by several authors.[104,109,110] The rationale for this approach is supported by the fact that normal venous drainage has been rerouted due to venous hypertension in the diseased sinus. By combining surgical skeletonization and excision, this approach provides the most effective possibilities for permanent cure.[104] Usually, it involves extensive cauterization of the entire dural surface, followed by excision of the nidus and associated veins.[53,83,108–112] Although red veins can be divided with relative impunity, those that are venous must be preserved.[110] When the sinuses are contributing to normal tissue drainage, stepwise transvenous occlusion is optimum to allow for reequilibration. Once this has been achieved, resection is less dangerous.[84] In the pediatric population, Morita and colleagues[84] assumed that total surgical resection is currently the only definitive treatment and should be considered in severe symptomatic patients. Other authors have criticized this approach as excessive given the fact that less invasive approaches work as well. When there is no question that the fistula is dural and when the outflow is through a single cortical vein, it is not necessary to completely excise the malformation.[113] In reality, although excision is extremely effective, the surgical risk is high because this method often requires sinus wall resection, an extensive craniotomy, and in some cases significant brain retraction.[110] When the fistula involves the entire sigmoid sinus down to the cranial base we caution against attempts at curative skeletonization or excision. Near the jugular foramen, vagal nerve fibers become interspersed in dura and excision can lead to disabling dysphagia.

Sinus Packing

Dr. Mullan pioneered the field of sinus packing and has contributed immensely to our understanding of dural AVFs.[79,95,114,115] His work in this area has been the impetus for advances in venous embolization. Packing is a simple procedure, which for many fistulas does not involve opening the dura. In effect, this technique is surgically less invasive and technically less demanding. The rationale is essentially the same as with excision. When the existing venous outflow is occluded, the fistula thromboses immediately. Added is the reality that feeders are often adjacent to the sinus and even may run in the wall. According to Mullan, whenever the entire venous outflow of a dural fistula, regardless of how complex it is, can be occluded, the fistula will be cured.[113] Furthermore, provided that alternative pathway of venous return from the brain exists, therapy proceeds safely with staged sinus occlusion.[84] Thus, in the presence of retrograde flow in the involved sinus, occlusion is safe without causing a venous stroke.[116] Some authors consider that even when sinuses are draining normal tissue, stepwise transvenous occlusion of the sinus may allow reequilibration.[84] Practically, when it is demonstrated preoperatively that the hemispheric drainage has found alternate pathways, occlusion could be safely undertaken. However, the hazard that exists in this assumption is that the high-flow fistulous washout, if it was not visualized, could obscure some significant hemispheric drainage.[115]

When there are innumerable feeders, embolization of the affected sinus or venous sac or both is useful to diminish flow.[84] Because they are adjacent to the sinus and may even run in the walls, they cannot be obliterated by the transarterial route.[117] In this case, transvenous obliteration has been reported to be effective.[95,117]

With both this technique and sinus excision care must be taken to ensure that the segment of the sinus that is being sacrificed does not drain normal brain tissue. Given the invasiveness of both techniques the likelihood of cure based on angiographic anatomy should be calculated prior to surgery to assess the value of intervention. Despite being less demanding, this technique is extremely meticulous. Unless the coils are placed across the entire involved portion, the fistula will not thrombose. Any small unoccluded segment will continue to allow flow, and with time, the residual fistula will probably enlarge. Coils must not be placed where there are normal veins, especially close to the vein of Labbé, whenever antegrade drainage occurs into the sinus.[116]

Unfortunately, in many instances it is unrealistic to isolate the sinus. Thus, despite offering many advantages, this technique has certain limitations and hazards. Obliteration rates with craniotomy and direct transvenous glue or coil embolization are not as high as with extensive resection.[113] Particularly, in some instances, it is impossible to exclude some minimal drainage that could be obscured by the high fistulous flow. Another limitation occurs in the case of a single cortical venous outflow, where transvenous approach cannot access the lesion successfully.[113] One feared complication is when thrombosis extends beyond what is optimal to occlude and leads to deep cerebral venous thrombosis. Another technical pitfall may be faced when the fistula is located at the vein of Labbé, and venous drainage occurs into the sinus. In this case, neither occlusion nor excision can handle the problem without occlusion of this vessel, and the transarterial approach might be useful.

Draining Vein Interruption

More recently several authors have explored draining vein interruption as close to the fistula as possible.[81,94,118] This technique, pioneered for spinal AVFs, seems ideally suited to the treatment of fistulas with cortical/leptomeningeal drainage that are inaccessible to a transvenous approach.[85,119–122] When the sinus is thrombosed and venous outflow occurs entirely toward the cortical veins, the definitive therapy is surgical. Because the sinus is already occluded, its removal is not necessary.[116] Interruption of the draining veins is curative. Hoh et al[113] reported such an approach in five patients with

highly favorable results and low morbidity. When the exiting venous outflow is occluded, sinus thrombosis is initiated.[95] It is believed that occlusion of "arterialized" venous outflow is safe as long as normal antegrade venous drainage is not compromised. In fact, because draining veins have inverted their flow, their occlusion at their dural origin is not followed by venous engorgement.[104] Following this procedure, they become thrombosed, and usually this phenomenon remains hemodynamically insignificant.[94,123] When performing direct clipping of the draining vein, it is advisable to remain as close as possible to the dural fistula and to cauterize extensively the dural base.[113] Particularly in dural AVFs, when venous outflow is occluded before the arterial inflow, bleeding does not occur, presumably because these lesions are imbedded within the dura and therefore protected from rupture.

In neonates with heart failure, attempted complete occlusion has uniformly led to volume overload and even to death from cardiac decompensation. Even partial occlusion may stress an already ischemic and maximally dilated heart.[124,125] In this case, volume status and cardiac function need to be monitored closely.[35] In older children without or with mild cardiac failure, this complication is of much less concern, and occlusion can usually be achieved through a single procedure.

Arterial Ligation

Because dural AVFs frequently recur if treated only by arterial ligation, this approach alone cannot be considered curative.[95,104,113,116] Occasionally, despite ligating the feeding vessels and excising the fistulous communication, there is surprisingly poor response to treatment, and filling might occur through different branches.[126] Nevertheless, it has an important role in decreasing the flow through the fistula, for palliative or symptomatic treatment, and to simplify the architecture of complex lesions prior to surgery.[97,98,102,111,117,127,128] For cases where sinus packing is an option, endovascular approaches can achieve high cure rates.

Arteriovenous Fistula–Varix Combination

In the case of AVF–varix combination, surgical therapy is used to isolate the fistula from its vascular supply.[1] The varix can remain in situ and its removal is not usually undertaken unless it is causing symptoms from mass effect.[2,4,35,48] Therefore, treatment is deemed successful when it results in the elimination of the shunt as well as a collapse or thrombosis of the varix. Further credence to this contention is provided by previous reports of progressive collapse after feeder clipping.[35] It is our recommendation that feeders should be followed to their entrance into the venous varix where they should be clipped. The varix can change from red to blue immediately after feeder closure, and decreased turgor can also be observed.

Varices are not typically easy to treat. With an endovascular approach, there is always the risk of embolizing the varix and compromising the venous outflow.[107] They also may continue to refill from other branches, and this arterial supply may be enough to prevent their thrombosis.[1]

In some instances, particularly in bleeding and hematoma formation, a separation of the varix from the adjacent brain tissue may occur, and removal is made easier. Barnwell et al[1] has reported a case where he was able to remove the varix. Separation from the adjacent area of normal brain was eased by the surgical plane carved by the hemorrhage.

Given the complex nature of pediatric AVFs certain patients will not be candidates for curative procedures. When venous hypertension cannot be treated by endovascular approaches or the aforementioned techniques, bypass procedures from the sinuses to the jugular veins may provide some palliation and decrease symptoms.

> **PEARL** Because dural AVFs frequently recur if treated only by arterial ligation, this approach alone cannot be considered curative.

> **PEARL** In neonates with heart failure, attempted complete occlusion has uniformly led to volume overload and even to death from cardiac decompensation. Even partial occlusion may stress an already ischemic and maximally dilated heart.

■ Illustrative Cases

Case 1

A 4-year-old boy presented to a pediatrician with headaches, vomiting, and unsteady gait. Enhanced CT was performed due to the concern about the possibility of a posterior fossa tumor. This study (**Fig. 8–2**) was felt to show a homogeneously enhancing tumor. At an outside institution the lesion was surgically exposed and biopsied (with impressive results). Fortunately, the surgical incision could be closed with 4–0 suture after torrential bleeding was controlled. After transfer, angiography disclosed a direct distal posterior inferior cerebellar artery AVF emptying into a massive varix. The lesion was treated by surgical trapping with excellent results.

Case 2

A 6-year-old girl was treated in another state for a severe dural AVF supplied by bilateral cavernous carotid branches and bilateral posterior cerebral artery (PCA) branches. She had been treated with several surgical and endovascular procedures to pack the massively dilated superior sagittal sinus. Her clinical situation was stable until she collapsed into coma in a supermarket. She was found to have severely elevated intracranial pressure that was not manageable medically. After transfer to our institution, repeat radiological studies were performed (**Fig. 8–3**). MRI showed continued patency of the massive sinus with preservation of brain anatomy (**Fig. 8–3A**). Repeat angiography showed persistent flow via cavernous branches and PCA branches (**Fig. 8–3B,C**). The surprise finding was in the venous phase. Both transverse sinuses were occluded and her sole venous outflow was via sluggish deep brain venous structures ultimately emptying into the supratentorial system (**Fig. 8–3D,E**).

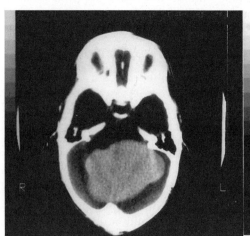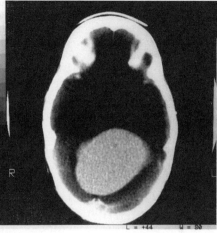

FIGURE 8–2 Enhanced computed tomographic scan on a 4-year-old child. Initial interpretation was posterior fossa tumor. Subsequent angiography demonstrated distal posterior inferior cerebellar artery arteriovenous fistula with giant varix.

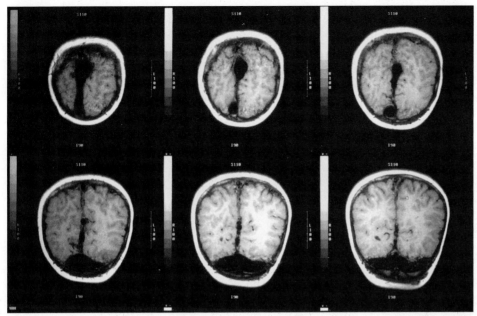

A

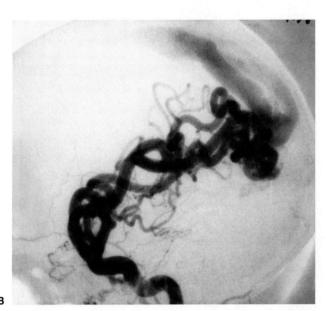

B

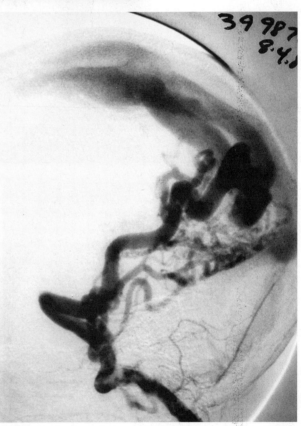

C

FIGURE 8–3 Six-year-old girl with complex arteriovenous fistula referred after sudden unconsciousness 4 days before. **(A)** Magnetic resonance imaging shows a patent superior sagittal sinus with massive dilation. **(B,C)** Carotid and vertebral angiography showed filling of the falcine fistula via cavernous carotid and posterior cerebral artery branches.

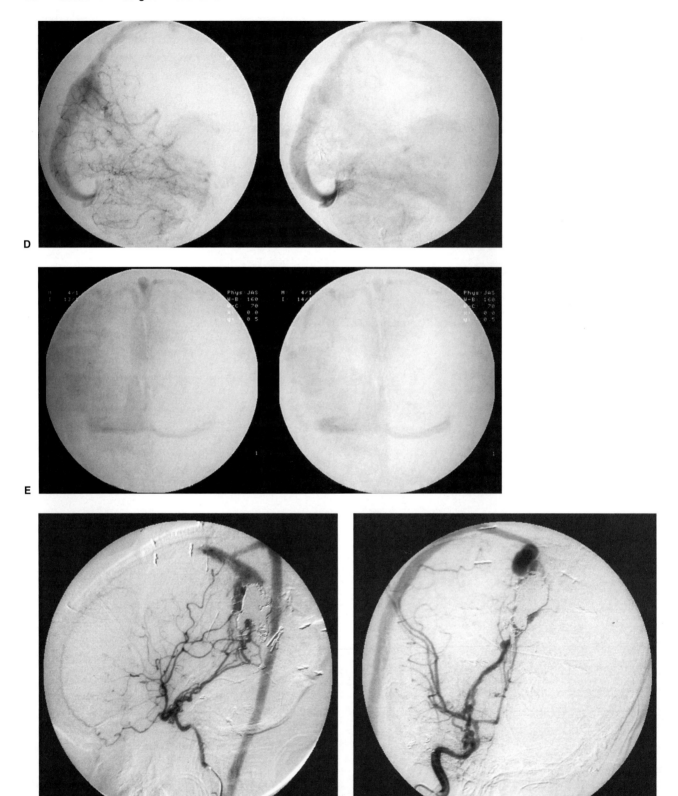

FIGURE 8–3 *(Continued)* **(D,E)** Venous phase studies showed occlusion of both transverse sinuses with slow egress of brain venous drainage into sphenoparietal and facial veins. **(F,G,H)** Postoperative angiography confirmed patency of a saphenous vein graft from the superior sagittal sinus into the external jugular vein.

We considered many options and ultimately tried a novel strategy that had been discussed a few years earlier by Dr. Cole Giller (personal communication). Because her real problem was venous hypertension we decided to leave the arterial input alone and put a saphenous vein graft into the right transverse sinus vein and restore drainage into the external jugular external vein. The first attempt failed with graft occlusion. We returned to the operating room the next day and used the superior sagittal sinus instead. This "bypass" gave beautiful and immediate reduction in ICP (**Figs. 8–3F–H**). Her level of consciousness began to improve also. One week later we returned to surgery to repair a large pseudomeningocele from the initial attempt. During the uneventful repair she suffered a sudden cardiac arrest from which she could not be saved. Subsequent autopsy was unrevealing as to the cause of death.

■ Complications and Avoidance

Surgery for AVFs is associated with a variety of complications, and any patient being considered for such an approach should undergo careful assessment.

Closure of a big fistula results in a shift of a significant portion of the blood volume from the venous to the arterial side. This may result in an abrupt increase in peripheral resistance with circulatory overload.[47] Thus close cardiac monitoring is essential in the operative as well as the postoperative period to control possible cardiac decompensation. Such complications can be avoided or decreased by staging the procedures, and with close

control of the intra- and postoperative blood pressure.[107] Surgery may be associated with rapid blood loss that can be life threatening.[110] Particularly in infants, blood loss is a special concern. This risk may be decreased by preoperative embolization allowing an extensive resection without the loss of a large volume of blood.[19,104] This treatment modality should be targeted to the specific area of shunting that is thought to be the most responsible for the patient's symptoms.[30] Although associated with a high rate of recurrence, it results in transient symptomatic improvement. Whenever it is thought to be of help, it should be kept in mind that it may isolate the involved sinus making further transvascular attempts difficult or impossible.[30]

Thrombosis in the outflow drainage is another feared complication. Its propagation from the lesion might lead to venous infarction and neurological injury. Another possibility is the initiation of thrombosis in the outflow drainage due to passage of embolic material.[53,129,130] Thus it may be advisable to transect the connections with the draining sinus. This may also prevent thrombosis from expanding into the normal draining veins.[1] There is a potential risk of venous infarction if the occlusion of a sinus causes obstruction of the outflow of a vein draining normal cerebral tissue.[85] Thus it should be remembered that venous embolization is most indicated for cases in which the involved sinus is already compromised and no longer contributes to the drainage of normal tissue.[97,127]

After clipping feeders, the altered hemodynamic state may result in the development of the normal perfusion pressure breakthrough (NPPB) phenomenon.[131,132] Delayed postoperative hemorrhage, when it occurs, may be related to the sudden diversion of rapid flow into the surrounding brain where vessels are unable to contain the pressure.[6,131] Therefore, it is often preferable to stage the closure of large fistulas.

Monitoring of transcranial Doppler (TCD) velocities may indicate impairment of autoregulation or hyperemia after fistula obliteration, and therefore can be performed serially because NPPB may occur immediately[133] or in a delayed fashion.[52] After resection of AVMs, changes have been noted in NPPB[134] and have been used to detect and to follow their treatment.

These complications can also be minimized by other strategies such as controlled intraoperative and postoperative hypotension.[2,4,48–50] Despite being associated with relatively good outcomes,[6,107] there are no data regarding any values that should be used. Furthermore, hypotension may disturb regional flow from the maximally dilated arteries.[107]

Risk might also be reduced when balloon test occlusion is tolerated. In the absence of this trial there is no reliable measure to determine the risks associated with acute fistula closure. Giller et al[135] reported the use of

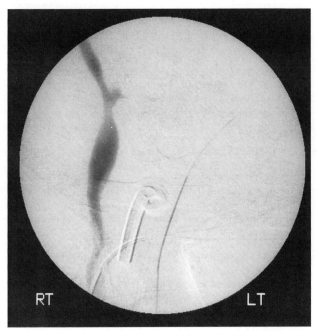

RT   LT

H

single photon emission tomography (SPECT) and TCD studies to assess the occurrence of hyperemia during balloon test occlusion in high-flow fistulas. This combination proved helpful in preoperative counseling of therapeutic risk and in the formulation of a treatment plan. By showing the immediate ability of the surrounding brain to compensate, and in the absence of significant hemodynamic changes, it allows direct fistula obliteration and avoids staged procedures. It might also be helpful in distinguishing the neurological deficit arising from NPPB from that of ischemia or from venous occlusion. Qualitative information from SPECT studies can be used to make side by side comparisons at baseline and during balloon occlusion to detect altered cerebral hemodynamics.[135] However, a delayed occurrence of NPPB cannot be evaluated by any of these hemodynamic tests. Intraoperative angiography can be helpful. It visualizes the arterial patterns and allows more accurate and specific treatment.[6] It is also an essential exam after the operation to document complete obliteration.[1]

When multifocal dural shunts involve nearly all the major dural sinuses, they cannot be cured immediately by any technique. When surgery is still believed to be associated with high risk, embolization may be used for the palliation of symptoms.[98,127,136–138] The morbidity of an erroneous occlusion could reroute the fistulous output and overload a dural sinus.

Recurrence has been observed after surgical approaches. For example Robinson and Sedzimir reported a 19-month-old boy with an aneurysmal sac draining into an enormously dilated transverse sinus. It was fed by a large left posterior auricular artery running through a skull defect. After ligation of the ECA at the skull entry point and behind the sternocleidomastoid artery, it was excised. One month later, angiography showed shunting from the right ECA, cervical vertebral artery, and suboccipital arterial plexus.[126]

▪ Conclusion

Pediatric AVFs are often multiple and more complex than their adult counterparts. It is our belief that the wide variation of this disease cannot be approached with any single strategy. Therefore, treatment should be based on careful preoperative evaluation and should be addressed specifically on a case by case basis. Incompletely occluded fistulas maintain the potential for aggressive behavior and evolution toward more complex lesions.[105,111]

Cure can be achieved only after understanding of the overall architecture of the lesion. We also stress careful coordination of endovascular and surgical techniques. Multiple procedures are inconvenient, but if they enhance safety by any fraction beyond the morbidity of infection, then this approach should be considered.

REFERENCES

1. Barnwell SL, Ciricillo SF, Halbach VV, Edwards MS, Cogen PH. Intracerebral arteriovenous fistulas associated with intraparenchymal varix in childhood: case reports. Neurosurgery 1990;26: 122–125
2. Carrillo R, Carreira LM, Prada J, Rosas C, Egas G. Giant aneurysm arising from a single arteriovenous fistula in a child: case report. J Neurosurg 1984;60:1085–1088
3. Tomlinson FH, Piepgras DG, Nichols DA, Rufenacht DA, Kaste SC. Remote congenital cerebral arteriovenous fistulae associated with aortic coarctation: case report. J Neurosurg 1992;76:137–142
4. Vinuela F, Drake CG, Fox AJ, Pelz DM. Giant intracranial varices secondary to high-flow arteriovenous fistulae. J Neurosurg 1987; 66:198–203
5. Willinsky RA, Lasjaunias P, Terbrugge K, Burrows P. Multiple cerebral arteriovenous malformations (AVMs): review of our experience from 203 patients with cerebral vascular lesions. Neuroradiology 1990;32:207–210
6. Tomlinson FH, Rufenacht DA, Sundt TM Jr, Nichols DA, Fode NC. Arteriovenous fistulas of the brain and the spinal cord. J Neurosurg 1993;79:16–27
7. Morgan MK, Sundt TM Jr, Houser OW. Arterio-inferior sagittal sinus fistulae: case report. Neurosurgery 1989;25:971–975
8. Lasjaunias PL, Magufis A, Goulao R, Suthipongchai S, Rodesch R, Alvarez H. Anatomoclinical aspects of dural arteriovenous shunts in children. Intervent Neuroradiol 1996;2:179–191
9. Ushikoshi S, Kikuchi Y, Miyasaka K. Multiple dural arteriovenous shunts in a 5-year-old boy. AJNR Am J Neuroradiol 1999;20: 728–730
10. Garcia-Monaco R, Rodesch G, Terbrugge K, Burrows P, Lasjaunias P. Multifocal dural arteriovenous shunts in children. Childs Nerv Syst 1991;7:425–431
11. Luessenhop A. Dural arteriovenous malformations. In: Wilkins LH, ed. Neurosurgery. New York: McGraw-Hill; 1985:1473–1477
12. Newton TH, Cronqvist S. Involvement of dural arteries in intracranial arteriovenous malformations. Radiology 1969;93: 1071–1078
13. Houser OW, Campbell JK, Campbell RJ, Sundt TM Jr. Arteriovenous malformation affecting the transverse dural venous sinus— an acquired lesion. Mayo Clin Proc 1979;54:651–661
14. Coubes P, Humbertclaude V, Rodesch G, Lasjaunias P, Echenne B, Frerebeau P. Total endovascular occlusion of a giant direct arteriovenous fistula in the posterior fossa in a case of Rendu-Osler-Weber disease. Childs Nerv Syst 1996;12:785–788
15. Garcia-Monaco R, Taylor W, Rodesch G, et al. Pial arteriovenous fistula in children as presenting manifestation of Rendu-Osler-Weber disease. Neuroradiology 1995;37:60–64
16. Kikuchi K, Kowada M, Sasajima H. Vascular malformations of the brain in hereditary hemorrhagic telangiectasia (Rendu-Osler-Weber disease). Surg Neurol 1994;41:374–380
17. Oyesiku NM, Gahm NH, Goldman RL. Cerebral arteriovenous fistula in the Klippel-Trénaunay-Weber syndrome. Dev Med Child Neurol 1988;30:245–248
18. Benhaiem-Sigaux N, Zerah M, Gherardi R, Bellot J, Hurth M, Poirier J. A retromedullary arteriovenous fistula associated with the Klippel-Trénaunay-Weber syndrome: a clinicopathologic study. Acta Neuropathol (Berl) 1985;66:318–324
19. Albright AL, Latchaw RE, Price RA. Posterior dural arteriovenous malformations in infancy. Neurosurgery 1983;13:129–135
20. Roman G, Fisher M, Perl DP, Poser CM. Neurological manifestations of hereditary hemorrhagic telangiectasia (Rendu-Osler-Weber disease): report of 2 cases and review of the literature. Ann Neurol 1978;4:130–144
21. Kelly JJ Jr, Mellinger JF, Sundt TM Jr. Intracranial arteriovenous malformations in childhood. Ann Neurol 1978;3:338–343

22. Hanigan WC, Brady T, Medlock M, Smith EB. Spontaneous regression of giant arteriovenous fistulae during the perinatal period: case report. J Neurosurg 1990;73:954–957

23. Santosh C, Teasdale E, Molyneux A. Spontaneous closure of an intracranial middle cerebral arteriovenous fistula. Neuroradiology 1991;33:65–66

24. Mabe H, Furuse M. Spontaneous disappearance of a cerebral arteriovenous malformation in infancy: case report. J Neurosurg 1977;46:811–815

25. Pascual-Castroviejo I, Pascual-Pascual JI, Blazquez MG, Lopez-Martin V. Spontaneous occlusion of an intracranial arteriovenous malformation. Childs Brain 1977;3:169–179

26. Omojola MF, Fox AJ, Vinuela FV, Drake CG. Spontaneous regression of intracranial arteriovenous malformations: report of three cases. J Neurosurg 1982;57:818–822

27. Pasqualin A, Vivenza C, Rosta L, Scienza R, Da Pian R, Colangeli M. Spontaneous disappearance of intracranial arterio-venous malformations. Acta Neurochir (Wien) 1985;76:50–57

28. Friedman AH. Etiologic factors in intracranial dural arteriovenous malformations. In: Awad IA, Barrow DL, eds. Dural Arteriovenous Malformations. Park Ridge, IL: AANS Publications Committee; 1993:35–47

29. Lasjaunias PL, Rodesch G. Lesions types, hemodynamics, and clinical spectrum. In: Awad IA, Barrow DL, eds. Dural Arteriovenous Malformations. Park Ridge, IL: AANS Publications Committee; 1993:49–79

30. Kincaid PK, Duckwiler GR, Gobin YP, Vinuela F. Dural arteriovenous fistula in children: endovascular treatment and outcomes in seven cases. AJNR Am J Neuroradiol 2001;22:1217–1225

31. Chaloupka J. Endovascular therapy of dural arteriovenous fistulae. Semin Intervent Radiol 1994;11:1–13

32. Pellegrino PA, Milanesi O, Saia OS, Carollo C. Congestive heart failure secondary to cerebral arterio-venous fistula. Childs Nerv Syst 1987;3:141–144

33. Amacher AL, Shillito J Jr. The syndromes and surgical treatment of aneurysms of the great vein of Galen. J Neurosurg 1973;39:89–98

34. Gold AP, Ransohoff J, Carter S. Vein of Galen malformation. Acla Neurol Scand Suppl 1964;40(Suppl 2):1–31

35. Godersky JC, Menezes AH. Intracranial arteriovenous anomalies of infancy: modern concepts. Pediatr Neurosci 1987;13:242–250

36. De Marco JK, Dillon WP, Halback VV, Tsuruda JS. Dural arteriovenous fistulas: evaluation with MR imaging. Radiology 1990;175:193–199

37. Chen JC, Tsuruda JS, Halbach VV. Suspected dural arteriovenous fistula: results with screening MR angiography in seven patients. Radiology 1992;183:265–271

38. Davies MA, TerBrugge K, Willinsky R, Coyne T, Saleh J, Wallace MC. The validity of classification for the clinical presentation of intracranial dural arteriovenous fistulas. J Neurosurg 1996;85:830–837

39. Hugosson R, Bergstrom K. Surgical treatment of dural arteriovenous malformation in the region of the sigmoid sinus. J Neurol Neurosurg Psychiatry 1974;37:97–101

40. Kuhner A, Krastel A, Stoll W. Arteriovenous malformations of the transverse dural sinus. J Neurosurg 1976;45:12–19

41. Lasjaunias P, Lopez-Ibor L, Abanou A, Halimi P. Radiological anatomy of the vascularization of cranial dural arteriovenous malformations. Anat Clin 1984;6:87–99

42. Ojemann RG, Heros RC, Crowell RM. Dural arteriovenous malformations. In: Ojemann RG, Heros RC, Crowell RM, eds. Surgical Management of Cerebrovascular Disease, 2nd ed. Baltimore, MD: Williams and Wilkins; 1988:415–425

43. Malek, 2nd ed AM, Halbach VV, Higashida RT, Phatouros CC, Meyers PM, Dowd CF. Treatment of dural arteriovenous malformations and fistulas. Neurosurg Clin N Am 2000;11:147–166

44. Holden AM, Fyler DC, Shillito J Jr, Nadas AS. Congestive heart failure from intracranial arteriovenous fistula in infancy: clinical and physiologic considerations in eight patients. Pediatrics 1972;49:30–39

45. Cumming GR. Circulation in neonates with intracranial arteriovenous fistula and cardiac failure. Am J Cardiol 1980;45:1019–1024

46. Lakier JB, Milner S, Cohen M, Levin SE. Intracranial arteriovenous fistulas in infancy: haemodynamic considerations. S Afr Med J 1982;61:242–245

47. Levine OR, Jameson AG, Nellhaus G, Gold AP. Cardiac complications of cerebral arteriovenous fistula in infancy. Pediatrics 1962;30:563–575

48. Vinuela F, Fox AJ, Kan S, Drake CG. Balloon occlusion of a spontaneous fistula of the posterior inferior cerebellar artery: case report. J Neurosurg 1983;58:287–290

49. Aoki N, Sakai T, Oikawa A. Intracranial arteriovenous fistula manifesting as progressive neurological deterioration in an infant: case report. Neurosurgery 1991;28:619–622

50. Halbach VV, Higashida RT, Hieshima GB, Hardin CW, Dowd CF, Barnwell SL. Transarterial occlusion of solitary intracerebral arteriovenous fistulas. AJNR Am J Neuroradiol 1989;10:747–752

51. Morgan MK, Johnston IH, Sundt TM Jr. Normal perfusion pressure breakthrough complicating surgery for the vein of Galen malformation: report of three cases. Neurosurgery 1989;24:406–410

52. Smith RR, Burt T. Hypoperfusion after carotid endarterectomy managed by removable clamp. J Neuroimag 1993;3:16–19

53. Awad IA, Little JR, Akarawi WP, Ahl J. Intracranial dural arteriovenous malformations: factors predisposing to an aggressive neurological course. J Neurosurg 1990;72:839–850

54. Barrow DL. Unruptured cerebral arteriovenous malformations presenting with intracranial hypertension. Neurosurgery 1988;23:484–490

55. Bousser MG, Chiras J, Bories J, Castaigne P. Cerebral venous thrombosis: a review of 38 cases. Stroke 1985;16:199–213

56. Brainin M, Samec P. Venous hemodynamics of arteriovenous meningeal fistulas in the posterior cranial fossa. Neuroradiology 1983;25:161–169

57. Dobbelaere P, Jomin M, Clarisse J, Laine E. Prognostic importance of the study of venous drainage in cerebral arteriovenous aneurysms [in French]. Neurochirurgie 1979;25:178–184

58. Garcia JH, Williams JP, Tanaka J. Spontaneous thrombosis of deep cerebral veins: a complication of arteriovenous malformation. Stroke 1975;6:164–171

59. Hassler W, Thron A, Grote EH. Hemodynamics of spinal dural arteriovenous fistulas: an intraoperative study. J Neurosurg 1989;70:360–370

60. Merland JJ, Riche MC, Chiras J. Intraspinal extramedullary arteriovenous fistulae draining into the medullary veins. J Neuroradiol 1980;7:271–320

61. Teng MM, Chang T, Pan DH, et al. Brainstem edema: an unusual complication of carotid cavernous fistula. AJNR Am J Neuroradiol 1991;12:139–142

62. Vassilouthis J. Cerebral arteriovenous malformation with intracranial hypertension. Surg Neurol 1979;11:402–404

63. Yasargil MG. Microneurosurgery, Vol 3: Clinical Considerations and Microsurgery of the Arteriovenous Racemose Angiomas. New York: Thieme; 1987:193–211

64. Brown RD Jr, Wiebers DO, Nichols DA. Intracranial dural arteriovenous fistulae: angiographic predictors of intracranial hemorrhage and clinical outcome in nonsurgical patients. J Neurosurg 1994;81:531–538

65. Wilms G, Demaerel P, Lagae L, Casteels I, Mombaerts I. Direct caroticocavernous fistula and traumatic dissection of the ipsilateral internal carotid artery: endovascular treatment. Neuroradiology 2000;42:62–65

66. Ciesielski T, Stefanowicz E, Brzozowski E. A case of post-traumatic carotid-cavernous fistula in a 9-year-old girl [in Polish]. Neurol Neurochir Pol 1984;18:65–67

67. Polomisova L, Fusek I, Bret J, Havrankova J. Pulsating exophthalmos associated with a post-traumatic carotid-cavernous fistula in a child [in Czechoslovakian]. Cesk Oftalmol. 1983;39:327–331

68. Keller HM, Imhof HG, Valavanis A. Persistent cervical intersegmental artery as a cause of recurrence of a traumatic carotid-cavernous fistula: case report, with emphasis on Doppler ultrasound diagnosis. Neurosurgery 1982;10:492–498

69. Sanders MD, Hoyt WF. Hypoxic ocular sequelae of carotid-cavernous fistulae: study of the causes of visual failure before and after neurosurgical treatment in a series of 25 cases. Br J Ophthalmol 1969;53:82–97

70. Barrow DL, Spector RH, Braun IF, Landman JA, Tindall SC, Tindall GT. Classification and treatment of spontaneous carotid-cavernous sinus fistulas. J Neurosurg 1985;62:248–256

71. Debrun GM, Vinuela F, Fox AJ, Davis KR, Ahn HS. Indications for treatment and classification of 132 carotid-cavernous fistulas. Neurosurgery 1988;22:285–289

72. Peeters FL, Kroger R. Dural and direct cavernous sinus fistulas. AJR Am J Roentgenol 1979;132:599–606

73. Vinuela F, Fox AJ, Debrun GM, Peerless SJ, Drake CG. Spontaneous carotid-cavernous fistulas: clinical, radiological, and therapeutic considerations: experience with 20 cases. J Neurosurg 1984;60:976–984

74. Pang D, Kerber C, Biglan AW, Ahn HS. External carotid-cavernous fistula in infancy: case report and review of the literature. Neurosurgery 1981;8:212–218

75. Kerber CW, Bank WO, Cromwell LD. Cyanoacrylate occlusion of carotid-cavernous fistula with preservation of carotid artery flow. Neurosurgery 1979;4:210–215

76. Conley FK, Hamilton RD, Hosobuchi Y. Successful surgical treatment of bilateral carotid-cavernous fistulas. J Neurosurg 1975;43:357–361

77. Black P, Uematsu S, Perovic M, Walker AE. Carotid-cavernous fistula: a controlled embolus technique for occlusion of fistula with preservation of carotid blood flow: technical note. J Neurosurg 1973;38:113–118

78. Parkinson D. Carotid cavernous fistula: direct repair with preservation of the carotid artery: technical note. J Neurosurg 1973;38:99–106

79. Mullan S. Experiences with surgical thrombosis of intracranial berry aneurysms and carotid cavernous fistulas. J Neurosurg 1974;41:657–670

80. Day JD, Fukushima T. Direct microsurgery of dural arteriovenous malformation type carotid-cavernous sinus fistulas: indications, technique, and results. Neurosurgery 1997;41:1119–1124

81. Thompson BG, Doppman JL, Oldfield EH. Treatment of cranial dural arteriovenous fistulae by interruption of leptomeningeal venous drainage. J Neurosurg 1994;80:617–623

82. Iizuka Y, Rodesch G, Garcia-Monaco R, et al. Multiple cerebral arteriovenous shunts in children: report of 13 cases. Childs Nerv Syst 1992;8:437–444

83. Barnwell SL, Halbach VV, Dowd CF, Higashida RT, Hieshima GB, Wilson CB. A variant of arteriovenous fistulas within the wall of dural sinuses: results of combined surgical and endovascular therapy. J Neurosurg 1991;74:199–204

84. Morita A, Meyer FB, Nichols DA, Patterson MC. Childhood dural arteriovenous fistulae of the posterior dural sinuses: three case reports and literature review. Neurosurgery 1995;37:1193–1199

85. Roy D, Raymond J. The role of transvenous embolization in the treatment of intracranial dural arteriovenous fistulas. Neurosurgery 1997;40:1133–1141

86. Bitoh S, Sakaki S. Spontaneous cure of dural arteriovenous malformation in the posterior fossa. Surg Neurol 1979;12:111–114

87. Hansen JH, Sogaard I. Spontaneous regression of an extra- and intracranial arteriovenous malformation: case report. J Neurosurg 1976;45:338–341

88. Olutola PS, Eliam M, Molot M, Talalla A. Spontaneous regression of a dural arteriovenous malformation. Neurosurgery 1983;12:687–690

89. Lownie S, Duckwiler G, Fox A, Drake C. Endovascular therapy of non-Galenic cerebral arteriovenous fistulas. In: Vinuela F, Halbach VV, Dion J, eds. Interventional Neuroradiology: Endovascular Therapy of the Central Nervous System. New York: Raven; 1992:87–106

90. Nelson K, Nimi Y, Lasjaunias P, Berenstein A. Endovascular embolization of congenital intracranial pial arteriovenous fistulas. Neuroimag Clin North Am 1992;2:309–317

91. Miller PD, Albright AL. Posterior dural arteriovenous malformation and medulloblastoma in an infant: case report. Neurosurgery 1993;32:126–130

92. Rosenbloom S, Edwards MSB. Dural arteriovenous malformations. In: Edwards MSB, Hoffman HJ, eds. Cerebral Vascular Disease in Children and Adolescents. Baltimore: Williams and Wilkins; 1989:343–365

93. Chan ST, Weeks RD. Dural arteriovenous malformation presenting as cardiac failure in a neonate. Acta Neurochir (Wien) 1988;91:134–138

94. Collice M, D'Aliberti G, Talamonti G, et al. Surgical interruption of leptomeningeal drainage as treatment for intracranial dural arteriovenous fistulas without dural sinus drainage. J Neurosurg 1996;84:810–817

95. Mullan S. Reflections upon the nature and management of intracranial and intraspinal vascular malformations and fistulae. J Neurosurg 1994;80:606–616

96. Versari PP, D'Aliberti G, Talamonti G, Branca V, Boccardi E, Collice M. Progressive myelopathy caused by intracranial dural arteriovenous fistula: report of two cases and review of the literature. Neurosurgery 1993;33:914–919

97. Borden JA, Wu JK, Shucart WA. A proposed classification for spinal and cranial dural arteriovenous fistulous malformations and implications for treatment. J Neurosurg 1995;82:166–179

98. Cognard C, Gobin YP, Pierot L, et al. Cerebral dural arteriovenous fistulas: clinical and angiographic correlation with a revised classification of venous drainage. Radiology 1995;194:671–680

99. Djindjian R, Merland JJ. Super-selective Arteriography of the External Carotid Artery. Berlin: Springer-Verlag; 1978:405–537

100. Houser OW, Baker HL Jr, Rhoton AL Jr, Okazaki H. Intracranial dural arteriovenous malformations. Radiology 1972;105:55–64

101. Malik GM, Pearce JE, Ausman JI, Mehta B. Dural arteriovenous malformations and intracranial hemorrhage. Neurosurgery 1984;15:332–339

102. Picard L, Bracard S, Islak C, et al. Dural fistulae of the tentorium cerebelli: radioanatomical, clinical and therapeutic considerations. J Neuroradiol 1990;17:161–181

103. Aminoff MJ, Kendall BE. Asymptomatic dural vascular anomalies. Br J Radiol 1973;46:662–667

104. Collice M, D'Aliberti G, Arena O, Solaini C, Fontana RA, Talamonti G. Surgical treatment of intracranial dural arteriovenous fistulae: role of venous drainage. Neurosurgery 2000;47:56–66

105. Lalwani AK, Dowd CF, Halbach VV. Grading venous restrictive disease in patients with dural arteriovenous fistulas of the transverse/sigmoid sinus. J Neurosurg 1993;79:11–15

106. Lasjaunias P, Chiu M, ter Brugge K, Tolia A, Hurth M, Bernstein M. Neurological manifestations of intracranial dural arteriovenous malformations. J Neurosurg 1986;64:724–730

107. Drake CG. Cerebral arteriovenous malformations: considerations for and experience with surgical treatment in 166 cases. Clin Neurosurg 1979;26:145–208

108. Barnwell SL, Halbach VV, Higashida RT, Hieshima G, Wilson CB. Complex dural arteriovenous fistulas: results of combined endovascular and neurosurgical treatment in 16 patients. J Neurosurg 1989;71:352–358

109. Sundt TM Jr, Piepgras DG. The surgical approach to arteriovenous malformations of the lateral and sigmoid dural sinuses. J Neurosurg 1983;59:32–39

110. Sundt TM Jr, Nichols DA, Piepgras DG, Fode NC. Strategies, techniques, and approaches for dural arteriovenous malformations of the posterior dural sinuses. Clin Neurosurg 1991;37:155–170

111. Awad IA. Intracranial dural arteriovenous malformations. In: Wilkins RH, Rengachary SS, eds. Neurosurgery. New York: McGraw-Hill; 1966:2519–2527

112. Lewis AI, Tomsick TA, Tew JM Jr. Management of tentorial dural arteriovenous malformations: transarterial embolization combined with stereotactic radiation or surgery. J Neurosurg 1994;81:851–859

113. Hoh BL, Choudhri TF, Connolly ES Jr, Solomon RA. Surgical management of high-grade intracranial dural arteriovenous fistulas: leptomeningeal venous disruption without nidus excision. Neurosurgery 1998;42:796–804

114. Mullan S. Treatment of carotid-cavernous fistulas by cavernous sinus occlusion. J Neurosurg 1979;50:131–144

115. Mullan S, Johnson DL. Combined sagittal and lateral sinus dural fistulae occlusion. J Neurosurg 1995;82:159–165

116. Barnwell SL, Nesbit GM. Dural arteriovenous malformations of the transverse and sigmoid sinuses. In: Loftus CM, Batjer HH, eds. Techniques in Neurosurgery. Vol 2. Philadelphia, PA: Lippincott-Raven; 1995:53–65

117. Halbach VV, Higashida RT, Hieshima GB, Mehringer CM, Hardin CW. Transvenous embolization of dural fistulas involving the transverse and sigmoid sinuses. AJNR Am J Neuroradiol 1989;10:385–392

118. Grisoli F, Vincentelli F, Fuchs S, et al. Surgical treatment of tentorial arteriovenous malformations draining into the subarachnoid space: report of four cases. J Neurosurg 1984;60:1059–1066

119. Kendall BE, Logue V. Spinal epidural angiomatous malformations draining into intrathecal veins. Neuroradiology 1977;13:181–189

120. Oldfield EH, Doppman JL. Spinal arteriovenous malformations. Clin Neurosurg 1988;34:161–183

121. Oldfield EH, Di Chiro G, Quindlen EA, Rieth KG, Doppman JL. Successful treatment of a group of spinal cord arteriovenous malformations by interruption of dural fistula. J Neurosurg 1983;59:1019–1030

122. Symon L, Kuyama H, Kendall B. Dural arteriovenous malformations of the spine: clinical features and surgical results in 55 cases. J Neurosurg 1984;60:238–247

123. Halbach VV, Higashida RT, Hieshima GB, Wilson CB, Hardin CW, Kwan E. Treatment of dural fistulas involving the deep cerebral venous system. AJNR Am J Neuroradiol 1989;10:393–399

124. Hoffman HJ, Chuang S, Hendrick EB, Humphreys RP. Aneurysms of the vein of Galen: experience at the Hospital for Sick Children, Toronto. J Neurosurg 1982;57:316–322

125. Jedeikin R, Rowe RD, Freedom RM, Olley PM, Gillan JE. Cerebral arteriovenous malformation in neonates: the role of myocardial ischemia. Pediatr Cardiol 1983;4:29–35

126. Robinson JL, Sedzimir CB. External carotid-transverse sinus fistula: case report. J Neurosurg 1970;33:718–720

127. Urtasun F, Biondi A, Casaco A, et al. Cerebral dural arteriovenous fistulas: percutaneous transvenous embolization. Radiology 1996;199:209–217

128. Gobin YP, Rogopoulos A, Aymard A, et al. Endovascular treatment of intracranial dural arteriovenous fistulas with spinal perimedullary venous drainage. J Neurosurg 1992;77:718–723

129. Miyasaka Y, Yada K, Ohwada T, et al. Hemorrhagic venous infarction after excision of an arteriovenous malformation: case report. Neurosurgery 1991;29:265–268

130. Spetzler RF, Selman WR. Pathophysiology of cerebral ischemia accompanying arteriovenous malformations. In: Wilson CB, Stein BM, eds. Intracranial Arteriovenous Malformations. Baltimore: Williams and Wilkins; 1984:24–31

131. Spetzler RF, Wilson CB, Weinstein P, Mehdorn M, Townsend J, Telles D. Normal perfusion pressure breakthrough theory. Clin Neurosurg 1978;25:651–672

132. Kondoh T, Tamaki N, Takeda N, Suyama T, Oi SZ, Matsumoto S. Fatal intracranial hemorrhage after balloon occlusion of an extracranial vertebral arteriovenous fistula: case report. J Neurosurg 1988;69:945–948

133. Halbach VV, Higashida RT, Hieshima GB, Norman D. Normal perfusion pressure breakthrough occurring during treatment of carotid and vertebral fistulas. AJNR Am J Neuroradiol 1987;8:751–756

134. Batjer HH, Purdy PD, Giller CA, Samson DS. Evidence of redistribution of cerebral blood flow during treatment for an intracranial arteriovenous malformation. Neurosurgery 1989;25:599–605

135. Giller CA, Batjer HH, Purdy P, Walker B, Mathews D. Interdisciplinary evaluation of cerebral hemodynamics in the treatment of arteriovenous fistulae associated with giant varices. Neurosurgery 1994;35:778–782

136. Halbach VV, Higashida RT, Hieshima GB, Reicher M, Norman D, Newton TH. Dural fistulas involving the cavernous sinus: results of treatment in 30 patients. Radiology 1987;163:437–442

137. Halbach VV, Higashida RT, Hieshima GB, Goto K, Norman D, Newton TH. Dural fistulas involving the transverse and sigmoid sinuses: results of treatment in 28 patients. Radiology 1987;163:443–447

138. Hirabuki N, Mitomo M, Miura T, Hashimoto T, Kawai R, Kozuka T. External carotid artery embolization of dural arteriovenous malformations involving the cavernous sinus: outcome and role of venous thrombosis. Acta Radiol 1990;31:197–201

9

Surgical Treatment of Arteriovenous Malformations in Children

MICHAEL A. HORGAN, JEFFREY FLORMAN, AND ROBERT F. SPETZLER

Arteriovenous malformations (AVMs) are distinguished from other types of cerebral vascular malformations by their direct anastomosis between arterial and venous channels without any intervening capillaries. Since the first complete excision of a cerebral AVM in 1932 by Olivecrona,[1] surgery has become a mainstay in the management of AVMs. However, the therapeutic options are becoming increasingly complex. Although there remains a clear role for neurosurgery in the management of pediatric AVMs, a multidisciplinary approach including endovascular adjuncts and radiosurgery is often appropriate and now widely available. Successful management depends upon many factors, including the presentation, clinical condition, and age of the child. Additionally, neuroanatomical features of the AVM are paramount, including the size, location, and angioarchitecture of the lesion. This chapter reviews the clinical features and management of parenchymal AVMs in children with a focus on the role of open surgical techniques.

■ Clinical Features

Cerebral AVMs are uncommon lesions with a prevalence in the general population of 0.5 to 1%.[2,3] Between 10 and 20% of AVMs are diagnosed in children and adolescents, resulting in a prevalence between 0.014 and 0.028% in the pediatric population.[4] The annual incidence of AVM rupture in children is one per 100,000 population.[5] The vast majority occur sporadically, although familial cases have been reported[6] and there are a few syndromes associated with a predisposition for AVMs. The risk for AVM in children with hereditary hemorrhagic telangiectasia (Osler-Weber-Rendu disease) is 7.9%,[7] and this syndrome should be strongly considered in patients with multiple AVMs.[8] Wyburn-Mason's syndrome has the unique association of AVMs of the visual pathway and midbrain with frequent occurrence of an ipsilateral facial nevus.[9]

Although AVMs are believed to have a congenital origin, the mean age at diagnosis is nearly 30 years, with up to 20% of AVMs becoming symptomatic under the age of 15 years.[2,10–12] No consistent gender predilection has been reported in children or adults with AVMs.[13,14] Most AVMs are located in the supratentorial compartment and 10 to 20% of AVMs in children are located infratentorially.[12,15] The average size of AVMs in children may be greater than in the adult population.[12]

The most common presentations for AVMs in both adults and children are hemorrhage and seizures. These points are illustrated in a study of 1289 patients with AVM by Hofmeister et al in which 53% presented with hemorrhage and 40% presented with seizure.[10] In the pediatric population, hemorrhage is recorded more commonly than in the adult population.[2,11,16–18] The presentations associated with pediatric AVMs include ~70 to 75% hemorrhage and 10 to 15% seizures.[12,18,19] Other clinical manifestations of AVMs, including headache, focal neurological deficit, and progressive neurological decline, are seen in all age groups.[10] AVMs with large arteriovenous shunts can also present with heart failure in the infant population.

> **PEARL** The most common presentations for AVMs are hemorrhage and seizures.

■ Natural History

The natural history of AVMs is typically not benign and there is a significant risk of recurrent symptoms. Although AVMs may be found incidentally, the majority present with symptoms of hemorrhage or seizures, and eventual neurological decline and morbidity are common. The risk of hemorrhage from an unruptured AVM is 1.5 to 3% per year.[20,21] This translates into a 30 to 40% risk of serious morbidity and a 10 to 15% risk of mortality per decade.[21] These data predict an aggressive and threatening course for AVMs presenting in the pediatric population.

The greatest risk to a child with an AVM is hemorrhage. Without treatment, the risk for rehemorrhage is nearly 6% during the first year after the initial hemorrhage, with a return to 1.5 to 3% per year thereafter.[13,22,23] Children may have a higher risk for rebleeding than adults.[24,25] In a general population of patients with AVMs, each hemorrhage carries a 10% mortality and 30 to 50% morbidity.[26] However, many authors describe a worse prognosis in children, with mortality after hemorrhage above 20%.[16,17,27,28] Efforts have been directed at identifying subsets of patients with AVMs who may be at increased risk for hemorrhage. Correlations have been identified between the risk for hemorrhage and the presence of aneurysms,[20] size of the AVM,[29] depth in the brain,[14] and venous drainage pattern.[30]

> **PEARL** The lifetime risk of morbidity or mortality in a child with an AVM is extremely high and should be considered when contemplating treatment.

Most seizures attributed to AVMs are generalized.[10] The proposed mechanisms for seizures in the presence of an AVM include focal cerebral ischemia secondary to arteriovenous shunting, gliosis of the surrounding brain, and secondary epileptogenesis in the temporal lobe.[31] A thorough evaluation of an epileptic child with an AVM should include the input of an epileptologist. Optimizing postoperative seizure control may occasionally necessitate neocortical resection in addition to AVM resection.

■ Radiological Evaluation

Computed tomography (CT) should generally be the first radiological study in a child suspected of having an AVM. This may demonstrate hemorrhage or hydrocephalus, and noncontrast head CT may suggest the presence of an AVM by showing calcifications or dilated vessels.

Contrasted CT will often demonstrate the nidus. Magnetic resonance imaging (MRI) is more sensitive and specific but can be more difficult to obtain in children. CT and magnetic resonance angiography may not only identify the lesion but may offer information about the angioarchitecture; however, they lack the sensitivity and resolution to negate the need for formal angiography. Catheter angiography remains the gold standard study for AVMs and may be obtained with minimal risk in the pediatric population. Sedation and potentially general anesthesia may be necessary for the study. Aggressive efforts should be made to demonstrate the complete anatomy, including imaging of the extracranial circulation in addition to the anterior and posterior intracranial circulation. Angiography will also demonstrate any associated arterial aneurysms or venous restrictions.

■ Management

The decision to pursue a therapeutic intervention in a child must be carefully considered and predicated upon the natural history of the lesion. The primary goals of therapy for children with AVMs are to eliminate the risk of future hemorrhage, control seizures, and relieve symptoms related to vascular steal. Surgical excision is considered by many to be the treatment of choice for parenchymal AVMs in children,[2,4,15,16,25,32–35] and the prognosis for surgically treated AVMs in children has been superior to conservative outcomes for well over a decade.[15,18]

Prior to surgical intervention, the risk of expectant management must be weighed against the risk of surgery. We use the five-grade system of Spetzler and Martin[36–38] to predict the risk of surgical intervention. This five-grade system assigns points to the size (1 for <3 cm, 2 for 3–6 cm, 3 for >6 cm), the pattern of venous drainage (0 for superficial, 1 for deep), and the eloquence of surrounding brain (0 for noneloquent, 1 for eloquent). The sum of the points determines the grade from I to V. Prospective evaluation of this grading system in patients undergoing complete resection of their AVMs with or without preoperative embolization suggest a morbidity approaching 20% for grade IV or V lesions. Although these numbers may be lower when considering children (Spetzler, personal communication), they need to be weighed against the natural history of the disease. Surgery is usually recommended for grade I and II lesions, whereas grade III lesions are dealt with case by case, with most undergoing surgery in the pediatric population. Surgery on grade IV and V lesions is still reserved for those patients with significant or repetitive hemorrhage or progressive neurological instability.[37]

The timing of surgical intervention will depend primarily upon the presentation and clinical status of the child. Immediate surgery is indicated for patients with intracerebral hemorrhage and associated progressive neurological deficit or brain stem compression. In such a life-threatening event, it is often infeasible to obtain an angiogram prior to surgery, and preoperative diagnostic evaluation is limited to CT with and without contrast. The primary goal of surgery becomes decompression of the hematoma and hemostasis. Attempt at AVM resection is sometimes considered if the AVM appears small and the child's clinical condition has stabilized. However, most surgeons will delay AVM resection for 2 to 4 weeks after a hemorrhage or until the patient's condition is optimized. This will allow for complete investigation and stabilization of the patient prior to pursuit of complete surgical obliteration.

Contemporary management strategies for AVMs must include consideration of embolization. Improved control of intraoperative bleeding after embolization has translated into safer surgeries with improved hemostasis.[39] This notion takes on even greater importance when considering the pediatric population. Most embolization is performed preoperatively, although intraoperative embolization has been used when the nidus is diffuse or the target vessels are difficult to approach via endovascular techniques. Although preoperative embolization should be strongly considered in all pediatric AVMs, embolization of small superficial AVMs should be avoided. The risk of surgery alone in these AVMs is minor compared with morbidity and mortality from embolization of up to 10% and 6%, respectively.[40] As an isolated treatment, embolization of AVMs achieves a cure rate of only ~5%,[41] and incomplete embolization is not considered protective against hemorrhage.[17,42] Thus embolization of AVMs is generally reserved as an adjunct and may be performed as a single or staged procedure. Multiple-staged procedures with cure as the end point are reserved for large AVMs with considerable arteriovenous shunting where the risk of normal perfusion pressure breakthrough bleeding is considered to be high. The exception is children with high-grade, diffuse AVMs regarded as inoperable, in whom embolization has been used alone with limited success.[40]

Radiosurgery alone or in combination with other treatment modalities has become an important tool in managing AVMs. The precise role for radiosurgery in the pediatric population, however, is unclear. The long-term effect of radiosurgery in the pediatric population remains incompletely defined, although in selected children radiosurgery has been used successfully to manage AVMs.[43] The major determinants of successful radiosurgical obliteration are the size of the lesion and the dose delivered. However, complications of radiosurgery are also a function of the size of the lesion and the dose delivered.[43] Although there is limited experience with childhood AVMs, complete obliteration in children has been reported in 80% of AVMs less than 3 mL and 59% of larger lesions.[43] A major concern is the latency between radiosurgical treatment and obliteration during which no protection is gained from hemorrhage.[6]

■ Surgical Considerations and Techniques

The operative goal for AVMs is complete excision, with preservation of the normal circulation and surrounding parenchyma. Greatly aiding in the pursuit of this goal is the continued advancement of microsurgical instrumentation and techniques and the judicious use of magnified vision. Contemporary microscopes offer optimal illumination and magnification and have greatly improved the safety and feasibility of resection of deep and small lesions.

Also greatly aiding in the success of surgical resection of AVMs are advances in neuroanesthesia. The optimal care of the pediatric neurosurgical patient should involve an anesthesiology team specializing in neuroanesthesia and knowledgeable in the unique needs of the pediatric patient. Invasive arterial blood pressure monitoring, central venous access, and electroencephalography (EEG) are routinely used during pediatric craniotomies for AVM. These measures are invaluable in the event of significant blood loss, prolonged surgeries, and induced blood pressure augmentation. This invasive monitoring also facilitates the use of barbiturate EEG burst suppression, which is felt to be cerebroprotective.[44] Recently, propofol burst suppression has been used successfully for EEG burst suppression with the advantage of a short half-life. It must be noted that propofol is generally not recommended below the age of 3 years and little literature is available on its use in this setting. The use of mild intraoperative hypothermia is also regularly used because this may afford additional cerebroprotection.[45]

Preparation for the craniotomy in the pediatric patient should include the same standard technical considerations as in the adult. The choice of head immobilization will depend on the age of the child. In children older than 6 years of age, standard three-pin fixation is used. In those younger than 6 years, pediatric head pins are used and only 40 pounds of pressure per pin are applied. Under the age of 2 years, craniotomy should be performed on a well-padded head holder without the use of pins. A radiolucent head frame should be used if intraoperative angiography is anticipated.

Planning the craniotomy is often assisted by frameless stereotaxy, and the bony and dural opening should be thoughtful of meningeal vascular contributions to the AVM. The exposed AVM at the surface of the brain should be inspected. Circumferential dissection should

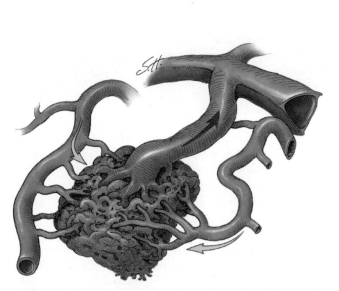

FIGURE 9–1 Arteriovenous malformation schematic depicting feeders *en passant* on the left of the malformation and a direct feeder on the right (see Color Plate 9–1).

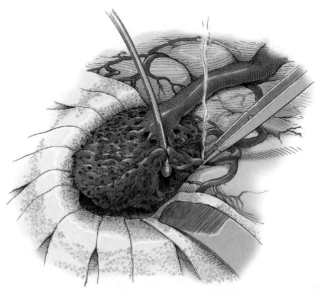

FIGURE 9–2 A malleable suction is used to retract the arteriovenous malformation to expose individual feeders, which are then coagulated with a bipolar cautery and subsequently cut. Circumferential dissection is performed, leaving the draining vein intact until the end of the resection (see Color Plate 9–2).

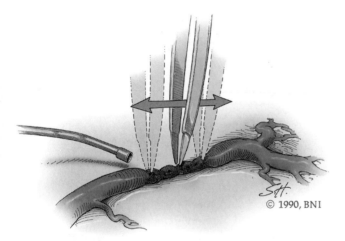

© 1990, BNI

FIGURE 9–3 Bipolar forceps are used to coagulate the feeding vessel back and forth to ensure total coagulation of the vessel prior to cutting (see Color Plate 9–3).

be pursued with careful identification of the plane between normal parenchyma and the AVM. The presence of a hematoma may assist the dissection because they often track along the margin of the AVM. Prior to sacrifice of any arterial feeder, its dedication to the malformation should be certain. One or two of the major draining veins should be maintained during the resection. After the AVM has been otherwise devascularized, the remaining venous drainage and the nidus can be removed. The angiographic anatomy should be correlated to the intraoperative findings throughout the procedure.

The AVM is often friable, and bleeding may be encountered with even minor manipulations. The pursuit of meticulous hemostasis is achieved with a combination

of electrocautery, topical hemostatic agents, and gentle tamponade. Irrigating or Teflon-coated bipolar cautery is crucial because it minimizes adherence to the vessels (**Figs. 9–1, 9–2,** and **9–3**).

Once the lesion is felt to be completely excised and hemostasis achieved, a brief trial of induced hypertension can be considered, along with direct inspection of the resection bed. In the event of focal bleeding, residual AVM should be suspected and careful scrutiny of the region should be performed. At closure, the blood pressure is normalized and strict avoidance of hypertension should be prioritized.

■ Complications

Intraoperative

The most common intraoperative complication during AVM resection is hemorrhage. In the pediatric population, blood loss greater than 25% of the blood volume can result in shock. This translates into ~20 mL/kg of blood loss, or only 200 mL in the average 1-year-old and 340 mL in the average 5-year-old. Although tachycardia will usually accompany the early blood loss, the compensatory mechanisms in children begin to fail after 35 to 45% blood loss.[46] Frequent interactions between the anesthesiologist and surgeon are paramount to the successful surgery on pediatric AVMs. Avoiding significant blood loss begins with hemostasis during the craniotomy and dural opening. Despite attention to the general principles of resection, bleeding may occur due to the often friable nature of the vessels. Wandering into the nidus during the resection may lead to hemorrhage, which is difficult to control. Also, premature sacrifice of veins can lead to engorgement of the nidus and may lead to intraoperative rupture. Preoperative embolization, strict attention to meticulous hemostasis, a carefully circumscribed dissection, and maintenance of the major venous outflow during the resection will all help to avoid significant blood loss.

> **PEARL**   Attention to hemostasis is paramount. As little as 200 mL of blood loss in the average 1-year-old may lead to shock.

Parenchymal injury during the surgery may occur as a result of sacrifice of *en passage* vessels, brain retraction, hemorrhage, and unnecessary cortical resection. Careful study of the preoperative angiogram with correlation to the intraoperative findings will aid in the identification of *en passage* vessels that supply normal brain and should be preserved. Thoughtful attention to the anatomy coupled with technical precision will help to minimize inadvertent brain injury. Similarly, avoiding incomplete resection of AVMs relies on the surgical technique and correlation of the intraoperative findings with the radiological studies. In the case of intraoperative uncertainty or a complex nidus, intraoperative angiography should be considered. Additionally, frameless stereotaxis can substantially aid in the resection and may help to avoid leaving a remnant of AVM.

Postoperative

The most common and morbid postoperative complication is hemorrhage. The most concerning source is residual AVM, although insecure intraoperative hemostasis or perfusion pressure breakthrough coupled with postoperative hypertension is a potential contributor. Postoperative hemorrhage usually occurs during the first few hours after surgery. Angiography should be obtained in the setting of postoperative hematoma formation. Residual AVMs should be reexplored and resected, at which time frameless stereotaxis and intraoperative angiography should be considered.

Normal perfusion pressure breakthrough can occur after AVM resection when the blood flow that was directed through the AVM is redistributed into the adjacent normal cerebrovasculature. If the perfusion pressure is greater than the autoregulatory capacity of the surrounding brain, swelling or hemorrhage may occur.[47] This rare complication may be avoided by staged embolization or staged resection of large AVMs.

> **PEARL**   Serious consideration should be given to preoperative embolization to prevent intraoperative hemorrhage as well as diminish the chance of postoperative normal perfusion pressure breakthrough bleeding.

Seizures may occur in the early postoperative period, although immediate postoperative epilepsy is rare. The incidence of new-onset seizures after AVM resection is ~15%, and long-term epilepsy occurs in 7%.[48] A therapeutic level of anticonvulsant should be maintained perioperatively. In the event of a postoperative seizure, a search for a structural lesion should be pursued, such as hematomas, edema, and infarction. Other potential postoperative complications include vasospasm and retrograde vascular occlusion with either venous or arterial thrombosis.

Avoidance of postoperative complications relies on intensive postoperative monitoring. All children should be observed in an intensive care setting with invasive arterial blood pressure monitoring and serial neurological examinations. The assistance of a pediatric intensivist and nurses familiar with caring for children should not be underestimated.

■ Outcome

Children now represent ~12 to 18% of surgical AVM series in experienced centers, and overall outcomes are improving.[16,49–51] The precise prognostic value of age remains unclear. Some authors have reported better outcomes in children than in adults,[49] whereas others have reported better outcomes in adults than in children.[18,24,28] Excellent or good outcomes can now be achieved in 95% of pediatric AVMs,[52] with complete angiographic obliteration achieved in over 90%.[52] In most pediatric series, severe complications are reported in ~10% and operative mortality is between 0 and 8%.[4,15,17,33,53]

Of the factors that influence surgical outcomes for AVM surgery, Spetzler and Martin grading[37] has been highly predictive.[36,48,54] The precise relationship between AVM grade and outcome in children is not known and in some studies the outcome has not correlated directly. Better than expected outcomes in children with grade IV AVMs was reported in a recent series by Di Rocco et al,[17] and some surgeons have successfully managed pediatric AVMs without emphasizing the Spetzler and Martin grading system.[33]

In the pediatric population, the neurological status may be one of the most predictive factors of outcome.[17] However, the gravity of a child's clinical condition must be weighed carefully because pediatric patients are capable of better outcomes than might be expected in the adult population.[15–17,53] In a series of 20 deeply comatose children with an acutely ruptured AVM, Meyer et al[55] achieved 60% survival with a good functional outcome in the survivors.

> **PEARL** The gravity of a child's clinical condition must be weighed carefully because pediatric patients are capable of better outcomes than might be expected in the adult population.

Nearly 50% of patients with preoperative seizures are eventually seizure-free and off anticonvulsants after AVM resection.[48] Similarly, in patients who present with epilepsy, significant improvement in seizure control is achieved in as many as 86% of patients postoperatively.[56] Correlations have been made between patient age at seizure onset and postoperative seizure control, as well as between the duration of the seizure disorder and the control rate. In one study, younger patients (<30 years old) presenting with epilepsy who underwent early surgery (<1 year of epilepsy) had the greatest chance of seizure control.[57]

Defining AVM obliteration is ideally done with angiography; however, MRI has been used in the pediatric population.[43] Although MRI is less expensive, noninvasive, and associated with minimal risk, angiography remains the only modality that can confirm cure, and the risk of neurological complications is minuscule in patients less than 50 years of age.[58] Serial radiological examination of children after AVM resection is mandated. Even though postoperative recurrence of an AVM is rare, children may be at the highest risk. Delayed regrowth after apparent complete surgical removal has been reported.[50,59] In their series of 808 patients with

complete excision confirmed by early postoperative angiography, Kader et al[50] reported five patients with recurrence. Because all of these cases of recurrence were in children under 15 years of age, late postoperative angiography should be considered in all children.

Although aggressive surgical therapy is often advocated, a combined surgical, radiosurgical, and endovascular approach to managing pediatric AVMs is likely to improve outcome.[52] Each patient must be considered individually and the merits of the interventional tools carefully measured. The combination of endovascular treatment and surgery has resulted in excellent cure rates,[60] and embolization should be used liberally when low morbidity and mortality can be achieved. Radiosurgery should be considered in unruptured, small AVMs that are deep seated, and also in small residual AVMs. In spite of substantial recent advances in microsurgery, radiosurgery, and interventional neuroradiology, limited options for therapy still exist for ~10% of cases.[33] The prognosis for children who cannot undergo treatment remains grim.[14,17]

■ Illustrative Cases

Case 1

A 15-year-old female presented obtunded with a left hemiparesis. Initial CT revealed a right thalamic hemorrhage with intraventricular extension (**Fig. 9–4A**). Ventriculostomy was placed with poor control of intracranial pressure. Angiography performed later that day revealed a Spetzler-Martin grade III AVM (**Figs. 9–4B–D**). She was brought to the operating room for right frontal

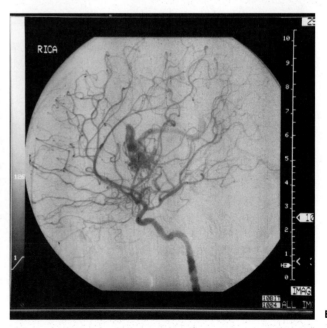

A

B

FIGURE 9–4 (A) (B) Case 1 of 15-year-old female who presented obtunded with a left hemiparesis. (**A**) Initial CT scan showing right thalamic hemorrhage with intraventricular extension. (**B,C,D**) Initial angiograms revealing Spetzler–Martin grade III arteriovenous malformation.

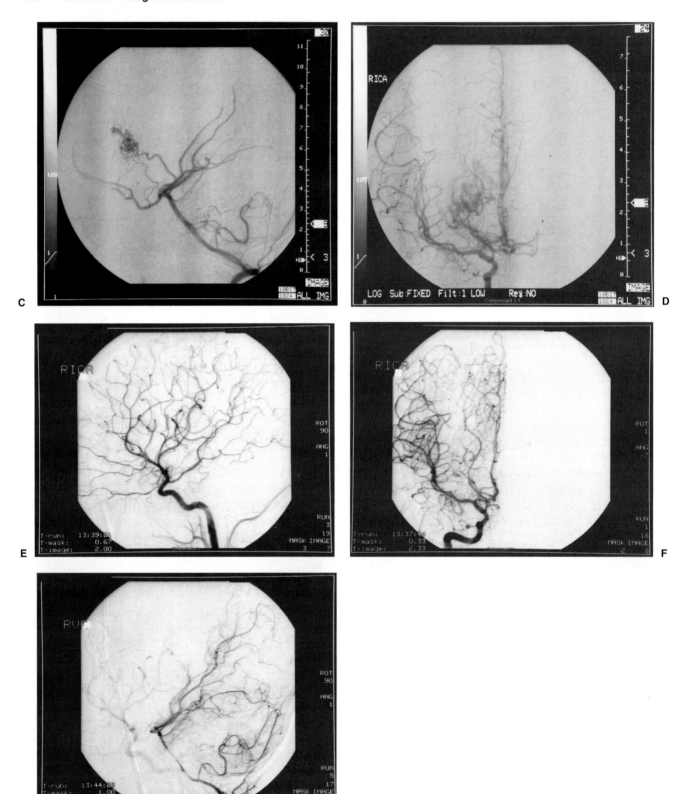

FIGURE 9–4 (*Continued*) (E,F,G) Postoperative angiograms.

craniotomy, evacuation of hematoma, and excision of the AVM (**Figs. 9–4E–G**). Postoperatively her hemiparesis was unchanged. Over the course of 2 to 3 days, she became alert and awake and at 3-month follow-up, she was ambulating with a walker, her hemiparesis moderately improved.

Case 2

An 11-year-old male presented with sudden-onset headache and obtundation. Initial CT revealed hydrocephalus and right cerebellar hemorrhage (**Fig. 9–5A**). A ventriculostomy was placed and within 1 to 2 hours, the patient became alert and awake without deficit. Angiography performed the following morning revealed a Spetzler-Martin grade III AVM of the right cerebellar hemisphere (**Fig. 9–5B–D**). He underwent posterior fossa craniotomy later that morning to evacuate the hemorrhage and resect the AVM (**Fig. 9–5E,F**). He made an excellent recovery and was discharged in normal neurological condition 5 days later.

Case 3

A 17-year-old female presented after sudden collapse following a 2-day history of headache. On initial exam, her

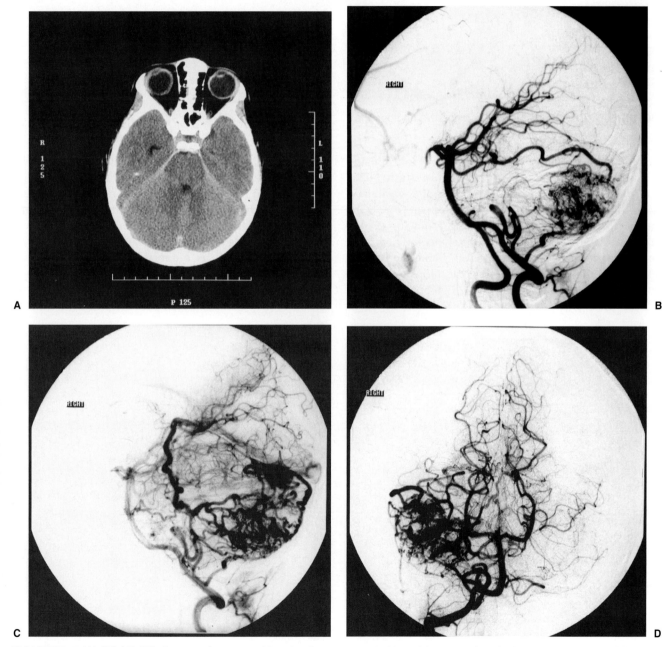

FIGURE 9–5 (A) (B) (C) (D) Case 2 of 11-year-old male who presented with sudden-onset headache and obtundation. (**A**) Initial CT scan. (**B,C,D**) Initial angiograms showing Spetzler–Martin grade III arteriovenous malformation.

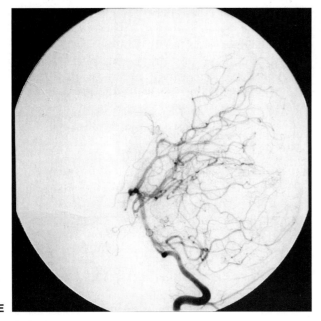

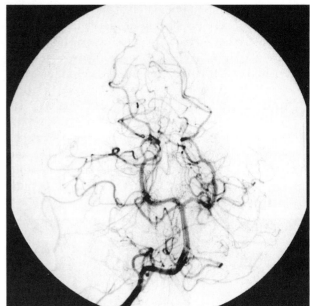

E

F

FIGURE 9–5 (*Continued*) (E, F) Postoperative angiograms.

Glasgow coma scale was 3. Her pupils were 3 to 4 mm and nonreactive and she displayed decerebrate posturing bilaterally. CT scan revealed extensive posterior fossa hemorrhage (**Fig. 9–6A**). A ventriculostomy was placed and she was brought directly to the operating room for decompression. After craniotomy and dural opening, a large amount of bleeding was encountered. The bone flap was left out and the hematoma rapidly reaccumulated. Immediate cerebral angiography revealed a Spetzler-Martin grade II AVM (**Fig. 9–6B–D**). On repeat examination, she displayed nonspecific flexion in her right upper extremity. She was taken directly back to the operating room where the AVM was excised (**Fig. 9–6E,F**) and the hematoma evacuated (**Fig. 9–6G**). The patient made a slow recovery over the following 3 to 6 months and required ventriculoperitoneal as well as a fourth ventricular shunt. At 9-month follow-up, she was cognitively normal, preparing to take her college entrance exams. She was ambulatory

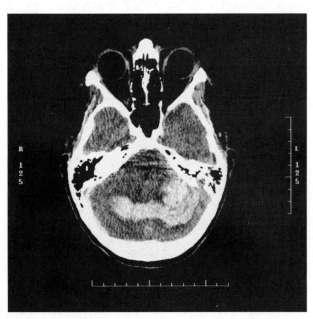

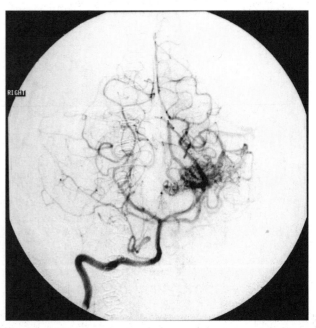

A

B

FIGURE 9–6 (A) (B) Case 3 of a 17-year-old female who presented after a sudden collapse following a 2-day headache. **(A)** Initial CT scan. **(B,C,D)** Cerebral angiography revealing Spetzler–Martin grade II arteriovenous malformation.

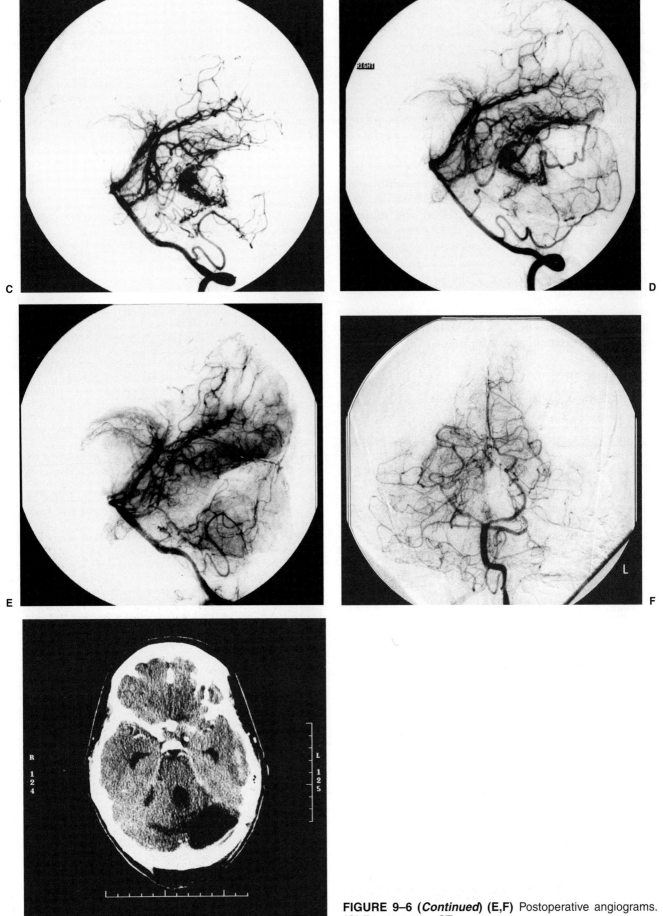

FIGURE 9–6 (*Continued*) (E,F) Postoperative angiograms. **(G)** Postoperative CT scan.

with crutches but displayed moderately severe ataxia of gait and dysmetria of her left upper extremity.

■ Conclusions

The natural history of AVMs in the pediatric population combined with long life expectancy justifies special consideration. AVMs have a malignant natural history, and surgical excision offers excellent protection from hemorrhage and the opportunity for cure. Additionally, postoperative seizure control is achieved in most patients. The overall rates of morbidity and mortality from surgery for AVMs in children have improved with refinements in microsurgical technique, and surgery should be considered the optimal therapy for AVMs in children. The ultimate goal is the normal life of the child. Each child and each lesion must be carefully evaluated. Contemporary management strategies can optimize the outcome by considering the roles of surgery, embolization, and radiosurgery.

REFERENCES

1. Forster DMC, Steiner L, Hakanson S. Arteriovenous malformations of the brain: a long-term clinical study. J Neurosurg 1972;37:562–570
2. Millar C, Bissonnette B, Humphreys RP. Cerebral arteriovenous malformations in children. Can J Anaesth 1994;41:321–331
3. Partington MD, Davis DH, Kelly PJ. Stereotactic resection of pediatric vascular malformations. Pediatr Neurosci 1989;15:217–222
4. Garza-Mercado R, Cavazos E, Tamez-Montes D. Cerebral arteriovenous malformations in children and adolescents. Surg Neurol 1987;27:131–140
5. Schoenberg BS, Mellinger JF, Schoenberg DG. Cerebrovascular disease in infants and children: a study of the incidence, clinical features, and survival. Neurology 1978;28:763–768
6. Aberfeld DC, Rao KR. Familial arteriovenous malformation of the brain. Neurology 1981;31:184–186
7. Roman G, Fisher M, Perl DP. Neurological manifestations of hereditary hemorrhagic telangiectasia (Rendu-Osler-Weber disease): report of 2 cases and review of the literature. Ann Neurol 1978;4:130–144
8. Willinsky RA, Lasjaunias P, Terbrugge K, Burrows P. Multiple cerebral arteriovenous malformations (AVMs): review of our experience from 203 patients with cerebral vascular lesions. Neuroradiology 1990;32:207–210
9. Wyburn-Mason R. Arteriovenous aneurysms of midbrain and retina, facial naevi and mental changes. Brain 1943;66:12–203
10. Hofmeister C, Stapf C, Hartmann A, et al. Demographic, morphological, and clinical characteristics of 1289 patients with brain arteriovenous malformation. Stroke 2000;31:1307–1310
11. Jomin M, Lesoin F, Lozes G. Prognosis for arteriovenous malformations of the brain in adults based on 150 cases. Surg Neurol 1985;23:362–366
12. Yasargil MG. AVM of the Brain, Clinical Considerations, General and Special Operative Techniques, Surgical Results, Nonoperated Cases, Cavernous and Venous Angiomas, Neuroanesthesia. New York: Thieme; 1988. Microneurosurgery; vol IIIB
13. Graf CJ, Perret GE, Torner JC. Bleeding from cerebral arteriovenous malformations as part of their natural history. J Neurosurg 1983;58:331–337
14. Itoyama Y, Uemura S, Ushio Y, et al. Natural course of unoperated intracranial arteriovenous malformations: study of 50 cases. J Neurosurg 1989;71:805–809
15. Humphreys RP, Hendrick BE, Hoffman HJ. Arteriovenous malformations of the brainstem in childhood. Childs Brain 1984;11:1–11
16. Celli P, Ferrante L, Palma L, Cavedon G. Cerebral arteriovenous malformations in children: clinical features and outcome of treatment in children and in adults. Surg Neurol 1984;22:43–49
17. Di Rocco C, Tamburrini G, Rollo M. Cerebral arteriovenous malformations in children. Acta Neurochir (Wien) 2000;142:145–158
18. Gerosa MA, Capelloto P, Licata C. Cerebral arteriovenous malformations in children (56 cases). Childs Brain 1981;8:356–371
19. Martin NA, Edwards MSB. Supratentorial arteriovenous malformations. In: Edwards MSB, Hoffman HJ, eds. Cerebral Vascular Disease in Children and Adolescents. Baltimore: Williams and Wilkins; 1989:283–308
20. Brown RD Jr, Wiebers DO, Forbes G. The natural history of unruptured intracranial arteriovenous malformations. J Neurosurg 1988;68:352–357
21. Samson DS, Batjer HH. Preoperative evaluation of the risk/benefit ratio for arteriovenous malformations of the brain. In: Wilkins RH, Rangachary SS, eds. Neurosurgery Update II. New York: McGraw-Hill; 1991:119–125
22. Fults D, Kelly DL Jr. Natural history of arteriovenous malformations of the brain: a clinical study. Neurosurgery 1984;15:658–662
23. Heros RC, Tu YK. Is surgery therapy needed for unruptured arteriovenous malformations? Neurology 1987;37:279–286
24. Sheikh BY, Hassounah M, Al-Moutare K, Ammar A, Enazi A. Childhood intracranial arteriovenous malformations in Saudi Arabia. Childs Nerv Syst 1999;15:262–266
25. So SC. Cerebral arteriovenous malformations in children. Childs Brain 1978;4:242–250
26. Ondra SL, Troupp H, George ED. The natural history of symptomatic arteriovenous malformations of the brain: a 24-year followup assessment. J Neurosurg 1990;73:387–391
27. Kondziolka D, Humphreys RP, Hoffman HJ, Hendrick BE, Drake JM. Arteriovenous malformations of the brain in children: a forty-year experience. Can J Neurol Sci 1992;19:40–45
28. Mori K, Murata T, Hashimoto N. Clinical analysis of arteriovenous malformations in children. Childs Brain 1980;6:13–25
29. Spetzler RF, Hargraves RW, McCormick PW, Zambramski JM, Flom RA, Zimmerman RS. Relationship of perfusion pressure and size to risk of hemorrhage form arteriovenous malformations. J Neurosurg 1992;76:918–923
30. Miyasaka Y, Yada K, Ohwada T, Kitahara T, Kurata A, Irikura K. An analysis of the venous drainage system as a factor in hemorrhage from arteriovenous malformations. J Neurosurg 1992;76:239–243
31. Yeh HS, Kashiwagi S, Tew JM Jr, Berger TS. Surgical management of epilepsy associated with cerebral arteriovenous malformations. J Neurosurg 1990;72:216–223
32. Caldarelli M, Di Rocco C, Iannelli A, Rollo M, Tamburrini G, Velardi F. Combined management of intracranial vascular malformations in children. J Neurosurg Sci 1997;41:315–324
33. Humphreys RP, Hoffman H, Drake M, Rutka J. Choices in the 1990s for the management of pediatric cerebral arteriovenous malformations. Pediatr Neurosurg 1996;25:277–285
34. Malik GM, Sadasivan B, Knighton RS, Ausman JI. The management of arteriovenous malformations in children. Childs Nerv Syst 1991;7:43–47
35. Ventureyra EC, Herder S. Arteriovenous malformations of the brain in children. Childs Nerv Syst 1987;3:12–18
36. Hamilton MG, Spetzler RF. The prospective application of a grading system for arteriovenous malformations. Neurosurgery 1994;34:2–7
37. Spetzler RF, Martin NA. A proposed grading system of arteriovenous malformations. J Neurosurg 1986;65:476–483

38. Spetzler RF, Martin NA, Carter LP, et al. Surgical management of large AVMs by staged embolization and operative excision. J Neurosurg 1987;67:17–28

39. Marciano FF, Vishteh AG, Apostolides PJ, Spetzler RF. Arteriovenous malformations—supratentorial. In: Kay AH, Black PMcL, eds. Operative Neurosurgery. London: Churchill Livingstone; 2000: 1070–1091

40. Wikholm G, Lundqvist C, Svendsen P. Embolization of cerebral arteriovenous malformations, I: Technique, morphology and complications. Neurosurgery 1996;39:448–459

41. Frizzel RT, Fisher WS III. Cure, morbidity and mortality associated with embolization of brain arteriovenous malformations: a review of 1246 patients in 32 series over a 35-year period. Neurosurgery 1995;37:1031–1040

42. Guo WY, Karlsson B, Ericson K, Lindqvist M. Even the smallest remnant of an AVM constitutes a risk for further bleeding. Acta Neurochir (Wien) 1993;121:212–215

43. Levy EI, Niranjan A, Thompson TP, et al. Radiosurgery for childhood arteriovenous malformations. Neurosurgery 2000;47:834–842

44. Nehls DG, Todd MM, Spetzler RF, Drummond JC, Thompson RA, Johnson PC. A comparison of the cerebral protective effects of isoflurane and barbiturates during temporary focal ischemia in primates. Anesthesiology 1987;66:453–464

45. Spetzler RF, Hadley MN, Rigamonti D, et al. Aneurysms of the basilar artery treated with circulatory arrest, hypothermia, and barbiturate cerebral protection. J Neurosurg 1988;68:868–879

46. Ramenofsky ML. Infants and children as accident victims and their emergency management. In: O'Neill JA Jr, Rowe MI, Grosfeld JL, Fonkalsrud EW, Coran AG, eds. Pediatric Surgery. 5th ed. St. Louis: Mosby; 1998:235–243

47. Spetzler RF, Wilson CB, Weinstein P, Mehdorn M, Townsend J, Telles D. Normal perfusion pressure breakthrough theory. Clin Neurosurg 1978;25:651–672

48. Heros RC, Korosue K, Diebold PS. Surgical excision of cerebral arteriovenous malformations: late results. Neurosurgery 1990;26: 570–578

49. D'Aliberti G, Talamonti G, Versari PP, et al. Comparison of pediatric and adult cerebral arteriovenous malformations. J Neurosurg Sci 1997;41:331–336

50. Kader A, Goodrich JT, Sonstein WJ, Stein BM, Carmel PW, Michelsen WJ. Recurrent cerebral arteriovenous malformations after negative postoperative angiograms. J Neurosurg 1996;85: 14–18

51. Kahl W, Kessel G, Schwarz M, Voth D. Arteriovenous malformations in childhood: clinical presentation, results after operative treatment and long-term follow-up. Neurosurg Rev 1989;12:165–171

52. Hoh B, Ogilvy C, Butler W, Loeffler J, Putman C, Chapman P. Multimodality treatment of nongalenic arteriovenous malformations in pediatric patients. Neurosurgery 2000;47:346–358

53. Fong D, Chan S. Arteriovenous malformations in children. Childs Nerv Syst 1988;4:199–203

54. Steinberg GK, Chang SD, Levy RP, Marks MP, Frankel K, Marcellus M. Surgical resection of large incompletely treated intracranial arteriovenous malformations following stereotactic radiosurgery. J Neurosurg 1996;84:920–928

55. Meyer PG, Orliaguet GA, Zerah M, et al. Emergent management of deeply comatose children with acute rupture of cerebral arteriovenous malformations. Can J Anaesth 2000;47:758–766

56. Pellettieri L. Surgical versus conservative therapy of intracranial arteriovenous malformations: a study in surgical decision-making. Acta Neurochir (Wien) 1980;29:1–86

57. Yeh HS, Tew JM, Gartner M. Seizure control after surgery on cerebral arteriovenous malformations. J Neurosurg 1993;78:12–18

58. Heiserman JE, Dean BL, Hodak JA, et al. Neurologic complications of cerebral angiography. AJNR Am J Neuroradiol 1994; 15:1401–1407

59. Gabriel EM, Sampson JH, Wilkins RH. Recurrence of cerebral arteriovenous malformations after surgical excision: case report. J Neurosurg 1996;84:879–882

60. Westphal M, Cristante L, Grzyska U, et al. Treatment of cerebral arteriovenous malformations by neuroradiological intervention and surgical resection. Acta Neurochir (Wien) 1994;130:20–27

10

Surgical Treatment of Vein of Galen Malformations in Children

STEPHEN LAWRENCE HUHN, JEFF A. LEE, AND GARY K. STEINBERG

Vein of Galen malformations represent only a small percentage of intracranial vascular anomalies but have historically posed a significant surgical challenge. Aneurysmal dilatation of the vein of Galen predominantly occurs in the pediatric age range and accounts for ~1% of all cerebrovascular lesions.[1] In 1895 Steinheil described an arteriovenous malformation (AVM) involving the vein of Galen,[2] but the first report of attempted treatment was not until 1937 by Jaeger et al.[3] In 1947, Oscherwitz and Davidoff first attempted to treat a large calcified aneurysm located between the occipital lobes in a 27-year-old patient.[4] The surgical intervention consisted of little more than opening the aneurysm wall and packing it with Gelfoam for hemostasis. Remarkably, the patient's symptoms improved, but the case typifies the significant surgical challenge offered by these lesions not only in the past but in all surgical reports thereafter.

The combination of young age, systemic manifestations, complex vascular anatomy, and eloquent location makes vein of Galen malformations difficult to treat surgically. With the development of endovascular techniques, however, the poor prognosis associated with these lesions has changed considerably.[5] Primary surgical approaches are no longer advocated for most patients. However, improvements in microsurgical techniques, pediatric anesthesia, and better comprehension of the vascular anatomy suggest that surgery may be appropriate in select cases, particularly when used as an adjunct to endovascular therapy. This chapter reviews the history of surgical therapy for vein of Galen malformations and highlights the associated surgical indications, approaches, and outcomes.

■ Vascular Classification of Vein of Galen Malformations

Vein of Galen malformations are neither true aneurysms nor true AVMs. Dilatation of the vein of Galen is secondary to arteriovenous (AV) shunting of multiple fistulae with resultant "aneurysmal" expansion of the draining venous system. Unlike AVMs, which are located in the subpial space, vein of Galen malformations are located within the extracerebral subarachnoid space. A proper vein of Galen aneurysm or malformation consists of a central venous dilatation with AV fistulae contained within the wall of the dilated vein. Arterial participation tends to be bilateral and may involve both the anterior and posterior circulation.

The embryological origin of vein of Galen malformations is thought to be the median prosencephalic vein of Markowski.[6] This structure is the precursor to the vein of Galen and initially is responsible for venous drainage of the choroid plexus. The median prosencephalic vein of Markowski normally disappears by the eleventh week of embryonic development. The persistent arterial feeders associated with vein of Galen malformations correlate with the embryonic anatomy of the median prosencephalic vein, suggesting a developmental insult prior to 11 weeks of gestation. The persistence of the median prosencephalic vein accounts for the complex and often unrecognizable anatomy of the AV fistulae.

PEARL The median prosencephalic vein of Markowski is the embryological origin of the vein of Galen and is generally regarded as the true venous structure comprising the aneurysmal malformation.

Clinically, two separate angiographic classifications have been proposed for vein of Galen malformations. Garcia-Monaco, Lasjaunias, and Berenstein proposed a classification involving two subgroups depending on the location of the fistula.[7] "Mural" vein of Galen aneurysms have their predominant fistula located within the wall of the median prosencephalic vein and typically are supplied by collicular or posterior choroidal arteries. "Choroidal" vein of Galen aneurysms have fistulae located in the cistern of the velum interpositum, and the malformation is supplied by choroidal arteries, pericallosal arteries, and branches of the thalamoperforators.

Yasargil[8] used four subgroups to categorize vein of Galen malformations, also largely based on location of the fistula. Type I, the simplest malformation, is characterized by single or multiple pericallosal and posterior cerebral arteries feeding a cisternal fistula. Type II lesions involve communication with the thalamoperforators. Type III, a mixture of both type I and type II, is the subtype by which most malformations are classified. Type IV malformations are not considered "true" vein of Galen aneurysms but represent increased venous capacity in the vein of Galen from a true parenchymal AVM. In type IV malformations, there are no direct fistulae with the veinous wall.

Patient outcome is associated with the angiographic classification. If the Spetzler-Martin[9] grading system were applied to vein of Galen aneurysms, even the most straightforward lesion would receive a grade IV classification (two points for size, one point for deep venous drainage, and one point for eloquent location). Under this classification system, surgical morbidity rates for grade IV malformations may range from 20 to 30%.[8–10] Yasargil believed that types I, II, and III could be addressed with reasonable surgical risk in contrast to type IV, which carried significantly more neurological embarrassment.[10] Apart from the vascular complexity, other systemic factors can prohibit successful treatment. Unlike other AVMs of the central nervous system (CNS), vein of Galen lesions may exert considerable systemic cardiovascular manifestations. Cardiovascular compromise in combination with the patient's age can lead to a formidable surgical and anesthetic challenge.

■ Neuroradiological Evaluation

All of the standard neuroimaging techniques, including ultrasonography, computed tomography (CT), and magnetic resonance imaging (MRI), may be employed to evaluate vein of Galen malformations, including the less conventional fetal MRI. Transcranial ultrasonography may be used pre- and postnatally.[11–13] Vascular pulsations detected by ultrasonography may differentiate vein of Galen malformations from other possible midline structures. Color Doppler imaging helps to characterize blood flow within the malformation and can be used to delineate feeding and draining vessels.[14] CT usually reveals a round mass in the quadrigeminal cistern behind the posterior border of an anteriorly displaced third ventricle. Thrombosis of the vein of Galen aneurysm is suggested by high density within the lesion.[15] A contrast agent demonstrates dense homogeneous opacification of a vein of Galen malformation, adjacent tentorial vessels, and draining sinuses. If the malformation is thrombosed, contrast enhancement of the aneurysmal wall and opacification of small regions within the aneurysmal pouch are observed similar to a target sign.[16] Calcification of the malformation wall is seen in ~14% of patients but rarely before the age of 15.[17] MRI and magnetic resonance (MR) angiography are superior to CT because multiplanar imaging helps to characterize the position of large and medium-sized arterial and venous structures relative to the surrounding brain structures. MRI also identifies sinus abnormalities and venous drainage patterns that can facilitate therapeutic planning of transvenous or transtorcular endovascular approaches. Determining the most critical vessels to study angiographically is important in neonates where venous access may be difficult and total permissible intravenous contrast loads are limited.[18]

Cerebral angiography is the most important imaging modality for vein of Galen malformations and is necessary to plan definitive surgical or endovascular therapy. Angiography typically reveals an AV shunt with one of more feeding vessels draining into an enlarged vein of Galen complex. The arterial feeders originate from prosencephalic and mesencephalic vessels. Branches from the anterior cerebral, posterior pericallosal, and posterior lateral choroidal arteries represent the prosencephalic contribution. The mesencephalic group includes the posterior medial choroidal artery, the thalamoperforators, and the superior cerebellar artery. An arterioarterial complex is often interposed between the arterial feeders and the vein of Galen.[6] Hoffman recognized age-dependent patterns of angiographic findings that could be categorized into four groups and correlated with the dominant clinical presentation for that age.[19] In neonates the feeding vessels entered the malformation anteriorly and superiorly with moderate aneurysmal volume and enlarged dural sinuses. Infants were characterized by fewer feeding vessels that often entered inferiorly and laterally. The two remaining groups consisted of older infants and children. Older infants had posterior choroidal and anterior cerebral artery branches entering anteriorly and superiorly. More extensive angiomatous networks were observed in older children. In each group the angiographic pattern predicted the type of clinical presentation according to the degree of fistulous flow.

> **PEARL** Four-vessel cerebral angiography is the most important diagnostic modality for determining the need for definitive surgical and/or endovascular therapy.

The venous drainage consists of aneurysmal dilatation of the vein of Galen with subsequent flow into the straight, transverse, and sigmoid sinuses and eventually into the jugular sinus. Internal cerebral veins are visualized in 50% of cases and when present are seldom directly involved as part of the malformation. Drainage into an accessory falcine sinus, as well as thrombosis, stenosis, duplication, or absence of a straight sinus, also may be seen. Zeran et al observed that stenosis of the outflow tracts was commonly associated with ventricular enlargement and would produce congestion in alternative venous pathways.[20] Because the cavernous sinus is not fully patent until the age of 2 years, the high venous outflow is directed toward orbital, sphenoparietal, and middle cerebral veins, which further increases intracranial venous hypertension. The CNS morbidity related to ischemia and calcifications partially reflects the venous congestion and pressure, and the underdeveloped venous system makes the neonate particularly vulnerable to abnormal flow and pressures.

■ Clinical Presentation

Clinical presentation depends on age. In 1964, Gold and coworkers first observed the association between age and clinical presentation in patients with vein of Galen malformations.[21] Neonates and infants have a much higher incidence of fulminant congestive heart failure (CHF) than other age groups. As a child matures, compensated CHF, seizures, focal neurological deficits, macrocephaly/hydrocephalus, developmental delay, and hemorrhage (parenchymal and subarachnoid) become more common manifestations. The pathophysiology of the CHF and the mechanism of hydrocephalus represent the two relatively unique clinical conditions that can influence treatment options and timing.

> **PEARL** Optimal preoperative management of the CHF and ventriculomegaly associated with vein of Galen malformations requires understanding their unique pathophysiology.

Approximately 40% of patients with a vein of Galen aneurysm are diagnosed when they are neonates. The most common mode of presentation in this age group is CHF where the amount of vascular shunting may be greater than 25% of cardiac output.[22] Signs and symptoms of CHF include hypoxia, low cardiac output, tachycardia, and pulmonary edema. Chest radiography in these patients shows cardiomegaly and pulmonary congestion typical of neonatal CHF.

Although the AV shunt develops in utero, CHF typically develops only after the child is born because of the hemodynamic transition between the fetal and postnatal circulations. High-output cardiac failure has been reported in utero, but the low systemic vascular resistance in the fetal circulation typically dampens the systemic effects of blood flow through the vascular malformation.[23,24] In the fetal circulation, the placenta receives ~40% of the cardiac output and thereby decreases the absolute blood volume of the intracranial shunt.[19] Because the left and right cardiac ventricles function in parallel, any circulatory overload is shared during fetal circulation.

Upon birth, the circulation switches to the neonatal pattern wherein the ventricles support the entire circuit in series and the placental vascular bed is absent. The pulmonary capillary bed resistance changes, and cardiac output must increase to maintain systemic vascular flow. As a result pulmonary hypertension develops and maintains the ductus arteriosus, leading to further shunting from the right to the left chambers. Subsequently neonatal cyanosis develops.[25] The circulatory burden created by the low vascular resistance in the cranium maintains a fetal circulation pattern by preserving the open ductus arteriosus.[22]

The combination of high cardiac output necessary to compensate for the intracranial shunting, high subendocardial pressure, and increased diastolic flow to the malformation eventually reduce coronary artery perfusion. These factors ultimately combine to produce myocardial ischemia and infarction. In addition, the preferred flow through the malformation produces a "steal" phenomenon within the cerebrum. When coupled with increased venous pressure and cardiac dysfunction, the vascular steal leads to cerebral ischemia, leukomalacia, and diffuse microinfarction.[26] Of 16 patients with antenatal diagnoses, the death rate from acute heart failure and extensive brain damage was 25%.[13] Initial medical management of the heart failure is indicated, but full control of CHF is rarely possible without endovascular or surgical reduction of the intracranial fistula.

Macrocephaly and ventriculomegaly may occur in 50% of patients with a vein of Galen malformation. Typically seen in infants and children, the head enlargement has been attributed to obstructive hydrocephalus from occlusion of the aqueduct of Sylvius by the dilated vein of Galen in the setting of a distensible skull. However, both MRI studies and pathological series have shown that the aqueduct is patent in many of these patients.[20,27] Furthermore, common signs of increased intracranial pressure, including a tense fontanelle, nausea, vomiting, lethargy, and ocular deviation, are rare among these patients. Indeed, CT and MRI usually seldom reflect periventricular edema indicative of pathologically increased cerebrospinal fluid (CSF) pressure.

It is most likely that the increased ventricular volume and resultant macrocephaly are the result of altered CSF hydrodynamics from an increase in sagittal sinus pressure.[28,29] CSF absorption depends on the pressure gradient across the subarachnoid space and the sagittal sinus. Therefore, any increase in sinus pressures produced by the malformation would need to be matched by the CSF pathways. Ventricular enlargement occurs as a compensatory mechanism involved in increasing CSF pressure to maintain a gradient of 5 to 7 mm Hg.[30,31] Macrocephaly and ventriculomegaly reverse with endovascular obliteration of the fistula, supporting the theory that high venous sinus pressure is the main origin of hydrocephalus in these patients.[5,20] Thus ventriculoperitoneal shunts should be avoided in these patients in favor of surgical or intravascular obliteration of the AV shunting. Subsequently, reduction in venous hypertension is reduced and the ventriculomegaly normalizes.

■ Surgical Outcomes

Given the grim natural history of vein of Galen malformations, attempts at treatment are preferable to the outcome of untreated cases. The mortality rate of untreated malformations was well documented by Johnston et al[32] and Hoffman et al.[33] In a review of the literature, Johnston et al.[32] reported a mortality rate of 77.2% in 92 untreated patients. Hoffman and et al's report of 29 untreated cases, which were included as part of the series in Johnston's report,[32] had a mortality rate of 76.9%. Only 7.7% were described as normal.[33] In each series the highest mortality rate was in the neonatal subgroup. Left untreated, newborns with vein of Galen malformations have an almost uniformly poor outcome. The mortality rate was 96% in this particular age group.[29] Typically, younger age patients die from cardiovascular complications and older children from progressive cerebral vascular insults related to arterial steal and infarction. The poor outcome of untreated disease tends to place the risks of treatment, whether surgical, endovascular, or a combination thereof, into perspective for patients, families, and surgeons.

The obstacles to successful surgical treatment of vein of Galen malformations are considerable. Several factors make this lesion one of the most challenging problems a neurosurgeon can encounter. The location, size, and vascular complexity offer significant impediments to successful surgical treatment. Exposure of the arterial component of the malformation is often difficult because the lesion is often central and deep. The bilateral multiple feeders in surgically inaccessible positions also pose challenges. Potential vascular involvement of the thalamus and midbrain complicates isolation of the fistulae. In addition to the complexity posed by the vascular anatomy, a patient's cardiac integrity, age, and blood volume also contribute significantly to the surgical risk. These factors must be weighed before operative intervention is posed.

The history of the surgical treatment of vein of Galen malformations is at best cautionary and at worst justified attempts at endovascular solutions. Hoffman et al chronicled their experience with patients at the Hospital for Sick Children in Toronto between 1950 and 1980.[33] Twenty-nine patients were evaluated, and 14 of 16 neonates presented with heart failure. Altogether, 14 patients underwent a surgical attempt at obliteration of the malformation. The transcallosal route was used in 11 cases, followed by the subtemporal and transtentorial routes in the remaining patients. The overall surgical mortality rate was 57% and was highest (87%) in the neonatal subgroup. The authors cited myocardial infarction as the leading cause of death in the neonatal patients. In 1987 Johnston et al[32] reviewed the literature and collected the results of 126 surgical cases. Twenty-two patients were treated with a shunt insertion for hydrocephalus. The remaining 104 patients (which included the Toronto series reported by Hoffman et al[33]) had surgical procedures designed to address the vein of Galen malformation directly. The mortality rate for the patients undergoing shunt placement was 36.4% compared with 39.4% for patients undergoing direct procedures intended to obliterate the vein of Galen malformation. The mortality rate for neonates in the study by Johnston et al[32] was 78.9%. Similarly, Massey et al[34] reported a 66.6% mortality rate in neonates in 1982. Yasargil's series included five newborn patients and their death rate was 100%.[10] Five infants in the series from University of California–San Francisco treated by surgery before 1983 all died.[35] In each of these series, the mortality and morbidity rated decreased with age. The review by Johnston et al[32] cited a mortality rate between 15.4 and 36.8% in nonneonates and older children. In each series neonatal death was attributed to cardiovascular instability. Surgical morbidity rates in survivors was related to the poor myelination of the immature brain and ischemia from cerebral "steal" produced by the fistula.

> **PEARL** The overall mortality rate of surgery in most series is between 39 and 57% and increases to between 66 and 87% in the neonatal subgroup.

As a result of the poor outcomes associated with both untreated and surgically treated patients, the rationale for an alternative approach using endovascular techniques was developed. The results of endovascular treatments, including transarterial, transvenous, and transtorcular approaches, are superior to those from surgical series. However, the endovascular techniques carry a risk of significant complications. Freidman et al[36] reported a 0% mortality rate and a 45% morbidity rate in 11 patients using largely transarterial intervention. Lasjaunias et al documented an 8% mortality rate and 75% morbidity rate in 13 patients using transarterial embolizations.[5] Lylyk et al documented a 36% mortality rate and a 27% rate of postprocedure deterioration in survivors.[37] Ciricillo et al[35] reported a 25% mortality rate and a 50% morbidity rate in eight neonates treated with combined arterial and venous approaches.[35]

Only two authors have reported the merit of multimodal treatments involving the use of surgical obliteration combined with endovascular techniques. Wisoff et al reported a 31.4% mortality rate in a series of 35 patients managed by a multimodal strategy.[38] In 1993 Lylyk et al in 1993 also supported a multimodal approach to optimize outcomes, but only two cases (7% of the total series) underwent surgical treatment.[37] Indeed, the preference for endovascular strategies is evident by the predominance of endovascular reports over the past 15 years, compared with the last surgical series of patients published by Hoffman et al in 1982[33] and similarly by Johnston et al in 1987.[32]

■ Surgical Indications and Considerations

The indication for surgical treatment of vein of Galen malformation should include a careful review of the complexity of the vascular anatomy, location, size, and clinical status of the patient. The decision to operate should also be made in the setting of consultations from interventional endovascular neuroradiologists, pediatric intensive or neonatal critical care specialists, and pediatric anesthesiologists. The goals of therapy, regardless of approach, are to reverse neurological deterioration related to hydrocephalus or cerebrovascular sequelae and to reverse cardiac instability and CHF. The treatment strategy should consider several options, including direct surgical obliteration, management of symptomatic hydrocephalus, or a combination of the spectrum of endovascular and surgical techniques.

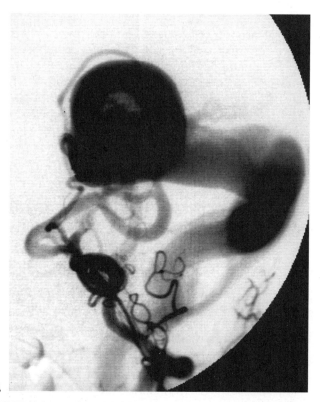

A

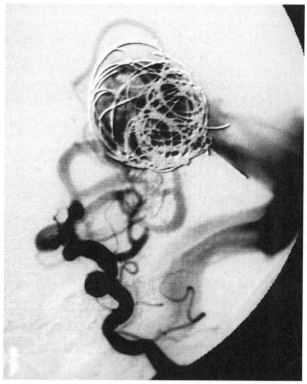

B

FIGURE 10–1 Complications of endovascular embolization techniques. Newborn with vein of Galen malformation. **(A)** Preembolization and **(B)** postembolization vertebrobasilar injection lateral angiograms. The postembolization study shows partial obliteration of the malformation.

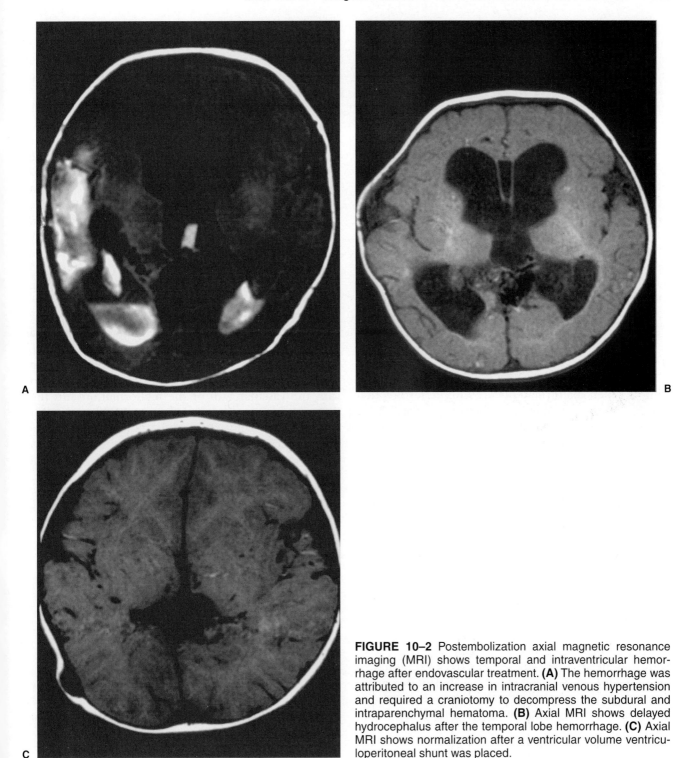

FIGURE 10–2 Postembolization axial magnetic resonance imaging (MRI) shows temporal and intraventricular hemorrhage after endovascular treatment. **(A)** The hemorrhage was attributed to an increase in intracranial venous hypertension and required a craniotomy to decompress the subdural and intraparenchymal hematoma. **(B)** Axial MRI shows delayed hydrocephalus after the temporal lobe hemorrhage. **(C)** Axial MRI shows normalization after a ventricular volume ventriculoperitoneal shunt was placed.

Because the integrity of the cardiovascular system can significantly influence outcome, the timing of definitive treatment is best undertaken after efforts to improve cardiopulmonary function.

In most cases endovascular obliteration of the malformation will be the first treatment option under consideration. Surgery may be indicated to treat vein of Galen malformations when endovascular methods are either unable to access the lesion or to effect a cure, or as an adjunct to endovascular treatment, particularly for neonatal patients suffering from CHF despite maximal medical and endovascular management.

The role for surgery alone, staged, or in combination with interventional techniques has not been well defined in the era of endovascular treatment failures or when only partial obliteration is possible. Because of the complexity or uncertainty of the vascular anatomy, direct surgical visualization and interruption may be necessary to preserve critical vessels for supplying parenchymal structures that might be threatened by unintended endovascular occlusion. Direct surgical clipping of large arterial feeders and of small arterial feeders inaccessible or unsafe for endovascular embolization may be feasible in medically optimized patients and become a necessity in the setting of refractory CHF. Other indications for surgery include evacuation of intraparenchymal, subdural, or subarachnoid hematomas associated with vein of Galen malformations or incomplete endovascular treatment, (**Figs. 10–1** and **10–2**).

■ Surgical Technique

Vein of Galen malformations are unique lesions that require careful consideration before proceeding to surgical intervention. The anatomy of the lesion itself and the patient's overall medical status must be understood. The poorly myelinated and delicate neonatal and infant brain is fragile and cannot withstand surgical manipulation as well as the brain of an older child. If CHF is present, every effort should be made to stabilize the patient's cardiovascular status and to delay surgery until cardiac function can be optimized. The risk of intraoperative blood loss is an important consideration when operating on children, particularly neonates and infants. The estimated total blood volume of children varies slightly with age and is ~90 mL/kg for neonates, 80 mL/kg for infants and children, and 65 to 78 mL/kg for adolescents.[39] Total blood volume also may be estimated as ~7 to 8% of body weight. An infant who weighs 10 kg would have a blood volume of only 800 mL. Typically, infants manifest a physiological nadir in total hemoglobin between 4 and 6 months of age as fetal hemoglobin

decreases and adult hemoglobin increases.[40] Surgical timing may be altered to avoid this period. Finally, any preoperative nutritional deficit should be addressed, particularly if CHF has resulted in unrecognized failure to thrive.

Surgically, vein of Galen malformations can be addressed by subtemporal, interhemispheric-transcallosal, occipital transtentorial, or supracerebellar-transtentorial approaches, either alone or in combination (**Fig. 10–3A–D**).[41] The approach should be planned to provide maximal exposure of the feeding vessels with minimal retraction. In the most likely scenario, surgery is be used as an adjunct to intravascular techniques, and surgical planning and exposure are affected by the postembolization vascular anatomy. A temporal craniotomy and subtemporal approach can be used to address vein of Galen malformations with feeders from the posterior choroidal arteries.

Care should be exerted to preserve the vein of Labbé during retraction of the temporal lobe. Bilateral posterior choroidal feeders may require staged bilateral subtemporal approaches. The choroidal vessels can be identified and traced directly to the connection with the vascular wall of the malformation and then ligated and interrupted. Supracerebellar-transtentorial approaches may be required to address arterial feeders located inferior and posterior to the malformation. Supracerebellar-infratentorial approaches have been used to treat large calcified aneurysms.[42] The use of these approaches or a combination thereof may be necessary, including the possibility of staged procedures.

> **PEARL**   Surgical access to the galenic region can include the subtemporal, interhemispheric-transcallosal, occipital-transtentorial, or supracerebellar-transtentorial approaches, either alone, staged, or in combination.

Staged obliteration of the arterial flow to vein of Galen malformations may offer several practical and theoretical advantages. Although arguments have been made against

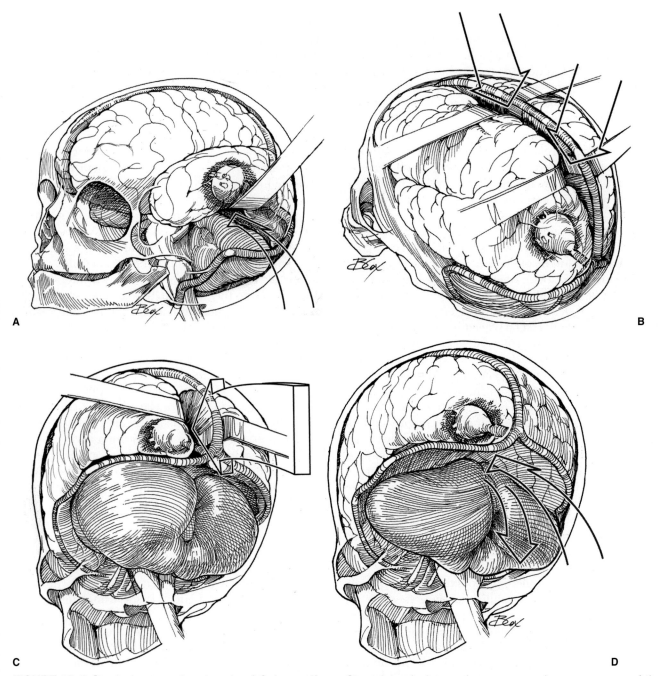

FIGURE 10–3 Surgical approaches to vein of Galen malformations: subtemporal (**A**), interhemispheric–transcallosal (**B**), occipital transtentorial (**C**), supracerebellar–transtentorial (**D**).

Staged surgical procedures may require one or more of the approaches shown to obliterate multiple and diverse fistulae.

staged treatment of vein of Galen malformations, the merits of less extensive surgery and gradual obliteration of large fistulae in the developing brain are worth considering.[43] Staged occlusion may allow the brain to adjust to the altered hemodynamics and protect against normal perfusion pressure breakthrough.[44–46] The theoretical risk should be considered in the treatment of any vascular malformation. After some vascular malformations have been obliterated, previously hypoperfused brain parenchyma may experience increased blood flow. Brain swelling, hemorrhage, and seizures can result. Staged treatment allows surgical ligation of arterial feeders not easily accessed by one particular exposure,[21] and enables a more gradual cardiac adjustment to the decreased output and increased afterload.

The approach most applicable to single-stage surgical obliteration and most often used is the posterior interhemispheric trajectory. Either a parietal or an occipital posterior interhemispheric approach can be used to gain access to the Galenic region and to expose the feeding arteries. The patient can be placed in the sitting, prone, or lateral position. The prone and lateral positions offer less risk of air embolus than the sitting position. When the modified park bench or lateral position is used, the head should be horizontal to the floor and the hemisphere of interest placed inferiorly. In this position, which is advocated by Hamilton et al,[47] the dependent hemisphere widens the interhemispheric space and provides the surgeon a more comfortable and natural working position. However, unusual head positions in neonates and infants are often problematic due to the risks associated with rigid pin fixation in the thin and the immature calvarium. In neonates and infants, straight positioning of the head in either the supine or prone positions, and proper padding of the face, is preferred to rigid fixation.

The craniotomy should be planned to provide ample access to the deep and midline arterial feeders. An approach similar to exposures for pineal region tumors involving an inferior paramedian opening usually is adequate to expose the thalamoperforating arteries common to Yasargil type II malformations. The anterior border of the craniotomy may need to be extended anteriorly to allow the feeders arising from the pericallosal arteries to be interrupted. Intracranial exposure of the contralateral structures can be obtained by sectioning the falx above the inferior sagittal sinus. However, deep branches of the posterior cerebral artery may require bilateral craniotomies to expose both sides of the interhemispheric fissure.

Unlike true AVMs and Yasargil type IV lesions, which have the nidus located in the brain parenchyma, true vein of Galen malformations occupy the subarachnoid spaces, theoretically enabling the surgeon to create broad exposure of the feeding vessels. Unfortunately, the size of the malformation often precludes easy dissection, and final exposure of the deep feeders usually cannot be accomplished until distention of the malformation is relieved by reducing blood flow through the aneurysm. The callosal, dorsal ambient, and quadrigeminal cisterns should be opened widely to provide the best exposure of the malformation and multiple fistulae. The posterior cerebral and superior cerebellar arteries within the lateral aspects of the ambient cistern are traced to the aneurysm. The junction of the artery with the aneurysm is then coagulated and divided. Surgical clips, including Sundt micro-AVM clips (Codman), Sundt mini-aneurysm clips, or small aneurysm clips may be used to ligate larger vessels. The anterior pericallosal artery feeders are likewise identified above the splenium, which is usually found anterior and superior to the vein of Galen malformation. As the major arterial feeders are obliterated, the vascular input to the malformation decreases as does the distension of the malformation. In turn, the residual anterior and inferior arterial feeders, often the most difficult to interrupt, are easier to expose.

Persistent turgor in the malformation may indicate unrecognized arterial feeders, usually from the less visible region anterior and inferior to the vein of Galen. With gentle technique, the vein of Galen may be retracted to allow identification of the deep feeders. Additional veins that may obstruct effective identification and manipulation of the residual feeders can be encountered at this part of the dissection. Yasargil believed that these veins could be interrupted without compromise because venous pressures and drainage were already significantly altered.[10] After pressure in the vein of Galen malformation is reduced following ligation of the arterial feeding vessels, the aneurysm can be reduced further by a large clip or series of clips. Resection of the aneurysm wall is unnecessary and can be dangerous. However, surgical resection may be indicated when mass effect persists from long-standing calcification.

Intraoperative angiography and direct intraoperative injection of acrylic glue also may be considered surgical adjuncts. However, intraoperative angiography is challenging in young patients and the quality of imaging is sometimes suboptimal. Direct operative intravascular injection may have an application in some vein of Galen malformations but requires intraoperative angiography to isolate the appropriate vessel for endovascular occlusion. Using either technique requires the participation of a highly experienced endovascular interventional neuroradiologist. Intraoperative surgical navigation using a frameless MR or CT angiographically guided tracking system may also be a useful surgical adjunct for localizing large feeding arteries. However, it is no substitute for a thorough preoperative understanding

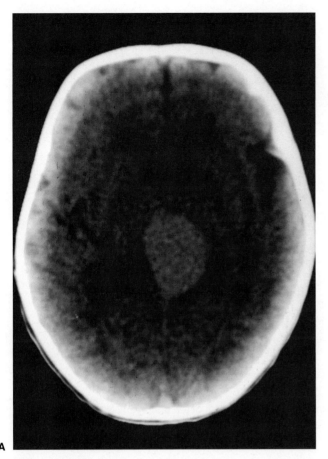 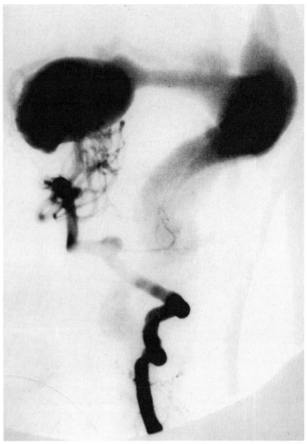

A   B

FIGURE 10–4 (A) Axial computed tomography and **(B)** vertebrobasilar lateral angiogram at initial presentation in newborn with vein of Galen malformation.

of the detailed anatomy involved with vein of Galen malformations.

■ Illustrative Case

A newborn female delivered at home via a midwife-assisted spontaneous vaginal route had Apgar scores of 8 and 9. The patient developed respiratory distress and signs of CHF at 10 days of life. A physical examination revealed a grade III/VI cardiac systolic murmur and a cranial bruit. CT and cerebral angiography demonstrated a vein of Galen aneurysm (**Fig. 10–4**). The CHF was treated successfully with digoxin, furosemide, and Aldactazide (Searle, Chicago, IL), and the infant was followed as an outpatient. At 11 months of age, MRI and angiography showed enlargement of the malformation and the onset of symptomatic hydrocephalus (**Fig. 10–5**). A ventriculoperitoneal shunt was placed. Her symptoms of CHF persisted. Transarterial balloon occlusion of a large posterior choroidal feeder was attempted but was unsuccessful

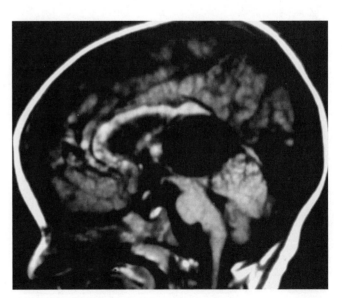

FIGURE 10–5 Sagittal magnetic resonance imaging shows enlargement of the malformation 11 months after the patient's initial presentation.

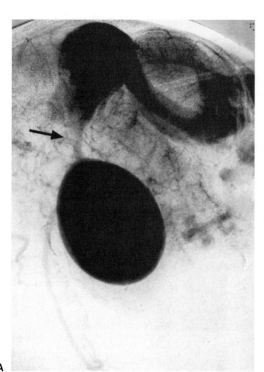
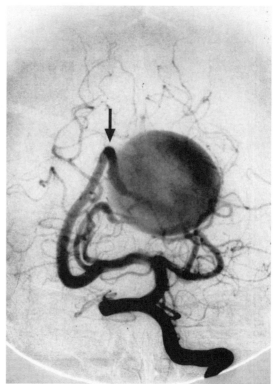

A

B

FIGURE 10–6 (A) Lateral and **(B)** vertebrobasilar angiograms demonstrate enlargement of the aneurysm. Note the stenosis of the straight sinus (arrow, **A**) and acute distal angle of the posterior choroidal feeder that prevented transarterial occlusion (arrow, **B**).

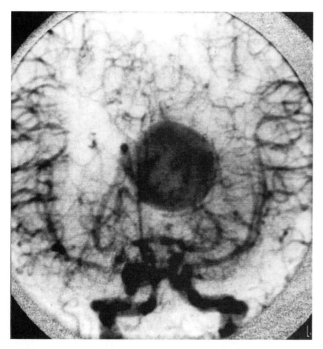

FIGURE 10–7 Anteroposterior view of intravenous digital subtraction angiogram obtained after the first craniotomy and clipping of right posterior cerebral artery feeders. The aneurysmal filling has slowed.

because a sharp turn in the distal part of the feeding vessel prevented further passage of the catheter (**Fig. 10–6**).

Three months after the unsuccessful endovascular procedures, the patient underwent a temporal craniotomy and a subtemporal approach. Four larger arterial feeders were clipped. This procedure reduced the AV shunt and her CHF resolved. She was discharged 1 week later off all cardiac medications. Postoperative angiography revealed slowed but persistent filling of the malformation (**Fig. 10–7**).

Six weeks after the first procedure the child returned to the operating room where a right parietal-occipital craniotomy and interhemispheric approach were utilized to occlude bilateral feeders. Her recovery was complicated by a frontal subdural hematoma that required evacuation 12 hours after surgery. Cerebral angiography performed on the sixth postoperative day revealed persistent filling but further degradation of blood flow. She was discharged neurologically intact on postoperative day 17.

Follow-up MRI and intravenous digital subtraction angiography 6 months after the second procedure showed complete obliteration of the vein of Galen malformation as well as thrombosis of the straight sinus. Intra-arterial digital angiography obtained 18 months later confirmed absence of blood flow through the malformation

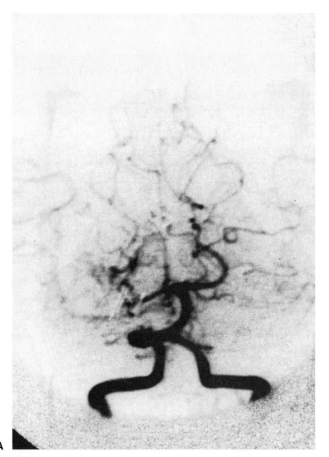
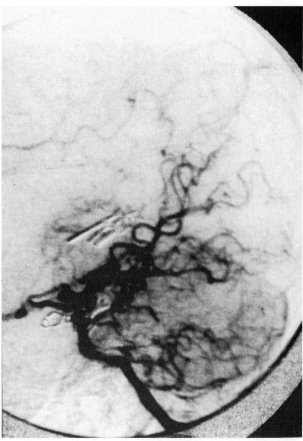

A   B

FIGURE 10–8 (A) Anteroposterior and **(B)** lateral vertebrobasilar angiograms obtained 18 months after the patient's second and final craniotomy showing complete thrombosis of the aneurysm.

(**Fig. 10–8**). At 6 years old the child remains free of neurological and cardiovascular dysfunction. Her physical and intellectual development are considered normal.[48]

■ Conclusions

Although endovascular treatment is the procedure of first choice, surgical management is appropriate in select cases, either as an adjunct to intravascular procedures or when endovascular techniques are infeasible. Understanding the cardiovascular effects of the vein of Galen malformation and management of the high output cardiac failure will reduce surgical risks. Staged and multimodal approaches should further decrease the mortality and morbidity rates associated with one of the most challenging neurosurgical disorders.

REFERENCES

1. Khayata M, Casasco A, Wakhloo A, Rekate H. Vein of Galen malformations: intravascular techniques. In: Carter LP, Spetzler RF, eds. Neurovascular Surgery. New York: McGraw-Hill; 1995: 1029–1039

2. Steinheil S. Ueber einen Fal von Varix Aneurysmaticus im bereit der Gehirngefoesse. Inaugural dissertation, Wurzburg, 1895. Cited by Dandy WE. Arteriovenous aneurysm of the brain. Arch Surg 1928;17:190–243; see 193, 240

3. Jaeger J, Forbes R, Dandy W. Bilateral congenital cerebral arteriovenous communication aneurysm. Trans Am Neurol Assoc 1937;63:173–176

4. Oscherwitz D, Davidoff L. Midline calcified intracranial aneurysm between occipital lobes: report of a case. J Neurosurg 1947;4: 539–541

5. Lasjaunias P, Garcia-Monaco R, Rodesch G, Ter Brugge K, Zerah M, de Victor D. Vein of Galen malformation: endovascular management of 43 cases. Childs Nerv Syst 1991;7:360–367

6. Raybaud C, Strother C, Hald J. Aneurysms of the vein of Galen: embryonic and anatomical features relating to the pathogenesis of the malformation. Neuroradiology 1989;31:109–128

7. Garcia-Monaco R, Lasjaunias P, Berenstein A. Therapeutic management of vein of Galen aneurysmal malformations. In: Vinuela F, Halbach VV, Dion JE, eds. Interventional Neuroradiology: Endovascular Therapy of the Central Nervous System. New York: Raven; 1992:113–127

8. Yasargil M. AVM of the Brain, Clinical Considerations, General and Special Operative Techniques, Surgical Results, Nonoperated Cases, Cavernous and Venous Angiomas, Neuroanesthesia. New York: Thieme; 1988. Microneurosurgery; vol IIIB

9. Spetzler RF, Martin NA. A proposed grading system for arteriovenous malformations. J Neurosurg 1986;64:476–483

10. Hamilton M, Spetzler R. The prospective application of a grading system for arteriovenous malfomations. Neurosurgery 1994;34:2–7

11. Jeanty P, Kepple D, Roussis P, Shah D. In utero detection of cardiac failure from an aneurysm of the vein of galen. Am J Obstet Gynecol 1990;163:50–51

12. Mendelsohn D, Hertzana Y, Butterworth A. In utero diagnosis of vein of Galen aneurysm by ultrasound. Neuroradiology 1984;26: 417–418

13. Rodesch G, Hui F, Alvarez H, Tanaka A, Lasjaunias P. Prognosis of antenatally diagnosed vein of galen aneurysmal malformations. Childs Nerv Syst 1994;10:79–83

14. Deeg K, Scarf J. Colour Doppler imaging of arteriovenous malformation of the vein of Galen in a newborn. Neuroradiology 1990;32: 60–63

15. Skirkhoda A, Whaley R, Boone S, Scatliff J, Schnapf D. Varied CT appearance of aneurysms of the vein of Galen in infancy. Neuroradiology 1981;21:265–270

16. Martelli A, Scotti G, Harwood-Nash D, Fitz C, Chuang S. Aneurysms of the vein of Galen in children: CT and angiographic correlations. Neuroradiology 1980;20:123–133

17. Chapman S, Hockley A. Calcification of an aneurysm of the vein of Galen. Pediatr Radiol 1989;19:541–542

18. Seidenwurm D, Berensteing A, Hyman A, Howalski H. Vein of Galen malformation: correlation of clinical presentation, arteriography and MR imaging. AJNR Am J Neuroradiol 1991;12: 347–354

19. Hoffman H. Malformations of the vein of Galen. In: Edwards MSB, Hoffman H, eds. Current Neurosurgical Practice: Cerebral Vascular Disease in Children and Adolescents. Baltimore: Williams and Wilkins; 1989:239–246

20. Zerah M, Garcia-Monaco R, Rodesch G, et al. Hydrodynamics in the vein of Galen malformations. Childs Nerv Syst 1992;8: 111–117

21. Gold A, Ransohoff J, Carter S. Vein of Galen malformations. Acta Neurol Scand 1964;40(Suppl 11):1–31

22. Cumming G. Circulation in neonates with intracranial arteriovenous fistula and cardiac failure. Am J Cardiol 1980;45:1019–1024

23. Hirsch J, Cyr D, Eberhardt H, Zunkel D. Ultrasonographic diagnosis of an aneurysm of the vein of Galen in utero by duplex scanning. J Ultrasound Med 1983;2:231–233

24. Johnson W, Berry J, Einzig S, Bass J. Doppler findings in nonimmune hydrops fetalis and cerebral arteriovenous malformation. Am Heart J 1988;115:1138–1140

25. Crawford J, Rossitch E, Oakes W, Alexander E. Arteriovenous malformation of the great vein of Galen associated with patent ductus arteriosus. Childs Nerv Syst 1990;6:18–22

26. Norman M, Becker L. Cerebral damage in neonates resulting from arteriovenous malformation of the vein of Galen. J Neurol Neurosurg Psychiatry 1974;37:252–258

27. Askenasy H, Herzberg E, Wijsenbeek H. Hydrocephalus with vascular malformations of the brain: a preliminary report. Neurology 1953;3:213–220

28. Hooper R. Hydrocephalus and obstruction of the superior vena cava in infancy: clinical study of the relationship between cerebrospinal fluid pressure and venous pressure. Pediatrics 1961;28: 792–799

29. Johnston I. Reduced C.S.F. absorption syndrome: reappraisal of benign intracranial hypertension and related conditions. Lancet 1973;2:418–420

30. De Lange S, de Vlieger M. Hydrocephalus associated with raised venous pressure. Dev Med Child Neurol Suppl 1970;12(Suppl 22): 28–32

31. Olivero W, Rekate H, Chizeck HJ, Ko W, McCormick JM. Relationships between intracranial and sagittal sinus pressure in normal and hydrocephalic dogs. Pediatr Neurosci 1988;14:196–201

32. Johnston I, Whittle I, Besser M, Morgan M. Vein of Galen malformation: diagnosis and management. Neurosurgery 1987;20:747–758

33. Hoffman H, Chuang S, Hendrick B, Humphreys R. Aneurysms of the vein of Galen. J Neurosurg 1982;57:316–322

34. Massey C, Carson L, Beveridge W. Aneurysms of the great vein of Galen: report of two cases and review of the literature. In: Smith R, Haerer A, Russell W, eds. Vascular Malformations and Fistulas of the Brain. New York: Raven; 1982:163–179

35. Ciricillo SF, Edwards MSB, Schmidt KG. Interventional neuroradiological management of vein of Galen malformations in the neonate. Neurosurgery 1990;27:22–28

36. Friedman D, Verma R, Madrid M, Wisoff J, Bernstein A. Recent improvement in outcome using transcatheter embolization techniques for neonatal aneurysmal malformations of the vein of Galen. Pediatrics 1993;91:583–585

37. Lylyk P, Vinuela F, Dion J, et al. Therapeutic alternatives for vein of Galen vascular malformations. J Neurosurg 1993;78:438–445

38. Wisoff J, Berenstein A, Choi I, Friedman D, Madrid M, Epstein F. Management of vein of Galen malformations. Concepts Ped Neurosurg. 1990;10:137–155

39. Landsman I, Cook D. Pediatric anesthesia. In: O'Neill J, Rowe M, Grosfeld J, Fonkalsrud E, Coran A, eds. Pediatric Surgery. Vol 1. 5th ed. St. Louis: Mosby; 1998:202–203

40. Hall S. Neuroanesthesia. In: McLone D, ed. Pediatric Neurosurgery: Surgery of the Developing Nervous System. 4th ed. Philadelphia: WB Saunders; 2001:1219–1220

41. Herman J, Hamilton A, Spetzler R. Vein of Galen malformations: surgical indications and techniques. In: Carter L, Spetzler R, eds. Neurovascular Surgery. New York: McGraw-Hill; 1995:1041–1047

42. de Morais J, Lemos S. Calcified aneurysm of the vein of Galen: successful removal. Surg Neurol 1982;17:304–306

43. Morgan M, Sundt T. The case against staged operative resection of cerebral arteriovenous malformations. Neurosurgery 1989;25: 429–436

44. Andrews B, Wilson C. Staged treatment of arteriovenous malformations of the brain. Neurosurgery 1987;21:314–323

45. Casasco A, Lylyk P, Hodes J, Kohen G, Aymard A, Merland J. Percutaneous transvenous catheterization and embolization of vein of Galen aneurysms. Neurosurgery 1991;28:260–266

46. Spetzler R, Martin N, Carter L, Flom R, Raudzens P, Wilkinsons E. Surgical management of large AVMs by staged embolization and operative excision. J Neurosurg 1987;67:17–28

47. Hamilton M, Herman J, Khayata M, Spetzler R. Aneurysms of the vein of Galen. In: Youmans J, ed. Neurological Surgery. Vol 2. Philadelphia: WB Saunders; 1996:1491–1510

48. Moriarity J, Steinberg G. Surgical obliteration for vein of Galen malformation: a case report. Surg Neurol 1995;44:365–370

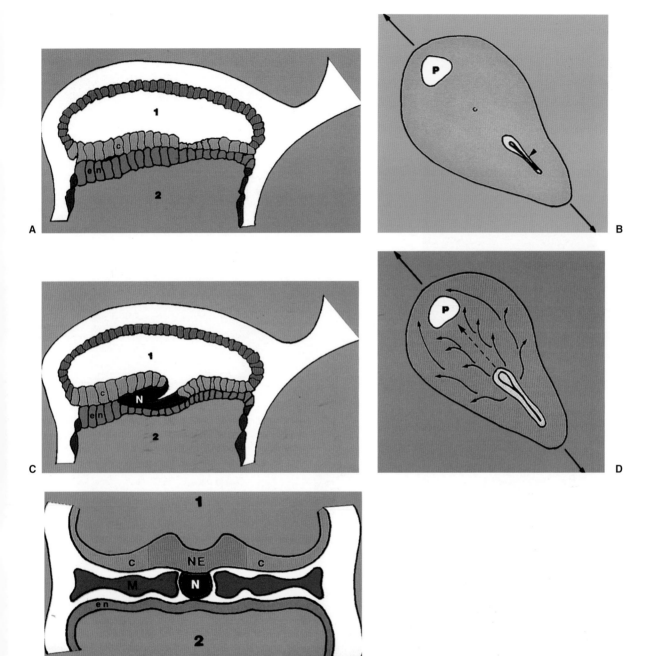

COLOR PLATE 1–1 (A,B,D) Bilaminar disk. The early embryo is a two-layered disk formed by the epiblastic cell layer (e), which faces the amnion (1) and the hypoblastic cell layer (h), which faces the yolk sac (2). The epiblast forms all of the future embryo. The hypoblast will form the extra-embryonic tissues. The disk is marked by the prochordal plate (p) at the future cephalic end of the embryo, and the primitive streak (arrowhead) in the caudal half of the disk. Hensen's node lies at the cephalic end of the primitive streak. **(C–E)** Trilaminar disk. Cells from the epiblast (e) migrate to the primitive streak (arrowhead), enter, and descend through it to form the future endoderm and mesoderm (gastrulation). The first cells to enter displace the hypoblast laterally and become the deep cell layer designated endoderm. The next-migrating cells pass between the epiblast and the new endoderm to form (from medial to lateral) the future paraxial mesoderm, intermediate mesoderm, and lateral mesoderm. The last-entering epiblastic cells ascend in the midline toward the prochordal plate to form the notochordal process (n) that will become the notochord. The epiblastic cells then spread out to become the ectoderm. By these processes, the bilaminar disk is converted to the trilaminar disk. Thereafter, under the influence of signaling, differentiation occurs into the central plate of the neural ectoderm (ne) overlying the notochord and the cutaneous ectoderm (c) laterally (see Figure 1–1, page 4). (Reprinted with permission from Naidich TP, Blaser SI, Delman BN, et al. Congenital anomalies of the spine and spinal cord: embryology and malformations. In: Atlas SW, ed. Magnetic Resonance Imaging of the Brain and Spine. Philadelphia: Lippincott Williams and Wilkins; 2002:1527–1537, Figs. 27.1 and 27.2, pp. 1528 and 1529.)

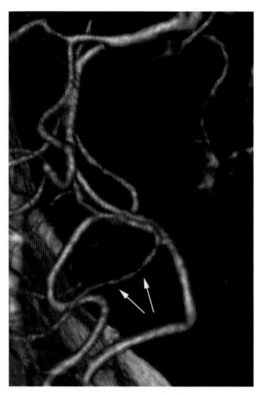

COLOR PLATE 3–10 Computed tomographic angiography of subtle vasculitic changes (arrows) in the distal middle cerebral artery (see Figure 3–10, page 44).

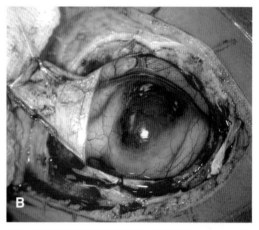

COLOR PLATE 5–3 (B) A gross intraoperative picture shows the hemorrhagic component of the cavernous malformation (see Figure 5–3B, page 67). (By permission from the Mayfield Clinic.)

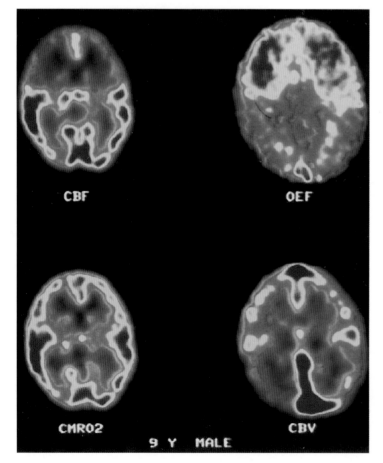

COLOR PLATE 6–2 Preoperative positron emission tomography images reveal a decrease in regional cerebral blood flow (rCBF) bilaterally in the frontal regions. However, regional cerebral metabolic rate of oxygen (CMR02) is relatively well preserved and the regional oxygen extraction fraction (rOEF) increases in these regions. Regional cerebral blood volume (rCBV) also markedly increases in the basal ganglia (see Figure 6–2, page 73).

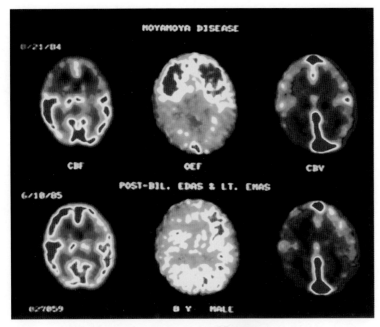

COLOR PLATE 6–8 Pre- and postoperative positron emission tomography (PET) images. Preoperative PET (upper row) reveals decrease in the regional cerebral blood flow (rCBF) bilaterally in the frontal regions. However, the CMR02 is relatively well preserved and oxygen exraction fraction (rOEF) is observed to increase in these regions. Cerebral blood volume (rCBV) also markedly increases in the basal ganglia. Postoperative PET (lower row) demonstrates an improvement, which includes an increase in the rCBF and a decrease in the rOEF in both frontal regions (see Figure 6–8, page 79). (Reprinted with permission from Matsushima T. Cerebral circulation in moyamoya disease and its surgical treatment. Fukuoka Acta Medica 1994;85:277–281.)

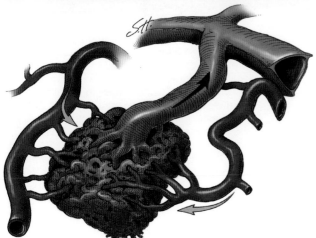

COLOR PLATE 9–1 Arteriovenous malformation schematic depicting feeders *en passant* on the left of the malformation and a direct feeder on the right (see Figure 9–1, page 107).

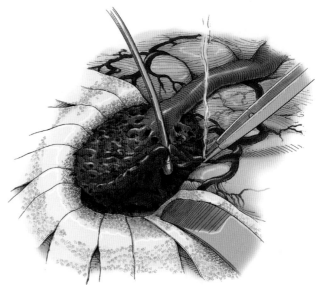

COLOR PLATE 9–2 A malleable suction is used to retract the arteriovenous malformation to expose individual feeders, which are then coagulated with a bipolar cautery and subsequently cut. Circumferential dissection is performed, leaving the draining vein intact until the end of the resection (see Figure 9–2, page 107).

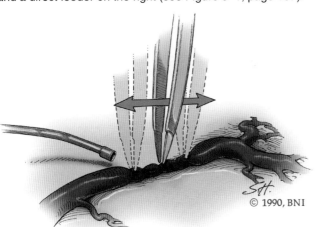

COLOR PLATE 9–3 Bipolar forceps are used to coagulate the feeding vessel back and forth to ensure total coagulation of the vessel prior to cutting (see Figure 9–3, page 107).

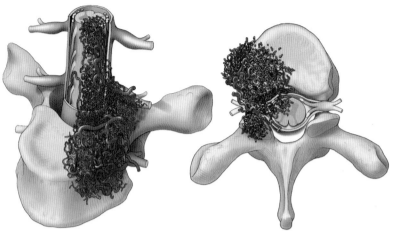

COLOR PLATE 11–1 Extradural-intradural spinal cord arteriovenous malformations (AVMs) have previously been described as juvenile spinal cord AVMs. These lesions can involve several adjacent tissue types, including spinal cord parenchyma, extradural soft tissues, the bony spine, and subcutaneous and cutaneous tissues. When the lesions are expansive enough to involve several tissue layers, they tend to be confined to one developmental metamere. Longitudinal and axial computer reconstructions demonstrate the expansive and infiltrative nature of these lesions involving several adjacent tissue types (see Figure 11–1, page 131). (Reprinted with permission from Spetzler RF, Detwiler PW, Riina HA, et al. Modified classification of spinal cord vascular lesions. J Neurosurg: Spine 2002;96(Suppl 2):145–156.)

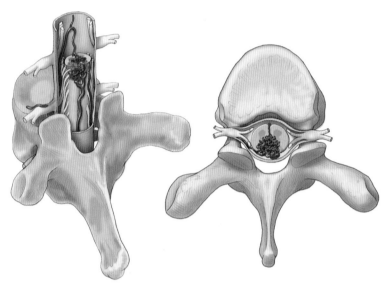

COLOR PLATE 11–2 Intramedullary spinal arteriovenous malformations (AVMs) were formerly referred to as glomus type spinal AVMs. These lesions intrinsically involve the spinal cord parenchyma, but they can extend to a pial surface. The nidus can be diffuse or compact. Longitudinal and axial computer reconstructions demonstrate an intramedullary spinal AVM with a compact nidus predominantly fed by dorsal arterial feeders (see Figure 11–2, page 131). (Reprinted with permission from Spetzler RF, Detwiler PW, Riina HA, et al. Modified classification of spinal cord vascular lesions. J Neurosurg: Spine 2002;96 (Suppl 2): 145–156.)

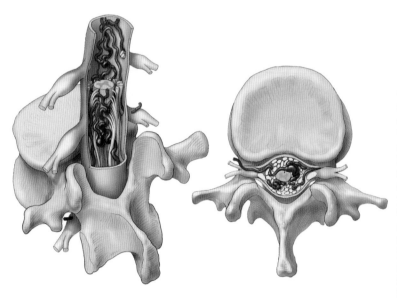

COLOR PLATE 11–3 Conus spinal arteriovenous AVMs) are a newly described classification for spinal AVMs reserved for lesions specifically involving the cauda equina and conus medullaris. These AVMs can spread to both extra- and intramedullary spaces with an arterial supply from the anterior and posterior spinal arteries. Longitudinal and axial computer reconstructions show an AVM diffusely involved with the tip of the conus and adjacent nerve roots (see Figure 11–3, page 132). (Reprinted with permission from Spetzler RF, Detwiler PW, Riina HA, et al: Modified classification of spinal cord vascular lesions. J Neurosurg: Spine 2002;96(Suppl 2): 145–156. With permission from the Journal of Neurosurgery.)

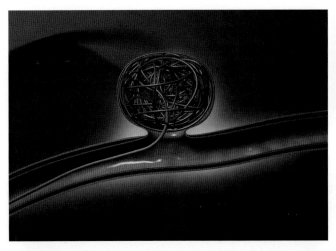

COLOR PLATE 13–1 A traditional saccular aneurysm with a small neck (<4 mm) and a dome to neck ratio of ≥2:1 is a good candidate for primary coil embolization without adjunctive devices (see Figure 13–1, page 146).

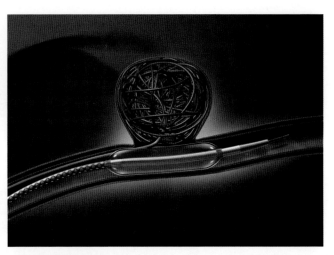

COLOR PLATE 13–2 Balloon assistance may be used with a compliant balloon for short intervals during the embolization of wider-necked aneurysms to place coils without herniation into the parent artery (see Figure 13–2, page 147).

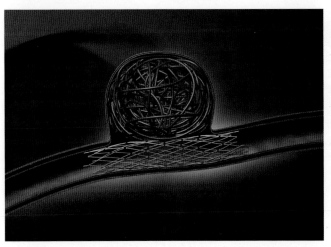

COLOR PLATE 13–3 Stent assistance for very wide-necked aneurysms protects against coil herniation and may redirect blood flow to some degree (see Figure 13–3, page 148).

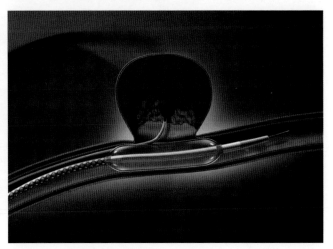

COLOR PLATE 13–4 Balloon-assisted liquid polymer embolization. A fast-polymerizing embolic agent is used to embolize the aneurysm with intermittent balloon inflation (see Figure 13–4, page 148).

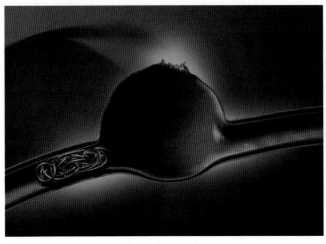

COLOR PLATE 13–5 In parent artery occlusion for fusiform and giant aneurysms, the artery is either occluded proximally or is occluded proximal and distal to the aneurysm and is effectively trapped (see Figure 13–5, page 149).

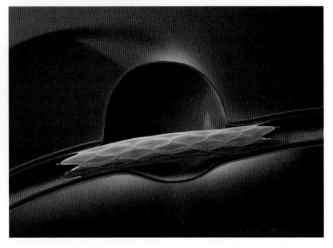

COLOR PLATE 13–6 For fusiform or dissecting aneurysms or pseudoaneurysms in the neck or at the skull base, a covered stent graft may reconstruct the artery internally, excluding the aneurysm but also occluding adjacent perforators (see Figure 13–6, page 149).

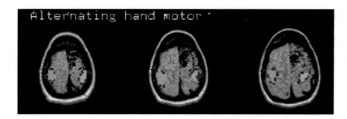

COLOR PLATE 15–1 Functional magnetic resonance imaging (fMRI) helps to localize functional regions such as motor and speech areas with respect to the arteriovenous malformation (AVM) nidus. Here the fMRI demonstrates this paracentral left frontal AVM nidus to be at least one gyrus anterior to the primary motor cortex activation for hand movement (see Figure 15–1, page 169).

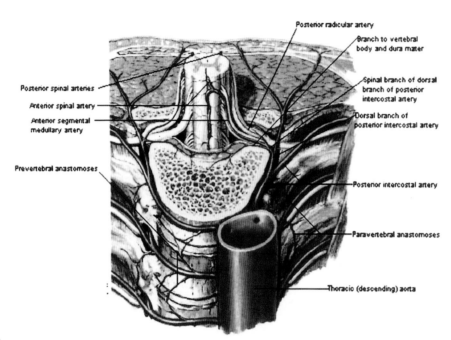

A

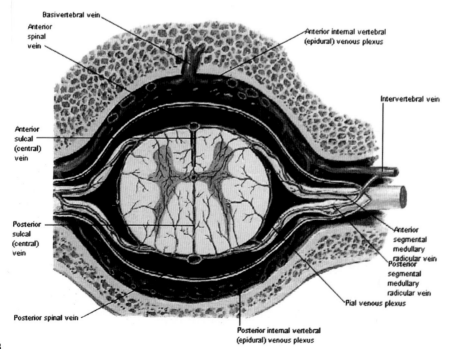

B

COLOR PLATE 17–1 (A) Axial illustration at the thoracic aorta level illustrates the arterial supply to the spinal cord and the origin of the intercostal arteries left and right from the aorta. Note the supply to the anterior spinal artery. **(B)** The venous drainage from the spinal cord in an axial cross section (see Figure 17–1, page 188).

11

Surgical Treatment of Spinal Vascular Malformations in Children

HOWARD A. RIINA, G. MICHAEL LEMOLE JR., AND ROBERT F. SPETZLER

Vascular lesions affecting the spine and spinal cord in the pediatric age group range from neoplastic vascular lesions to arteriovenous fistulae and arteriovenous malformations (AVMs). These lesions can be complex, and their successful treatment depends on a thorough understanding of their related anatomy. This treatment may require microneurosurgery, endovascular therapy, or a combination of both modalities to achieve successful obliteration. This multidisciplinary team is composed of vascular neurosurgeons, endovascular neurosurgeons, and interventional radiologists. Successful management is achieved by early diagnosis followed by implementation of appropriate therapy. Recent advances in imaging technologies have improved our ability both to diagnose and to treat such lesions. In this chapter the modified classification scheme proposed by the senior author for spinal cord vascular lesions is applied to these lesions in the pediatric age group. Pathophysiology as it relates to the components of diagnosis and successful treatment is also explored.

■ Neoplastic Lesions Affecting the Spinal Cord

As in the adult population, two types of vascular neoplastic lesions have been described in the pediatric age group: hemangioblastomas and cavernous malformations. Both lesions occur sporadically and with a familial pattern.[1–3]

Hemangioblastomas

Hemangioblastomas are highly vascular lesions that can occur in the substance of the spinal cord. They are composed of stromal, endothelial, and pericytic cells as well as the associated arteries and veins that feed and drain the lesion.[4] These arterial tributaries and draining veins can become quite prominent, creating the appearance of an AVM. In the spinal cord hemangioblastomas are predominantly intramedullary, but they often abut the pial surface. They have even been described as involving nerve root sheaths.[4,5]

Hemangioblastomas usually manifest secondary to mass effect on adjacent neuronal tissue. The mass effect causes myelopathy and symptoms related to compression at the level of spinal cord involvement. Spinal cord hemangioblastomas can be associated with a syrinx that causes myelopathic, radiculopathic, or myeloradiculopathic symptoms.[6,7]

The initial evaluation begins with magnetic resonance imaging (MRI), which shows a discrete mass that enhances after the administration of gadolinium. When the surrounding vasculature is engorged, flow voids may also be appreciated. The diagnosis can usually be made based solely on MRI; however, definitive diagnosis can be confirmed with digital subtraction angiography. Angiography is only necessary if preoperative embolization is to be attempted. As discussed later, embolization can be performed as long as the anterior spinal artery is protected. Injury or embolization of the anterior spinal artery can cause spinal cord infarction. Embolization can be undertaken preoperatively to facilitate resection, but surgery can be performed without it.

Cavernous Malformations

Many authors exclude cavernous malformations from the heading of neoplastic vascular lesions. Cavernous malformations are associated with a known and identifiable chromosomal abnormality.[3,8] They occur sporadically as well as in a familial pattern and can appear and grow spontaneously.[1-3] The true nature of these lesions is still being debated by the scientific community. From our perspective, however, these lesions and their behavior parallel that of neoplastic-type lesions. Consequently, we consider them as vascular lesions that affect the spinal cord.

> **PEARL** Care must be taken when resecting cavernous malformations to avoid injury to the venous angioma. Damage can cause a venous infarction in the normal territory drained by the venous anomaly.

Histologically, cavernous malformations are composed of sinusoids of endothelial-lined channels.[9] Cavernous malformations are often discovered incidentally or after a hemorrhage when their characteristic appearance is observed on MRI, computed tomography (CT), or both. On MRI, cavernous malformations appear as a focal area of abnormal signal surrounded by hemorrhage at various stages of absorption and resorption (methemoglobin).[10] The focal area is surrounded by a hemosiderin ring. Unenhanced CT scans show a high-density region associated with calcification.[10] Upon administration of contrast, the region may enhance.

A considerable number of patients have more than one cavernous malformation, and a venous angioma is often associated. Care must be taken when treating cavernous malformations to avoid injuring the venous angioma. Damage can cause a venous infarction in the normal territory drained by the venous anomaly. Cavernous malformations have also been described in children who have undergone spinal radiation to treat spinal cord tumors.[11]

■ Spinal Cord Arteriovenous Lesions

Traditionally, spinal vascular malformations have been divided as having either a dural or a pial supply. The dural-type lesions known to affect adults have not been observed in the pediatric population. Vascular lesions affecting the spinal cord in the pediatric age group are primarily pial based. Pial-based fistulas and pial-surface AVMs are restricted to the surface of the spinal cord whereas subpial AVMs involve the spinal cord parenchyma. Subpial intramedullary AVMs often have a diffuse nidus, but compact niduses have been observed as well. The nidus may be partially or totally imbedded in the spinal cord. In the senior author's modified classification of spinal vascular lesions, pial-based fistulas are called intradural arteriovenous fistulas and are further subdivided into dorsal and ventral subtypes. AVMs affecting the spine and spinal cord in children include extradural-intradural AVMs, intramedullary AVMs, and AVMs affecting the conus medullaris (**Table 11–1**).[12]

Extradural-Intradural Arteriovenous Malformations

Extradural-intradural lesions affect more than one type of tissue and can include an entire metamere (**Fig. 11–1**). Previously, these lesions have been described as metameric or juvenile AVMs. They often involve the vertebral column and have both an epidural and an intradural intramedullary component. When all tissue layers are involved (skin, extraspinal soft tissue, vertebrae, and spinal cord), the condition is referred to as Cobb's syndrome.[13] These lesions are rare but more common in children than in adults. Their treatment is complex and requires a multidisciplinary approach. The initial treatment of such lesions is intra-arterial embolization of the

TABLE 11–1 Clinical Summary of Arteriovenous Malformations

	Extradural-Intradural	Intramedullary	Conus
Pathophysiology			
	Compression	Hemorrhage	Venous hypertension
	Vascular steal	Compression	Compression
	Hemorrhage	Vascular steal	Hemorrhage
Presentation			
	Pain	Acute myelopathy	Progressive myelopathy
	Pain	Radiculopathy	Progressive myelopathy
Diagnostic Modality			
	MR imaging	MR imaging	MR imaging
	Angiography	Angiography	Angiography
	High flow		
	Multiple feeders		
Previous Nomenclature			
	Juvenile AVM	Classic AVM	None
	Metameric AVM	Glomus type	

AVM, arteriovenous malformation; MR, magnetic resonance. (Reprinted with permission from Spetzler RF, Detwiler PW, Riina HA, et al. Modified classification of spinal cord vascular lesions. J Neurosurg 2002;96(Suppl 2):145–156.)

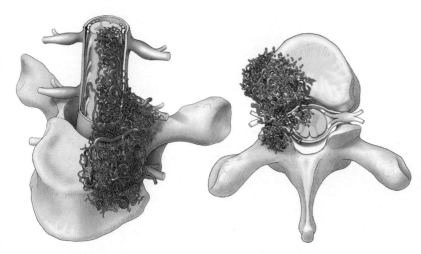

FIGURE 11–1 Extradural-intradural spinal cord arteriovenous malformations (AVMs) have previously been described as juvenile spinal cord AVMs. These lesions can involve several adjacent tissue types, including spinal cord parenchyma, extradural soft tissues, the bony spine, and subcutaneous and cutaneous tissues. When the lesions are expansive enough to involve several tissue layers, they tend to be confined to one developmental metamere. Longitudinal and axial computer reconstructions demonstrate the expansive and infiltrative nature of these lesions involving several adjacent tissue types (see Color Plate 11–1). (Reprinted with permission from Spetzler RF, Detwiler PW, Riina HA, et al. Modified classification of spinal cord vascular lesions. J Neurosurg: Spine 2002;96(Suppl 2):145–156.)

often multiple arterial feeders. Once embolization is performed surgical excision may follow. Surgery usually takes the form of staged resections, with complete resection being rare.

Intramedullary Arteriovenous Malformations

Intramedullary AVMs are subpial or reach the pial surface (**Fig. 11–2**). They involve the parenchyma of the spinal cord. As mentioned, their nidus is either diffuse or compact. Their arterial supply is derived from the spinal cord vasculature: the anterior and posterior spinal arteries. Intramedullary AVMs are characterized by high blood flow and high pressure. Because of these hemodynamics, the lesions often become symptomatic with hemorrhage or with myelopathy related to compression of the spinal cord by the dilated vasculature. Vascular steal can be a component of the initial symptomatology by causing ischemic myelopathy or spinal cord dysfunction.

> **PEARL**   In spinal AVMs that do not derive their blood supply from the anterior spinal artery, embolization can be performed prior to surgical excision.

The lesions can be diagnosed with MRI. Spinal angiography, however, is the best way to confirm the diagnosis and to determine the angioarchitecture of the malformation. In lesions that do not derive their blood supply from the anterior spinal artery, intra-arterial embolization can be attempted. Embolization is often followed by surgery. Lesions with a compact nidus tend

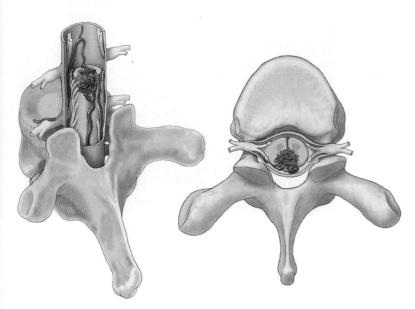

FIGURE 11–2 Intramedullary spinal arteriovenous malformations (AVMs) were formerly referred to as glomus type spinal AVMs. These lesions intrinsically involve the spinal cord parenchyma, but they can extend to a pial surface. The nidus can be diffuse or compact. Longitudinal and axial computer reconstructions demonstrate an intramedullary spinal AVM with a compact nidus predominantly fed by dorsal arterial feeders (see Color Plate 11–2). (Reprinted with permission from Spetzler RF, Detwiler PW, Riina HA, et al. Modified classification of spinal cord vascular lesions. J Neurosurg: Spine 2002;96(Suppl 2): 145–156.)

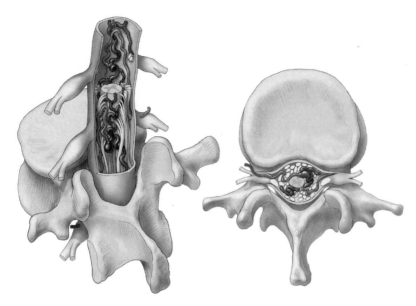

FIGURE 11–3 Conus spinal arteriovenous malformations (AVMs) are a newly described classification for spinal AVMs reserved for lesions specifically involving the cauda equina and conus medullaris. These AVMs can spread to both extra- and intramedullary spaces with an arterial supply from the anterior and posterior spinal arteries. Longitudinal and axial computer reconstructions show an AVM diffusely involved with the tip of the conus and adjacent nerve roots (see Color Plate 11–3). (Reprinted with permission from Spetzler RF, Detwiler PW, Riina HA, et al: Modified classification of spinal cord vascular lesions. J Neurosurg: Spine 2002;96(Suppl 2): 145–156. With permission from the Journal of Neurosurgery.)

to be more amenable to surgery than those with a diffuse nidus, and their complete resection is more likely. Lesions characterized by a diffuse nidus often require another operation to ensure their total resection.

Conus Arteriovenous Malformations

By definition, conus AVMs, arteriovenous lesions that affect the cauda equina and conus medullaris, are location specific (**Fig. 11–3**).[12] They have many of the components of the vascular lesions described earlier. They can have both extramedullary and intramedullary components as well as an arterial supply involving multiple arteriovenous shunts derived from the anterior and posterior spinal arteries. Involvement of the cauda equina can cause myeloradiculopathy, but radicular symptoms tend to predominate. The myelopathic component is related to venous congestion and compression. Patients may also become symptomatic with hemorrhage.

■ Diagnostic Imaging

All pediatric patients harboring vascular lesions of the spine and spinal cord should undergo MRI with and without gadolinium. The administration of gadolinium is useful but not mandatory to suggest the initial diagnosis. Cavernous malformations, with their characteristic appearance, can usually be diagnosed solely on MRI without further radiographic evaluation. Hemosiderin and methemoglobin staining (blood degradation products of various ages) can be appreciated as well as gliosis and calcification (**Fig. 11–4**). Cavernous malformations are angiographically occult.

Hemangioblastomas are highly vascular and can have both solid and cystic portions. The administration of gadolinium causes the solid portion of the lesion to enhance. MRI also may reveal surrounding edema and flow voids. Angiography confirms the diagnosis by demonstrating a tumor blush and prominent draining veins.

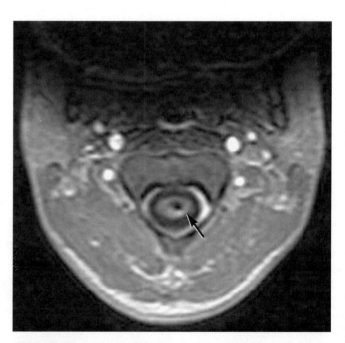

FIGURE 11–4 T1-weighted magnetic resonance imaging of a cervical spinal cord cavernous malformation shows a dorsal abnormality in a 15-year-old boy who presented with neurological decline. The signal intensity of the lesion (arrow) is consistent with blood and adjacent gliosis. The lesion appears to abut a pial surface dorsally.

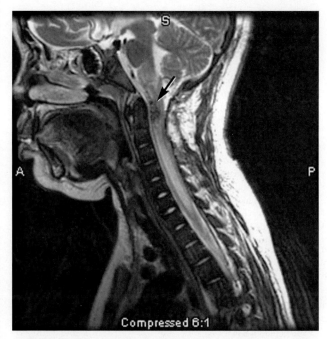

FIGURE 11–5 Sagittal T2-weighted magnetic resonance imaging showing a high cervical spinal cord arteriovenous malformation (AVM). The lesion (arrow) is located ventrally at the cervicomedullary junction and is denoted by multiple flow voids within the spinal cord parenchyma. Under the current classification scheme, this lesion would be considered an intramedullary spinal cord AVM. The patient, a 10-year-old girl, had presented after this AVM ruptured.

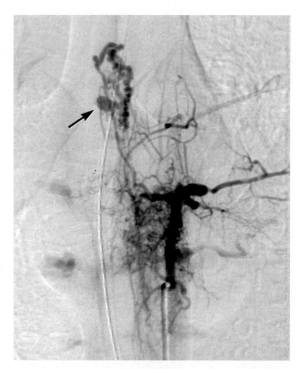

FIGURE 11–6 Anteroposterior spinal cord angiography with selective T6 radicular branch injection shows a diffuse extradural-intradural thoracic arteriovenous malformation (AVM). This 14-year-old girl presented with spinal cord hemorrhage from this lesion, which diffusely involved the spinal cord and adjacent spine. Note the pseudoaneurysm (arrow) at the rostral end of the AVM.

On MRI AVM lesions appear as regions of prominent and multiple flow voids (**Fig. 11–5**). Angiography can then be used to define the angioarchitecture of the lesion (**Fig. 11–6**).[14–16]

> **PEARL** Resection of spinal vascular malformations requires meticulous sharp dissection and preservation of the anterior spinal artery.

■ Treatment

Treatment of many vascular lesions of the spine and spinal cord requires careful planning and a multidisciplinary approach. Cavernous malformations may be resected when they are located in surgically accessible areas. This usually follows repeat hemorrhages and neurological decline. Care must be taken to preserve the often associated venous anomaly. Hemangioblastomas and arteriovenous lesions often require a combination of treatment modalities, including endovascular therapy and microneurosurgery. Preoperative embolization can decrease the vascular supply and facilitate surgical resection. Interventional procedures

are useful but not without risk; care must be taken to preserve and protect the anterior spinal artery. Postembolization hemorrhage has been known to occur. The use of intraoperative angiography can contribute to successful surgery by helping to identify regions of residual malformation. Microneurosurgical resection requires careful surgical planning including a thorough understanding of spinal anatomy and its relation to the angioarchitecture of the lesion. When undertaking surgical resection of a spinal cord vascular lesion, the tenets of vascular microneurosurgery must be followed: meticulous sharp dissection, preservation of the anterior spinal artery, and optimization of exposure. When necessary, staging the resection may be the best strategy to achieve complete resection of the lesion.

■ Conclusion

Pediatric spinal vascular malformations are complex lesions. Neurodiagnostic imaging, spinal angiography, endovascular therapy, and microneurosurgery all play important roles in their accurate diagnosis and successful treatment. The modified classification system as it applies to children is based on anatomy, operative observations, neuroimaging, and pathophysiology. It was designed to simplify communication among physicians and to facilitate the management of all surgically treated vascular lesions of the spinal cord in children. In the proper setting, microneurosurgery combined with preoperative embolization (in the case of arteriovenous lesions and hemangioblastomas) and as the sole therapy in the case of cavernous malformations offers effective treatment for many children with spinal cord vascular malformations.

REFERENCES

1. Malis LI. Intramedullary spinal cord tumors. Clin Neurosurg 1978;25:512–539
2. Rutka JT, Brant-Zawadzki M, Wilson CB, et al. Familial cavernous malformations: diagnostic potential of magnetic resonance imaging. Surg Neurol 1988;29:467–474
3. Anson JA, Spetzler RF. Surgical resection of intramedullary spinal cord cavernous malformations. J Neurosurg 1993;78:446–451
4. Ismail SM, Cole G. Von Hippel-Lindau syndrome with microscopic hemangioblastomas of the spinal nerve roots. J Neurosurg 1984; 60:1279–1281
5. Browne TR, Adams RD, Roberson GH. Hemangioblastoma of the spinal cord: review and report of five cases. Arch Neurol 1976;33: 435–441
6. Enomoto H, Shibata T, Ito A, et al. Multiple hemangioblastomas accompanied by syringomyelia in the cerebellum and the spinal cord. Surg Neurol 1984;22:197–203
7. Fox JL, Bashir R, Jinkins JR, et al. Syrinx of the conus medullaris and filum terminale in association with multiple hemangioblastomas. Surg Neurol 1985;24:265–271
8. Cosgrove GR, Bertrand G, Fontaine S, et al. Cavernous angiomas of the spinal cord. J Neurosurg 1988;68:31–36
9. McCormick PC, Michelsen WJ, Post KD, et al. Cavernous malformations of the spinal cord. Neurosurgery 1988;23:459–463
10. Furuya K, Sasaki T, Suzuki I, et al. Intramedullary angiographically occult vascular malformations of the spinal cord. Neurosurgery 1996;39:1123–1132
11. Maraire JN, Abdulrauf SI, Berger S, et al. De novo development of a cavernous malformation of the spinal cord following spinal axis radiation: case report. J Neurosurg 1999;90(Suppl 2):234–238
12. Spetzler RF, Detwiler PW, Riina HA, et al. Modified classification of spinal cord vascular lesions. J Neurosurg: Spine 2002;96(Suppl 2): 145–156
13. Mercer RD, Rothner AD, Cook SA, et al. The Cobb syndrome: association with hereditary cutaneous hemangiomas. Cleve Clin Q 1978;45:237–240
14. Doppman JL, Di Chiro G, Dwyer AJ, et al. Magnetic resonance imaging of spinal arteriovenous malformations. J Neurosurg 1987;66:830–834
15. Dormont D, Gelbert F, Assouline E, et al. MR imaging of spinal cord arteriovenous malformations at 0.5 T: study of 34 cases. AJNR Am J Neuroradiol 1988;9:833–838
16. Friedman DP, Flanders AE, Tartaglino LM. Vascular neoplasms and malformations, ischemia, and hemorrhage affecting the spinal cord: MR imaging findings. AJR Am J Roentgenol 1994;162:685–692

12

Radiosurgery in Children

RONNIE I. MIMRAN AND WILLIAM A. FRIEDMAN

The most devastating presentation associated with arteriovenous malformations (AVMs) of the brain is intracerebral hemorrhage. Numerous natural history studies have demonstrated a substantial (3 to 4% per year) risk of hemorrhage in patients harboring AVMs.[1–5] There are several treatment modalities (microsurgery, radiosurgery, or endovascular therapy) available that may eliminate the lesion before a hemorrhage can occur—or recur, in the case of a hemorrhagic presentation. When an AVM is amenable to safe microsurgical resection, this therapy is preferred because it offers immediate cure and elimination of hemorrhage risk. When the surgical morbidity is judged to be excessive, radiosurgery offers a reasonable expectation of delayed cure.

When an AVM is treated with radiosurgery, a pathological process appears to be induced that is similar to the response-to-injury model of atherosclerosis. Radiation injury to the vascular endothelium is believed to induce the proliferation of smooth-muscle cells and the elaboration of extracellular collagen, which leads to progressive stenosis and obliteration of the AVM nidus[6–10] and thereby eliminates the risk of hemorrhage.

> **PEARL** Although thrombosis of the lesion is achieved in the majority of cases, it commonly does not occur until 2 or 3 years after treatment.

The advantages of radiosurgery—compared with microsurgical and endovascular treatments—are that it is noninvasive, has minimal risk of acute complications, and is performed as an outpatient procedure requiring no recovery time for the patient. The primary disadvantage of radiosurgery is that cure is not immediate. Although thrombosis of the lesion is achieved in the majority of cases, it commonly does not occur until 2 or 3 years after treatment. During the interval between radiosurgical treatment and AVM thrombosis, the risk of hemorrhage remains. Another potential disadvantage of radiosurgery is possible long-term adverse effects of radiation. Finally, radiosurgery has been shown to be much less effective for lesions over 10 cc in volume. For these reasons, selection of an appropriate treatment modality is dependent on multiple variables, including perceived risks of surgery and predicted likelihood of hemorrhage for a given patient.

■ Arteriovenous Malformation Radiosurgery Technique

The technical methods of radiosurgery have been described at length in other publications,[11] but a brief description of radiosurgical techniques that apply specifically to AVM treatment is in order. The fundamental elements of any successful radiosurgical treatment include patient selection, head ring application, stereotactic image acquisition, treatment planning, dose selection, radiation delivery, and follow-up. All of these elements are critical, and poor performance of any step will result in suboptimal results.

Patient Selection

Open surgery is generally favored if an AVM is amenable to low-risk resection (e.g., low Spetzler-Martin grade; young, healthy patient) or is felt to be at high risk for hemorrhage during the latency period between radiosurgical treatment and AVM obliteration (e.g., associated aneurysm, prior hemorrhage, large AVM with diffuse morphology, venous outflow obstruction).

Radiosurgery is favored when the AVM nidus is small (<3 cm) and compact, when surgery is judged to carry a high risk or is refused by the patient, and when the risk of hemorrhage is not felt to be extraordinarily high.

Endovascular treatment, although rarely curative alone, may be useful as a preoperative adjunct to either microsurgery or radiosurgery.

The history, physical examination, and diagnostic imaging of each patient are evaluated and the various factors outlined here are weighed in combination to determine the best treatment approach for a given case.

Head Ring Application

The techniques for optimal head ring application for AVM radiosurgery are the same as those for other target lesions and are described in detail elsewhere.[11] In general, children 13 and older are able to tolerate head ring application under local anesthesia. Those younger are treated under general anesthesia.

Stereotactic Image Acquisition

The most problematic aspect of AVM radiosurgery is target identification. In some series (see later discussion), targeting error is listed as the most frequent cause of radiosurgical failure. The problem lies with imaging. Although angiography very effectively defines blood flow (feeding arteries, nidus, and draining veins), it does so in only two dimensions. Using the two-dimensional data from stereotactic angiography to represent the three-dimensional target results in significant errors of both overestimation and underestimation of AVM nidus dimensions.[12,13] Underestimation of the nidus size may result in treatment failure, whereas overestimation results in the inclusion of normal brain within the treatment volume. This can cause radiation damage to normal brain, which—when affecting an eloquent area—may result in a neurological deficit. To avoid such targeting errors, a true three-dimensional image database is required. Both contrast-enhanced computed tomography (CT) and magnetic resonance imaging (MRI) are commonly used for this purpose.

> **PEARL** Underestimation of the nidus size may result in treatment failure, whereas overestimation results in the inclusion of normal brain within the treatment volume.

Diagnostic (nonstereotactic) angiography is used to characterize the AVM, but because of its inherent inadequacies as a treatment planning database, stereotactic

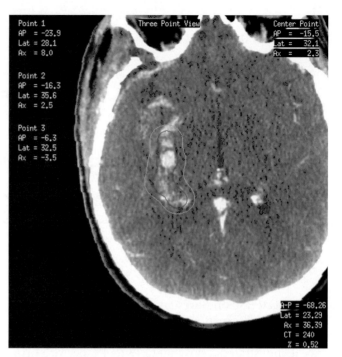

FIGURE 12–1 The goal of dosimetry is to create a treatment isodose line that conforms to the shape of the arteriovenous malformation (AVM). This AVM of the corpus callosum required multiple isocenters to generate the prescription isodose line (inner line). The outer line is 50% of the prescription isodose.

angiography has been largely abandoned at our institution. We use contrast-enhanced, stereotactic CT as a targeting image database for the vast majority of AVMs (**Fig. 12–1**). Our CT technique employs rapid infusion (1 mL/s) of contrast while scanning through the AVM nidus with 1 mm slices. The head ring is bolted to a bracket at the head of the CT table, assuring that the head ring–localizer complex remains immobile during the scan. This technique yields a very clear three-dimensional picture of the nidus. Alternative approaches use MRI and magnetic resonance angiography (MRA), as opposed to CT. Attention to optimal image sequences in both CT and MRI is essential for effective AVM radiosurgical targeting.

Treatment Planning

The primary goal of AVM radiosurgery treatment planning is to develop a plan with a target volume that conforms closely to the surface of the AVM nidus while maintaining a steep dose gradient (the rate of change in dose relative to position) away from the nidal surface to minimize the radiation dose to surrounding brain. Several treatment planning tools can be used to tailor the shape of the target volume to fit even highly irregular nidus shapes. Regardless of its shape, the entire nidus—not including the feeding arteries and draining veins—must lie within the target volume (the "prescription isodose shell"), with as little normal brain included as possible.

Another goal of dose planning is to manipulate the dose gradient such that critical brain structures receive the lowest possible dose of radiation to avoid disabling complications. In addition, many radiosurgeons strive to produce a treatment dose distribution that maximizes uniformity (homogeneity) of dose throughout the entire target volume. A detailed discussion of the methodology of dose planning is beyond the scope of this chapter but can be found elsewhere.[14]

> **PEARL** Minimum nidal doses lower than 15 Gy have been associated with a significantly lower rate of AVM obliteration, whereas doses above 20 Gy have been associated with a higher rate of permanent neurological complications.

Dose Selection

Various analyses of AVM radiosurgery outcomes (described in Surgical Outcomes) have elucidated an appropriate range of doses for the treatment of AVMs. Minimum nidal doses lower than 15 Gy have been associated with a significantly lower rate of AVM obliteration, whereas doses above 20 Gy have been associated with a higher rate of permanent neurological complications. We prescribe doses ranging from 15 Gy to as high as 22.5 Gy to the

margin of the AVM nidus, nearly always at the 70 or 80% isodose line. The selection of a dose within this range is made based on the volume of the nidus, as well as the eloquence and radiosensitivity of surrounding brain structures. Lower doses are prescribed for larger lesions and lesions in eloquent areas.

Radiation Delivery

The process of radiation delivery is the same for any radiosurgical target, but careful attention to detail and the execution of various safety checks and redundancies are necessary to ensure that the prescribed treatment plan is accurately and safely delivered.[11] When radiation delivery has been completed, the head ring is removed and the patient is observed for approximately 30 minutes and then discharged to resume normal activities.

Follow-Up

Standard follow-up after AVM radiosurgery typically consists of annual clinic visits with MRI/MRA to evaluate the effect of the procedure and monitor for neurological complications. Patients whose clinical status changes are followed more closely at clinically appropriate intervals.

Each patient is scheduled to undergo cerebral angiography at 3 years postradiosurgery, and a definitive assessment of the success or failure of treatment is made based on the results of angiography (**Fig. 12–2A,B**). If no flow is observed through the AVM nidus, the patient is pronounced cured and is discharged from follow-up. If the AVM nidus is incompletely obliterated, appropriate

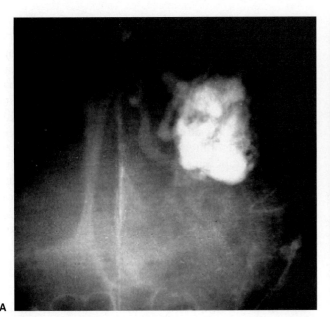
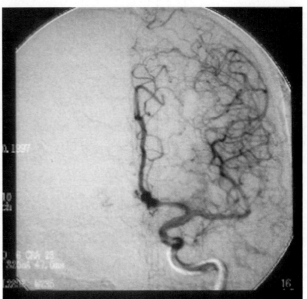

A   B

FIGURE 12–2 (A) Anteroposterior angiogram shows a large arteriovenous malformation (AVM) nidus. A peripheral dose of 1500 cGy was administered through multiple isocenters. **(B)** Angiogram 2 years later shows complete resolution of the AVM.

TABLE 12–1 Major Arteriovenous Malformation Radiosurgery Series[a]

First Author	Radiosurgical Device	Number of Patients	Angiographic Cure Rate	Permanent Radiation-Induced Complications	Hemorrhage
Yamamoto[29]	Gamma knife	40	65%	3 patients (7.5%)	None
Pollock[45]	Gamma knife	313	61%	30 patients (9%)	8 fatal
Karlsson[17]	Gamma knife	945	56%	5%	55 patients
Steinberg[25]	Proton beam	86	92%	11%	10 patients
Colombo[16]	LINAC	180	80%	4 patients (2%)	15 patients 5 fatal
Friedman[43]	LINAC	407	65%	7 patients (2%)	26 patients 5 fatal

[a]When a group had multiple reports, the most recent results are listed. LINAC, linear accelerator.

further therapy (most commonly repeat radiosurgery on the day of angiography) is prescribed, and the treatment/follow-up cycle is repeated.

■ Surgical Outcomes

Many series have evaluated rates of AVM thrombosis after radiosurgery.[10,13–30] Overall reported rates of successful angiographic AVM obliteration range from 56 to 92% (**Table 12–1**). The rate of obliteration is strongly correlated with AVM size. For example, among the 153 AVM radiosurgery patients that have undergone 3-year follow-up angiography at the University of Florida, rates of angiographic cure according to AVM volume were as follows: <1 cc, 82%; 1 to 4 cc, 81%; 4 to 10 cc, 73%; >10 cc, 42%. Similar trends have been reported by most groups.[14,15,20,25] Those few series that have specifically reported on AVM radiosurgery in children report similar results[11,30–33] (**Table 12–2**).

Between May 1988 and February 2000, 24 pediatric patients (ages up to 18) with AVMs were treated with stereotactic radiosurgery at the University of Florida. The patient details are listed in **Table 12–3**. Of the 20 patients with a follow-up of at lease 2 years, 13 (65%) have achieved a cure, as documented by angiogram or MRI. Of the remaining seven patients, four had a 75% or greater reduction in AVM nidus size and are candidates for retreatment. Three patients had posttreatment, radiation-induced neurological deficits (two transient, one permanent) and one patient experienced an intracranial hemorrhage.

TABLE 12–2 Pediatric Arteriovenous Malformation Series

First Author	Radiosurgical Device	Number of Patients	Angiographic Cure Rate
Baumann[31]	Gamma knife	27	33%
Kondziolka[32]	Gamma knife	39	75%
Tanaka[33]	Gamma knife	23	94%
Yamamoto[30]	Gamma knife	9	56%
Friedman[11]	LINAC	24	65%

LINAC, linear accelerator.

■ Why Does Radiosurgery Fail?

Synthesis of the published studies addressing etiologies of AVM radiosurgical failure[17,21,34–37] leads to several useful conclusions. The dose delivery to the periphery of the AVM (D_{min}) is the most significant predictor of successful obliteration, provided that the nidus is completely encompassed by the prescription isodose shell (targeting error is an important cause of failure and is commonly due to inadequate imaging/angiography). Larger lesion volume and high Spetzler-Martin grade are also predictors of failure, though less significant than D_{min}. The importance of AVM location and patient age is unclear. Based on our experience,[34] lower rates of AVM obliteration can be expected at peripheral doses below 15 Gy, and for lesion volumes greater than 10 cc.

■ Complications

Hemorrhage

The issue of AVM hemorrhage after radiosurgical treatment has been examined by several groups.[14,16,20,22,25,38–42] Although it has been reported that radiosurgery decreases the risk of hemorrhage even with incomplete AVM obliteration,[38] most reports have shown no postradiosurgical alteration in bleeding risk[43,44] from the 3 to 4% per year expected based on natural history.[1–5] This suggests that radiosurgery offers no protective effect unless complete obliteration is achieved.

Several groups have reported an increased risk of AVM hemorrhage with increasing AVM size or subtotal irradiation.[16,38,43] In our series,[43] a strong correlation between AVM volume and the risk of hemorrhage was also found. Ten of the 12 AVMs that bled were greater than 10 cc in volume. It is also noteworthy that in this study, neither age nor history of prior hemorrhage correlated with the incidence of hemorrhage.

Ten of the 12 AVMs that bled also had associated "angiographic risk factors" for bleeding, including arterial aneurysms, venous aneurysms, venous outlet obstruction, and periventricular location. Pollock et al[44]

TABLE 12–3 Data from Pediatric Patients Treated for AVMs with Stereotactic Surgery at the University of Florida from May 1988 to February 2000

Patient #	Age	Sex	Presentation	Location	Spetzler-Martin Grade	Volume (cc)	Dose (cGy)
1	16	M	Headache	Temporal	4	9.2	1500
2	16	F	Hemorrhage	Frontal	2	5.2	1500
3	17	M	Hemorrhage	Occipital	2	0.6	2000
4	9	M	Hemorrhage	Centrum	4	8.8	1500
5	18	M	Hemorrhage	Midbrain	3	14.3	1750
6	17	M	Headache	Thalamus	3	11.3	1500
7	17	M	Progressive deficit	Thalamus	4	11.9	1250
8	17	F	Hemorrhage	Centrum	3	1.3	2000
9	15	F	Hemorrhage	Centrum	3	2.6	2000
10	13	F	Headache	Occipital	3	5.4	1500
11	17	F	Headache	Occipital	2	1.2	1500
12	13	F	Seizure	Parietal	2	7.0	1500
13	18	M	Hemorrhage	Pontine	3	0.3	1500
14	7	F	Hemorrhage	Corpus callosum	3	3.9	1750
15	15	F	Seizure	Frontal	3	10.9	1250
16	14	M	Seizure	Parietal	4	11.4	1250
17	10	F	Seizure	Temporal	4	22.8	1000
18	17	F	Seizure	Frontal	2	6.7	1500
19	4	M	Hemorrhage	Occipital	3	1.7	2000
20	17	F	Hemorrhage	Sylvian	2	9.7	1750
21	12	M	Hemorrhage	Thalamus	3	2.0	1750
22	10	M	Seizure	Parietal	3	7.8	1750
23	14	F	Hemorrhage	Frontal	2	1.5	2000
24	8	F	Headache	Corpus callosum	4	5.0	1500

found a significant correlation between the incidence of postradiosurgical hemorrhage and presence of an unsecured proximal aneurysm, and recommended that such aneurysms be obliterated prior to radiosurgery.

The Pittsburgh group[45] also recently studied factors associated with bleeding risk of AVMs and found three AVM characteristics to be predictive of greater hemorrhage risk: (1) history of prior bleed, (2) presence of a single draining vein, and (3) diffuse AVM morphology. Based on the presence or absence of these risk factors, they stratified AVM patients with a high predicted hemorrhage risk would be considered less attractive candidates for radiosurgery due to their greater risk during the latency period between treatment and cure.

Radiation-Induced

Acute complications are rare after AVM radiosurgery. Several authors have previously reported that radiosurgery can acutely exacerbate seizure activity. Others have reported nausea, vomiting, and headache occasionally occurring after radiosurgical treatment.[46]

Delayed radiation-induced complications have been reported by all groups performing radiosurgery. Observed rates of permanent postradiosurgical neurological deficit range from 2 to 4%, and transient deficits have been observed in 3 to 9% of patients.[20,24,26,47] Symptoms are location-dependent and generally develop between 3 and 18 months after treatment. Symptomatic patients are commonly treated with steroids and nearly all improve (**Fig. 12–3A,B**). The use of peripheral doses greater than

20 Gy has been associated with a higher frequency of permanent neurological deficits.[47]

In addition to the well-established correlation between increasing radiosurgical target volume and increasing incidence of radiation necrosis,[40,48–50] the most important predictors of symptomatic radiation injury are lesion location and dose.[25,47,51] Radiation-induced changes appear frequently (20% in the Pittsburgh series) on postradiosurgery MRI.[52–54] These changes tend to be asymptomatic if the lesion is located in a relatively "silent" brain area, and symptomatic if the lesion is located in an "eloquent" brain area. This is further evidence that lesion location is an important consideration in radiosurgical treatment planning and dose selection.[48]

■ Conclusions

Many reports indicate that ~80% of AVMs in the "radiosurgery size range" will be angiographically obliterated 2 to 3 years after radiosurgical treatment. The likelihood of successful AVM obliteration decreases with increasing lesion volume and decreasing peripheral target dose. Accurate targeting is critical to successful AVM radiosurgery, and a three-dimensional image database (e.g., CT or MRI) is an indispensable element in the treatment planning process—stereotactic angiography alone is inadequate.

The major drawback of this treatment method is that patients are unprotected against hemorrhage during the 2- to 3-year latent period following treatment.

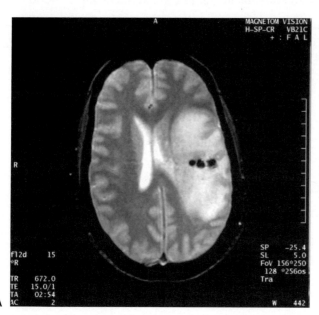

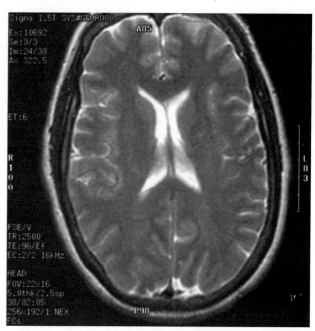

FIGURE 12–3 (A) This patient underwent radiosurgery for a small motor strip area arteriovenous malformation (AVM). Nine months posttreatment she presented with headache. This T2-weighted magnetic resonance imaging (MRI) scan shows a large area of edema around the treated AVM nidus. Oral steroid therapy was administered for 1 month. **(B)** MRI 3 months later shows complete resolution of the transient radiation-induced edema. Subsequent angiography revealed thrombosis of the AVM.

Radiosurgery does not significantly alter the natural rate of AVM hemorrhage until the lesion has completely thrombosed. Increasing AVM volume appears to be associated with a higher risk for hemorrhage, as are certain angiographic findings such as proximal aneurysms, venous outflow restriction, and periventricular location.

Radiation-induced neurological symptoms occur in 5 to 10% of patients, but the majority of these are transient—responding to steroid therapy. Permanent complications are rare (2 to 4%). The most significant predictors of radiation-induced complications are AVM volume, lesion location, and dose. Asymptomatic MRI changes are not uncommon.

REFERENCES

1. Brown RD, Wiebers DO, Forbes G. The natural history of unruptured intracranial arteriovenous malformations. J Neurosurg 1988; 68:352–357
2. Crawford PM, West CR, Chadwick DW. Arteriovenous malformations of the brain: natural history in unoperated patients. J Neurol Neurosurg Psychiatry 1986;49:1–10
3. Fults D, Kelly DL Jr. Natural history of arteriovenous malformations of the brain: a clinical study. Neurosurgery 1984;15:658–662
4. Graf CJ, Perret GE, Torner JC. Bleeding from cerebral arteriovenous malformations as part of their natural history. J Neurosurg 1983; 58:331–337
5. Ondra SL, Troupp H, George ED, et al. The natural history of symptomatic arteriovenous malformations of the brain: a 24-year follow-up assessment. J Neurosurg 1990;73:387–391
6. Chang SD, Shuster DL, Steinberg GK, Levy RP, Frankel K. Stereotactic radiosurgery of arteriovenous malformations: pathologic changes in resected tissue. Clin Neuropathol 1997;16: 111–116
7. Ogilvy CS. Radiation therapy for arteriovenous malformations: a review. Neurosurgery 1990;26:725–735
8. Schneider BF, Eberhard DA, Steiner LE. Histopathology of arteriovenous malformation after gamma knife radiosurgery [see comments]. J Neurosurg 1997;87:352–357
9. Szeifert GT, Kemeny AA, Timperley WR, Forster DM. The potential role of myofibroblasts in the obliteration of arteriovenous malformations after radiosurgery. Neurosurgery 1997;40:61–66
10. Yamamoto M, Jimbo M, Kobayashi M, et al. Long-term results of radiosurgery for arteriovenous malformation: neurodiagnostic imaging and histological studies of angiographically confirmed nidus obliteration. Surg Neurol 1992;37:219–230
11. Friedman WA, Buatti JM, Bova FJ, et al. LINAC Radiosurgery: A Practical Guide. Berlin: Springer-Verlag; 1988
12. Bova FJ, Friedman WA. Stereotactic angiography: an inadequate database for radiosurgery? Int J Radiat Oncol Biol Phys 1991;20: 891–895
13. Spiegelmann R, Friedman WA, Bova FJ. Limitations of angiographic target localization in radiosurgical treatment planning. Neurosurgery 1992;30:619–624
14. Betti OO, Munari C, Rosler R. Stereotactic radiosurgery with the linear accelerator: treatment of arteriovenous malformations. Neurosurgery 1989;24:311–321
15. Colombo F, Benedetti A, Pozza F, et al. Linear accelerator radiosurgery of cerebral arteriovenous malformations. Neurosurgery 1989;24:833–840
16. Colombo F, Pozza F, Chierego G, et al. Linear accelerator radiosurgery of cerebral arteriovenous malformations: an update. Neurosurgery 1994;34:14–21

17. Karlsson B, Lindquist C, Steiner L. Prediction of obliteration after gamma knife surgery for cerebral arteriovenous malformations. Neurosurgery 1997;40:425–431

18. Kemeny AA, Dias PS, Forster DM. Results of stereotactic radiosurgery of arteriovenous malformations: an analysis of 52 cases. J Neurol Neurosurg Psychiatry 1989;52:554–559

19. Loeffler JS, Alexander EI, Siddon RL, et al. Stereotactic radiosurgery for intracranial arteriovenous malformations using a standard linear accelerator. Int J Radiat Oncol Biol Phys 1989;17:673–677

20. Lunsford LD, Kondziolka D, Flickinger JC, et al. Stereotactic radiosurgery for arteriovenous malformations of the brain. J Neurosurg 1991;75:512–524

21. Pollock BE, Flickinger JC, Lunsford LD, Maitz A, Kondziolka D. Factors associated with successful arteriovenous malformation radiosurgery. Neurosurgery 1998;42:1239–1247

22. Pollock BE, Lunsford LD, Kondziolka D, et al. Patient outcomes after stereotactic radiosurgery for "operable" arteriovenous malformations. Neurosurgery 1994;35:1–8

23. Souhami L, Olivier A, Podgorsak EB, et al. Radiosurgery of cerebral arteriovenous malformations with they dynamic stereotactic irradiation. Int J Radiat Oncol Biol Phys 1990;19:775–782

24. Statham P, Macpherson P, Johnston R, et al. Cerebral radiation necrosis complicating stereotactic radiosurgery for arteriovenous malformation. J Neurol Neurosurg Psychiatry 1990;53:476–479

25. Steinberg GK, Fabrikant JI, Marks MP, et al. Stereotactic heavy-charged particle Bragg peak radiation for intracranial arteriovenous malformations. N Engl J Med 1990;323:96–101

26. Steiner L. Treatment of arteriovenous malformations by radiosurgery. In: Wilson CB, Stein BM, eds. Intracranial Arteriovenous Malformations. Baltimore/London: Williams and Wilkins; 1984:295–313

27. Steiner L. Radiosurgery in cerebral arteriovenous malformations. In: Fein JM, Flamm ES, eds. Cerebrovascular Surgery. Vol 4. Wien/New York: Springer-Verlag; 1985:1161–1215

28. Steiner L, Leksell L, Greitz T, et al. Stereotaxic radiosurgery for cerebral arteriovenous malformations: report of a case. Acta Chir Scand 1972;138:459–464

29. Yamamoto M, Jimbo M, Hara M, et al. Gamma knife radiosurgery for arteriovenous malformations: long-term follow-up results focusing on complications occurring more than 5 years after irradiation. Neurosurgery 1996;38:906–914

30. Yamamoto M, Jimbo M, Ide M, et al. Long-term follow-up of radiosurgically treated arteriovenous malformation in children: report of nine cases. Surg Neurol 1992;38:95–100

31. Baumann GS, Wara WM, Larson DA, et al. Gamma knife radiosurgery in children [abstract]. Pediatr Neurosurg 1996;24:193–201

32. Kondziolka D, Lunsford LD, Flickinger JC. Stereotactic radiosurgery in children and adolescents [abstract]. Pediatr Neurosurg 1990-91;16:219–221

33. Tanaka T, Kobayashi T, Kida Y, et al. Comparison between adult and pediatric arteriovenous malformations treated by gamma knife radiosurgery [abstract]. Stereotact Funct Neurosurg 1996;66:288–295

34. Ellis TL, Friedman WA, Bova FJ, Kubilis PS, Buatti JM. Analysis of treatment failure after radiosurgery for arteriovenous malformations. J Neurosurg 1998;89:104–110

35. Flickinger JC, Pollock BE, Konziolka D, et al. A dose-response analysis of arteriovenous malformation obliteration after radiosurgery. Int J Radiat Oncol Biol Phys 1996;36:873–879

36. Pollock BE, Kondziolka D, Lunsford LD, Bissonette D, Flickinger JC. Repeat stereotactic radiosurgery of arteriovenous malformations:

factors associated with incomplete obliteration. Neurosurgery 1996;38:318–323

37. Touboul E, Al Halabi A, Buffat L, et al. Single fraction stereotactic radiotherapy: a dose-response analysis of arteriovenous malformation obliteration. Int J Radiat Oncol Biol Phys 1998;41:855–861

38. Karlsson B, Lindquist C, Kihlstrom L, et al. Gamma knife surgery for AVM offers partial protection from hemorrhage prior to obliteration [abstract]. AANS Program Book 142, AANS Annual Meeting 1996

39. Kjellberg RN. Stereotactic Bragg peak proton beam radiosurgery for cerebral arteriovenous malformations. Ann Clin Res 1986;18(Suppl 47):17–19

40. Kjellberg RN, Hanamura T, Davis KR, et al. Bragg-peak proton-beam therapy for arteriovenous malformations of the brain. N Engl J Med 1983;309:269–274

41. Seifert V, Stolke D, Mehdorn HM, et al. Clinical and radiological evaluation of long-term results of stereotactic proton beam radiosurgery in patients with cerebral arteriovenous malformations. J Neurosurg 1994;81:683–689

42. Steiner L, Lindquist C, Adler JR, et al. Clinical outcome of radiosurgery for cerebral arteriovenous malformations. J Neurosurg 1992;77:1–8

43. Friedman WA, Blatt DL, Bova FJ, et al. The risk of hemorrhage after radiosurgery for arteriovenous malformations. J Neurosurg 1996;84:912–919

44. Pollock BE, Flickinger JC, Lunsford LD, et al. Hemorrhage risk after stereotactic radiosurgery of cerebral arteriovenous malformations. Neurosurgery 1996;38:652–661

45. Pollock BE, Flickinger JC, Lunsford LD, et al. Factors that predict the bleeding risk of cerebral arteriovenous malformations. Stroke 1996;27:1–6

46. Alexander E 3rd, Siddon RL, Loeffler JS. The acute onset of nausea and vomiting following stereotactic radiosurgery: correlation with total dose to area postrema. Surg Neurol 1989;32:40–44

47. Flickinger JC, Kondziolka D, Maitz AH, Lunsford LD. Analysis of neurological sequelae from radiosurgery of arteriovenous malformations: how location affects outcome. Int J Radiat Oncol Biol Phys 1998;40:273–278

48. Flickinger JC. An integrated logistic formula for prediction of complications from radiosurgery. Int J Radiat Oncol Biol Phys 1989;17:879–885

49. Flickinger JC, Schell MC, Larson DA. Estimation of complications for linear accelerator radiosurgery with the integrated logistic formula. Int J Radiat Oncol Biol Phys 1990;19:143–148

50. Kjellberg RN, Abbe M. Sterotactic Bragg peak proton beam therapy. In: Lunsford LD, ed. Modern Stereotactic Neurosurgery. Boston: Martinus Nijhoff; 1988:463–470

51. Karlsson B, Lax I, Soderman M. Factors influencing the risk for complications following gamma knife radiosurgery of cerebral arteriovenous malformations. Radiother Oncol 1997;43:275–280

52. Flickinger JC, Kondziolka D, Pollock BE, Maitz AH, Lunsford LD. Complications from arteriovenous malformation radiosurgery: multivariate analysis and risk modeling. Int J Radiat Oncol Biol Phys 1997;38:485–490

53. Kihlstrom L, Guo WY, Karlsson B, Lindquist C, Lindqvist M. Magnetic resonance imaging of obliterated arteriovenous malformations up to 23 years after radiosurgery [see comments]. J Neurosurg 1997;86:589–593

54. Marks MP, Delapaz RL, Fabrikant JI, et al. Intracranial vascular malformations: imaging of charged-particle radiosurgery, I: Results of therapy. Radiology 1988;168:447–455

▪ SECTION III ▪

Endovascular Treatments

13

Endovascular Treatment of Cerebral Aneurysms in Children

MICHAEL J. ALEXANDER

Although pediatric cerebral aneurysms are rare, their morphology and size can make them some of the more challenging aneurysms to treat. Aneurysms in children are more likely to be larger, dysmorphic, wide necked, and in less common locations.[1] Cerebral aneurysms at a young age are more likely to reflect an underlying connective tissue disorder or other vascular pathology.[2–5] Therefore successful treatment of these patients involves not only treating the aneurysm or aneurysms but also investigating the primary pathology.

As in adults, all ruptured cerebral aneurysms in children in which there is a reasonable chance of survival mandate therapy, either surgical or endovascular. This is due to the high morbidity and mortality associated with rerupture. Most unruptured aneurysms in children should also be highly considered for treatment because the number of years at risk for bleed is very high in these patients unless there is a severe underlying systemic disease that precludes treatment.

The basic treatment options for pediatric cerebral aneurysms are surgical, endovascular, or combined therapies. Because of the typically complex nature of pediatric cerebral aneurysms, these are best managed at tertiary care centers with an experienced neurovascular team to provide comprehensive treatment and management. This team should include a proficient neurovascular surgeon, a neurointerventionalist, a pediatric critical care intensivist, preferably with neurovascular experience, and a well-trained neuroanesthesia team.

Recent studies such as the International Subarachnoid Aneurysm Trial (ISAT trial) have lent more support for aneurysm embolization as a primary therapy for ruptured aneurysms.[6] Although this trial was performed in adults, it showed that there was a reduction in risk of the procedure (judged by modified Rankin scores) by 6.9% of majority morbidity and mortality in embolized patients, compared with those who had surgical clipping of their ruptured aneurysms. ISAT was the first prospective, randomized, multicenter trial that compared embolization to surgery for ruptured cerebral aneurysms. This study of 2143 patients showed a statistically significant reduction in death and dependency at 1 year in the embolized patients. The durability of coil embolization has been questioned by some, but in the long-term analysis of the ISAT patients, with over 8000 patient-years' follow-up data, it has been calculated that the benefit of the decreased morbidity/mortality in the endovascular group is not overshadowed by the rebleeding rate morbidity for a mean of over 70 years posttreatment.[7] Although it is difficult to extrapolate these data to children, this does imply that embolization should be a safe and effective treatment, even for the pediatric patient.

■ Aneurysm Embolization Principles

Cerebral aneurysms may occur in varied locations (anterior and posterior circulation), their relation to the artery may vary (sidewall vs bifurcation), their size may range from small to giant, their morphology may differ (saccular, fusiform, bilobed, etc.), and their presentation may differ (ruptured, mass effect, incidental). However, despite these multiple factors, the principles for embolization remain fairly constant.

First, all of our cerebral aneurysm embolization procedures performed in children are done under general anesthesia. Arterial access is obtained with a micropuncture needle. A 5 French femoral sheath is placed and a 5 French guide catheter is used for embolization. In some larger teenagers a 6 French guide catheter may be used, but a 5 French guide catheter is used in children, primarily due to the size of the arteries. Once access is obtained, we administer systemic intravenous heparin to obtain an activated clotting time in the 250 to 300 second range. Patients in which a stent placement is anticipated are loaded with antiplatelet medication in advance. A platelet function assay (PFA-100) is normally obtained prior to the procedure to ensure adequate antiplatelet effect.

The key to successful aneurysm embolization is to have an appropriate embolization plan based on the aneurysm size, location, and morphology. This plan may involve primary aneurysm embolization, balloon or stent assistance, parent artery occlusion, or other treatments. These treatment paradigms are discussed in further detail in the following sections.

■ Standard Coil Embolization Therapy

For cerebral aneurysms where the neck is not wide (<4 mm, and dome to neck ratio ≥2:1), and where the aneurysm is not integrally involved with a branch off the parent artery, standard coil embolization may be possible (**Fig. 13–1**). This is predicated on the fact that the neck of the aneurysm can be easily visualized and distinguished from the surrounding parent artery and branch vessels. Seeking the best embolization working view is often best accomplished by performing three-dimensional (3D) rotational angiography. Once the best working view is established, a microcatheter is advanced into the aneurysm dome under magnified roadmap guidance. The ideal catheter position is initially in the superior two thirds of the aneurysm but not against the aneurysm wall. A preshaped or steamed curve on the microcatheter may help stabilize the position within the aneurysm.

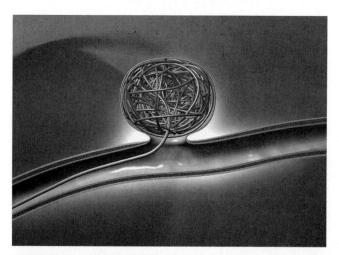

FIGURE 13–1 A traditional saccular aneurysm with a small neck (<4 mm) and a dome to neck ratio of ≥2:1 is a good candidate for primary coil embolization without adjunctive devices (see Color Plate 13–1).

Once the microcatheter is in position, an initial framing coil is used to provide a basket framework for the 3D circumference of the aneurysm. Subsequent to placing this coil, additional coils are then placed to fill the remainder of the aneurysm. Intraprocedural follow-up angiograms may be performed through the guide catheter during the embolization to assess the progress of the aneurysm filling. However, an angiogram is not necessary after each coil placement if the outer margin of the coils is unchanged because efforts must be made to keep the contrast load appropriate for the child's weight.

Aneurysms of the posterior circulation may be well suited for embolization in children, as in adults, because the morbidity associated with open surgery in posterior circulation aneurysms may be fairly high.[8–11] Open surgical treatment of posterior circulation aneurysms generally carries a higher risk for postoperative cranial nerve deficits, perforator infarctions, and other complications, such as cerebrospinal fluid leaks. In posterior circulation aneurysms with a relatively small neck, embolization avoids many of these complications. Similarly, aneurysms with aberrant anatomy or located at the skull base of the anterior circulation may be more easily dealt with via an endovascular approach.[12,13] The surgical approach to such aneurysms may require extensive bony dissection at the skull base, and may risk cranial nerves as in the posterior circulation. In such cases, again embolization may avoid many of the potential risks of surgery, particularly given that there are no significant perforator arteries in the petrous and cavernous carotid arteries, and the risk of aneurysm perforation during coiling of these extradural carotid aneurysms is minimal.

If the aneurysm is wide necked, a two-microcatheter technique may be employed to bridge the wide neck with two complex coils at the same time.[14] This may be more difficult to achieve in pediatric patients because either a larger shuttle-type guiding catheter is necessary or two separate guiding catheters, one for each microcatheter. Due to the smaller size of the pediatric vessels, this may be impractical. Likewise, this technique is often most safely performed with the assistance of a balloon in the parent artery.

A variety of coil systems currently exist on the market from a variety of vendors. Bare platinum coils have been the standard for many years since the development of the Guglielmi Detachable Coil (GDC) (Boston Scientific–Neurovascular, Fremont, CA) in the early 1990s. Since then, other bare platinum coils were introduced by Micrus Corporation (Sunnyvale, CA), Cordis Neurovascular (Miami Lakes, FL), Micro Therapeutics, Inc. (Irvine, CA), and MicroVention, Inc. (Aliso Viejo, CA).

PEARL   Bioactive coils used in aneurysm embolization may reduce long-term aneurysm recanalization and regrowth.

In 2002, Boston Scientific (Natick, MA) introduced the first polymer-coated coils in an effort to increase the healing response within the embolized aneurysms. Although bare platinum coils had been shown to be very safe, the long-term pathological studies demonstrated minimal healing across the neck of aneurysms embolized with bare platinum coils. It is thought that this lack of healing permitted delayed aneurysm recanalization or regrowth. The development of bioactive coils has been an attempt to augment the body's own healing response to promote increased healing and reduce long-term aneurysm recanalization or regrowth. The Matrix coil by Boston Scientific is a polyglycolic polylactic acid copolymer–coated coil. MicroVention has developed a polymer-coated Hydrocoil, which has an expanding hydrogel coating designed to increase the packing density of coiled aneurysms. And more recently, Micrus has introduced the Cerecyte coil, which has its polymer contained within the wrap of the platinum coil.

■ Balloon Assistance

When the neck of the aneurysm is somewhat wider (**Fig. 13–2**), balloon remodeling may be advisable. In this situation, a very compliant balloon, sized closely with the parent artery size, is inflated during the delivery of the coils into the aneurysm, a technique popularized by Moret and others.[15,16] As more coils are delivered into the aneurysm, there is complexity of the coils intertwining. By temporary inflation of the balloon during coil delivery into the aneurysm, there is remodeling of the coils at the neck of the aneurysm to conform to the curvature of the artery inner lumen. Creative balloon use is also possible at bifurcation aneurysms in which a "kissing balloon" technique may be used. In this situation, two balloons are used, one inflated in each branch artery of the bifurcation to remodel a complex neck. Use of balloon assistance in aneurysm embolization requires either the use of a large shuttle-type catheter to fit both the microcatheter and the balloon, or bifemoral access utilizing one guide catheter for the microcatheter and one guide catheter for the balloon.

The advantage of the balloon-assisted technique is that it generally does not require antiplatelet therapy following the procedure as is necessary in stent-assisted coiling. The disadvantage of the balloon remodeling technique is that is does not protect against delayed coil herniation once the balloon or the microwire is removed as a stent does. There have also been some reports of a higher incidence of embolic complications using a balloon compared with a standard aneurysm embolization.[17,18] It is unclear whether balloon assistance carries a higher risk of intraprocedural aneurysm rupture. Nevertheless, this is a widely used technique that has excellent applications in the aneurysm with an intermediate-sized neck.

■ Stent Assistance

When an aneurysm neck is very wide, the use of balloon assistance may not be feasible, but the use of stent assistance may allow for successful coil embolization. Even if the neck to dome ratio is 1:1, coil embolization can still be performed if a stent is used to contain the coils within the aneurysm. Stent-assisted aneurysm coiling may also allow for higher packing density of the aneurysm with coils and may, in fact, redirect flow from the aneurysm toward laminar flow in the parent artery.

Prior to the development of dedicated intracranial stents made of nitinol, balloon-expandable coronary stents were used to bridge wide-neck aneurysms for stent-assisted coiling. Cohen and colleagues have described balloon-expandable stent-assisted coiling of a large cavernous aneurysm in a 3-year-old child with excellent 2-year follow-up angiography.[13] These coronary stents do provide an option for wide-neck aneurysms, particularly close to the skull base; however, their stiffness and limited sizes limit their use.

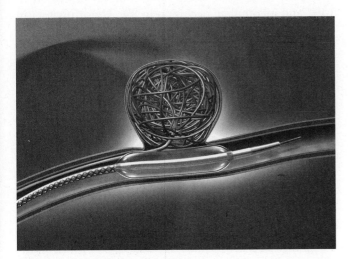

FIGURE 13–2 Balloon assistance may be used with a compliant balloon for short intervals during the embolization of wider-necked aneurysms to place coils without herniation into the parent artery (see Color Plate 13–2).

> **PEARL** The use of stent assistance in aneurysm embolization not only allows for better aneurysm packing but may also redirect flow away from the aneurysm.

The development of self-expanding ultrathin nitinol stents specifically for the treatment of wide-neck cerebral

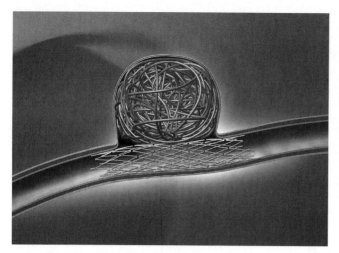

FIGURE 13–3 Stent assistance for very wide-necked aneurysms protects against coil herniation and may redirect blood flow to some degree (see Color Plate 13–3).

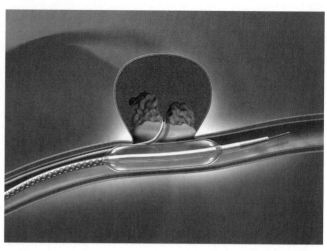

FIGURE 13–4 Balloon-assisted liquid polymer embolization. A fast-polymerizing embolic agent is used to embolize the aneurysm with intermittent balloon inflation (see Color Plate 13–4).

aneurysms was a revolution in the endovascular treatment of these complex aneurysms (**Fig. 13–3**). Like the coronary stents, these stents could be placed to cover the neck of the wide-neck aneurysm, then coil embolization of the sac of the aneurysm could proceed with more safety, although one would still need to guard against coil herniation into the parent artery.[19–21] However, unlike the coronary stents, these nitinol stents are extraordinarily flexible, more apt to treat aneurysms along a tight bend, and more trackable to distant locations in the cerebral circulation. Also, due to the self-expanding nature of the nitinol, these stents are less likely to perforate the artery with deployment. The long-term evaluation of these nitinol stents designed for aneurysms remains to be seen, but the midterm results at 1 to 2 years demonstrate these stents have much better patency rates than cerebral stents for atherosclerotic disease. In fact, a recent review of over 100 intracranial nitinol stents for aneurysm embolization with a mean follow-up of 12.1 months demonstrated a 98% patency rate.[22]

■ Balloon-Assisted Liquid Polymer Embolization

The development of quickly polymerizing nonadhesive polymers such as ethylene vinyl alcohol copolymer (Onyx, Micro Therapeutics, Inc., Irvine, CA) introduced the concept of polymer embolization without coils. In such situations, a protective balloon is inflated across the aneurysm neck while slow delivery of the liquid polymer is performed into the aneurysm via a microcatheter (**Fig. 13–4**). The liquid polymer is injected into the aneurysm gradually, in small aliquots, under balloon

protection while the liquid is polymerizing. The balloon is then deflated between injections to allow for cerebral perfusion intermittently during the procedure. This may be performed with or without stent assistance as well. The advantage of the liquid polymer is that it fills 100% of the aneurysm, versus coil systems, which generally fill only 20 to 60% of the aneurysm, relying on thrombosis to occur in the residual. The other advantage of the liquid polymer is that it can conform to very wide necks or irregularly shaped aneurysms.

The Cerebral Aneurysm Multicenter European Onyx (CAMEO) trial[23] was a study to evaluate Onyx liquid polymer in intracranial aneurysms. The early analysis at midterm angiographic follow-up showed complete occlusion in 79% of aneurysms, subtotal occlusion in 13%, and incomplete occlusion in 8%. Unfortunately, in this early series, there was also an issue with inadvertent delayed parent artery occlusion, which occurred in 13% (9/71) of the cases with angiographic follow-up at 12 months, though not all of these were symptomatic.

Further refinements in liquid and solid polymer technology will certainly make an impact in this aneurysm treatment paradigm in the future. The goal is to find the combination of filling ability and healing potential (at the aneurysm neck), with minimal embolic complications and minimal potential for parent artery stenosis or occlusion.

■ Parent Artery Occlusion

When an aneurysm cannot be treated through endovascular therapy by any of the foregoing methods and is not a surgical candidate, parent artery occlusion is an alternative

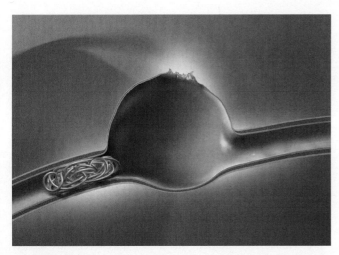

FIGURE 13–5 In parent artery occlusion for fusiform and giant aneurysms, the artery is either occluded proximally or is occluded proximal and distal to the aneurysm and is effectively trapped (see Color Plate 13–5).

salvage therapy. Parent artery occlusion may be achieved by occluding the artery proximal to the aneurysm with coils or with detachable balloons (**Fig. 13–5**). This strategy is similar to the surgical treatment of Hunterian ligation (i.e., proximal ligation) and is typically used for large or giant fusiform aneurysms.

In adults, permanent parent artery occlusion is typically only performed after the patient has passed a temporary balloon test occlusion of the parent artery. In this procedure, the patient is tested clinically during the temporary occlusion, and is usually tested by some perfusion test such as single photon emission tomography (SPECT) directly following the temporary occlusion to ensure that parent artery occlusion will not lead to ischemia or stroke in the vascular territory of interest.[24] If the patient fails temporary balloon test occlusion, then typically an extracranial-intracranial (EC-IC) bypass procedure is performed prior to permanent occlusion of the artery.

PEARL Balloon test occlusion is possible in children if perfusion testing, such as SPECT, is utilized.

In children, particularly younger children, clinical testing during temporary balloon occlusion is not practical. However, perfusion testing such as SPECT is still possible, even if the child is under general anesthesia for the test. If the child fails balloon test occlusion, then EC-IC bypass is still an option for treatment, followed by parent artery occlusion. In fact, some long-term information of patients who had EC-IC bypasses as children demonstrates these bypasses may stay patent over many years, even with marked growth and increase in height of the patient.[25]

Unfortunately, the risk of thromboembolic stroke is higher in deliberate parent artery occlusion than in standard embolization due to the stasis of flow. We typically will keep patients on a heparin drip overnight following occlusion, and attempt to keep the systolic blood pressure 110 to 120% of the patient's normal systolic blood pressure for 24 hours to promote collateral blood flow. It has also been reported in children that parent artery occlusion at an early age may be associated with possible aneurysm development or growth in other locations due to rerouted high-flow collaterals.[26–28]

Mycotic aneurysms, which may occur in children with coexisting heart defects, are also a type of aneurysm that may be treated endovascularly with parent artery occlusion. Mycotic aneurysms that are ruptured or growing on intravenous antibiotic therapy are candidates for treatment. In these circumstances, the aneurysm and the artery segment just at the aneurysm are either coiled or occluded with a liquid polymer such as n-butyl cyanoacrylate. The aneurysm is typically at a distal branch in which the artery is only occluded segmentally so that pial collateral vessels may supply the more distal artery retrograde.

■ Covered Stent Therapy

Many aneurysms are either too wide necked or are too large or fusiform to be treated by conventional embolization strategies. These patients may benefit from the use of a polymer-based, covered stent graft. This intervention serves to occlude the aneurysm while maintaining the patency of the parent artery (**Fig. 13–6**). Historically, covered stent grafts have been developed

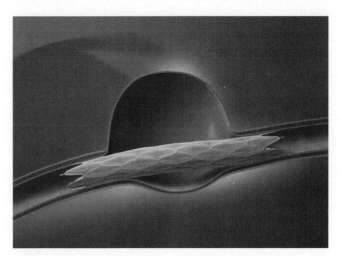

FIGURE 13–6 For fusiform or dissecting aneurysms or pseudoaneurysms in the neck or at the skull base, a covered stent graft may reconstruct the artery internally, excluding the aneurysm but also occluding adjacent perforators (see Color Plate 13–6).

for nonvascular pathologies such as tracheobronchial fistulas. However, over time, with the refinement of polymer and stent technologies, these stents have become available for intravascular use, primarily in the peripheral and coronary circulations.

Although no randomized trials have been performed utilizing this technology in the carotid or vertebral arteries, several case reports have demonstrated that this is a viable strategy in the neurovasculature. Alexander and coworkers were the first to describe the use of a self–expanding, nitinol-covered stent in the head for an iatrogenic pseudoaneurysm.[29] The Symbiot stent (Boston Scientific Scimed, Maple Grove, MN), used in this report, is an ePTFE polymer-covered stent based on a self-expanding nitinol platform. Less flexible, balloon-expandable, covered stents have also been reported for extracranial and intracranial aneurysms and pseudoaneurysms.[30–33] The JoStent by JoMed (Helsingborg, Sweden) is a balloon-expandable stainless steel stent within a stent construct, with a layer of ePTFE sandwiched between the stent layers. It was originally designed for coronary artery perforation treatment and is very stiff, but it has been used in the carotid and vertebral arteries for aneurysms, pseudoaneurysms, and fistulas as already noted. A benefit of these stent grafts is that they will usually exclude an aneurysm rupture, traumatic artery laceration, or dissection immediately. This can be a lifesaving therapy in patients who are actively bleeding. The incidence of endoleak is relatively rare with these stent grafts in the small arteries of the neurovasculature. But it is clear that these patients must be treated with an antiplatelet regimen postprocedurally to reduce the risk for acute stent graft thrombosis.

Covered stent grafts have limited use in that their primary role is at the skull base arteries. For arteries more distal in the anterior and posterior circulation, the occlusion of significant perforators by the stent graft becomes a significant issue. Therefore their use appears more promising in the carotid and vertebral arteries only.

■ Conclusions

Although pediatric cerebral aneurysms are very rare, they are usually challenging to treat. A tertiary or quaternary care hospital with an experienced multidisciplinary neurovascular team is best able to deal with these unusual aneurysms. Whether an individual child's aneurysm would best be treated by surgical, endovascular, or combined therapies is best decided based upon the aneurysm anatomy and an honest discussion of the risk factors by the surgeon and the interventionalist. Once treatment has been performed, these patients need close follow-up with magnetic resonance angiography or computed tomographic angiography of the treated aneurysm and potential de novo aneurysms because the development of a cerebral aneurysm at such a young age is typically a harbinger of future neurovascular problems.

REFERENCES

1. Humphreys RP, Hendrick EB, Hoffman HJ, Storrs BB. Childhood aneurysms: atypical features, atypical management. Concepts Pediatr Neurosurg 1985;6:213–229
2. Besbas N, Ozyurek E, Balkanci F, et al. Behçet's disease with severe arterial involvement in a child. Clin Rheumatol 2002;21:176–179
3. Vaicys C, Hunt CD, Heary RF. Ruptured intracranial aneurysm in an adolescent with Alport's syndrome: a new expression of type IV collagenopathy: case report. Surg Neurol 2000;54:68–72
4. Lilova MI, Petkov DL. Intracranial aneurysms in a child with autosomal recessive polycystic kidney disease. Pediatr Nephrol 2001;16:1030–1032
5. Diab KA, Richani R, Al Kutoubi A, Mikati M, Dbaibo GS, Bitar FF. Cerebral mycotic aneurysm in a child with Down's syndrome: a unique association. J Child Neurol 2001;16:868–870
6. Molyneux A, Kerr R, Stratton I, et al. International Subarachnoid Aneurysm Trial (ISAT) Collaborative Group. International Subarachnoid Aneurysm Trial (ISAT) of neurosurgical clipping versus endovascular coiling in 2143 patients with ruptured intracranial aneurysms: a randomised trial. Lancet 2002;360:1267–1274
7. Kerr R. New ISAT data. Presented at the AANS/CNS Cerebrovascular Section annual meeting. New Orleans, LA, February 2, 2005
8. Firat MM, Cekirge S, Saatci I, Akalan N, Balkanci F. Guglielmi detachable coil treatment of a partially thrombosed giant basilar artery aneurysm in a child. Neuroradiology 2000;42:142–144
9. Jones BV, Tomsick TA, Franz DN. Guglielmi detachable coil embolization of a giant midbasilar aneurysm in a 19-month-old patient. AJNR Am J Neuroradiol 2002;23:1145–1148
10. Hacein-Bey L, Muszynski CA, Varelas PN. Saccular aneurysm associated with posterior cerebral artery fenestration manifesting as a subarachnoid hemorrhage in a child. AJNR Am J Neuroradiol 2002;23:1291–1294
11. Massimi L, Moret J, Tamburrini G, Di Rocco C. Dissecting giant vertebro-basilar aneurysms. Childs Nerv Syst 2003;19:204–210
12. Al-Qahtani S, Tampieri D, Brassard R, Sirhan D, Mellanson D. Coil embolization of an aneurysm associated with an infraoptic anterior cerebral artery in a child. AJNR Am J Neuroradiol 2003;24:990–991
13. Cohen JE, Ferrario A, Ceratto R, Miranda C, Lylyk P. Reconstructive endovascular approach for a cavernous aneurysm in infancy. Neurol Res 2003;25:492–496
14. Baxter BW, Rosso D, Lownie SP. Double microcatheter technique for detachable coil treatment of large, wide-necked intracranial aneurysms. AJNR Am J Neuroradiol 1998;19:1176–1178
15. Moret J, Cognard C, Weill A, Castaings L, Rey A. Reconstruction technique in the treatment of wide-neck intracranial aneurysms: long-term angiographic and clinic results: apropos of 56 cases. J Neuroradiol 1997;24:30–44
16. Levy DI, Ku A. Balloon-assisted coil placement in wide-neck aneurysms: technical note. J Neurosurg 1997;86:724–727
17. Albayram S, Selcuk H, Kara B, et al. Thromboembolic events associated with balloon-assisted coil embolization: evaluation with diffusion-weighted MR imaging. AJNR Am J Neuroradiol 2004;25:1768–1777
18. Soeda A, Sakai N, Murao K, et al. Thromboembolic events associated with Guglielmi detachable coil embolization of asymptomatic cerebral aneurysms: evaluation of 66 consecutive cases with use of diffusion-weighted MR imaging. AJNR Am J Neuroradiol 2003;24:127–132

19. Benitez RP, Silva MT, Klem J, Veznedaroglu E, Rosenwasser RH. Endovascular occlusion of wide-necked aneurysms with a new intracranial microstent (Neuroform) and detachable coils. Neurosurgery 2004;54:1359–1367

20. Fiorella D, Albuquerque FC, Han P, McDougall CG. Preliminary experience using the Neuroform stent for the treatment of cerebral aneurysms. Neurosurgery 2004;54:6–16

21. Howington JU, Hanel RA, Harringan MR, Levy EI, Guterman LR, Hopkins LN. The Neuroform stent, the first microcatheter-delivered stent for use in the intracranial circulation. Neurosurgery 2004; 54:2–5

22. Alexander MJ, Zaidat OO, Tolbert M. Clinical outcome and technical feasibility of intracranial aneurysm therapy using Neuroform stent–assisted coil embolization [abstract]. J Neurosurg 2005; 102:A421

23. Molyneux AJ, Cekirge S, Saatci I, Gal G. Cerebral aneurysm multicenter European Onyx (CAMEO) trial: results of a prospective observational study in 20 European centers. AJNR Am J Neuroradiol 2004;25:39–51

24. Eckard DA, Purdy PD, Bonte FJ. Temporary balloon occlusion of the carotid artery combined with brain blood flow imaging as a test to predict tolerance prior to permanent carotid sacrifice. AJNR Am J Neuroradiol 1992;13:1565–1569

25. Zhang YJ, Barrow DL, Day AL. Extracranial-intracranial vein graft bypass for giant intracranial aneurysm surgery for pediatric patients: two technical case reports. Neurosurgery 2002;50:663–668

26. Yousaf I, Gray WJ, McKinstry CS, Choudhari KA. Development of posterior circulation aneurysm in association with bilateral internal carotid artery occlusion. Br J Neurosurg 2003;17: 471–472

27. Kaspera W, Majchrzak H, Kopera M, Ladzinski P. "True" aneurysm of the posterior communicating artery as a possible effect of collateral circulation in a patient with occlusion of the internal carotid artery: a case study and literature review. Minim Invasive Neurosurg 2002;45:240–244

28. Wolf RL, Imbesi SG, Galetta SL, Hurst RW, Sinson GP, Grossman RI. Development of a posterior cerebral artery aneurysm subsequent to occlusion of the contralateral internal carotid artery for giant cavernous aneurysm. Neuroradiology 2002;44:443–446

29. Alexander MJ, Smith TP, Tucci DL. Treatment of an iatrogenic petrous carotid artery pseudoaneurysm with a Symbiot covered stent: technical case report. Neurosurgery 2002;50:658–662

30. Saatci I, Cekirge HS, Ozturk MH, et al. Treatment of internal carotid artery aneurysms with a covered stent: experience in 24 patients with midterm follow-up results. AJNR Am J Neuroradiol 2004;25:1742–1749

31. Blasco J, Macho JM, Burrel M, Real MI, Romero M, Montana X. Endovascular treatment of a giant intracranial aneurysm with a stent-graft. J Vasc Interv Radiol 2004;15:1145–1149

32. Felber S, Henkes H, Weber W, Miloslavski E, Brew S, Kuhne D. Treatment of extracranial and intracranial aneurysms and arteriovenous fistulae using stent grafts. Neurosurgery 2004;55: 631–639

33. Burbelko MA, Dzyak LA, Zorin NA, Grigoruk SP, Golyk VA. Stent-graft placement for wide-neck aneurysm of the vertebrobasilar junction. AJNR Am J Neuroradiol 2004;25:608–610

14

Endovascular Treatment of Cerebral Arteriovenous Fistulas in Children

JAMES E. LEFLER AND VAN V. HALBACH

Pediatric neurovascular disease represents a large and diverse group of pathological entities involving the central nervous system. When compared with the adult population, pediatric neurovascular disease is relatively uncommon and, for several reasons, deserves special consideration. First and foremost, these pathological entities are usually different from those found in adults. Second, with regard to infants and children, the diagnostic evaluation and intervention are dramatically different from those for adults. Although pediatric cerebrovascular disease can be divided into conditions that result in intracranial hemorrhage and occlusive vascular disease, this chapter focuses on the former, with particular attention to pediatric dural arteriovenous malformations and fistulas, including the associated diagnostic and therapeutic options available for each entity.

■ Dural Arteriovenous Fistulas

Definition

Dural arteriovenous fistulas (AVFs) are defined as abnormal intracranial arteriovenous shunts within the substance of the dura mater, more specifically involving the walls of a dural sinus or an adjacent cortical vein.[1,2] Classically named for the involved sinus these are more commonly considered acquired lesions[3] and are usually found in middle-aged or older adults. The term *fistula* is used to differentiate this entity from arteriovenous malformation (AVM), which is a congenital abnormal tangle of vessels within brain parenchyma that is supplied by pial rather than dural feeding arteries and therefore does not involve a dural surface. Instead of a discrete

nidus as in AVMs, diffuse dural AVFs are composed of diffuse network of numerous arteriovenous microfistulae.

Incidence

Dural AVMs are exceedingly rare in the pediatric population. Fewer than 75 cases have been reported in the literature to date.[4–17] The largest case series (11 patients) was reported by Garcia-Monaco et al[18] in 1991, and most recently, Kincaid et al[19] described endovascular therapy and outcomes in seven children. In adults dural AVFs represent ~10 to 15% of all arteriovenous lesions.[1] However, with regard to the pediatric population, these lesions represent a lower percentage (10%) of intracranial arteriovenous lesions.[19]

Etiology

In adults, dural fistulas are considered acquired lesions, usually the result of some degree of venous obstruction.[20] Moreover, the exact etiology of these fistulas is unknown and probably multifactorial. Some conditions that have been associated with dural AVFs include intracranial venous hypertension,[21] previous sinus thrombosis, thrombophlebitis, neurosurgical procedures, and cranial trauma.[1,3,22,23] A recurring theme has been the observation of dural sinus thrombosis before the development of a lateral sinus dural AVF in the location of a preexisting thrombus.[3,22,23] It is postulated that some insult to the dural vasculature or some thrombus within the dural sinus enlarges or stimulates growth of normally present microscopic arteriovenous shunts in the wall of the sinus. As these microscopic arteriovenous shunts enlarge over time a dural AVF develops. The link between dural fistula development and dural sinus thrombosis may be bidirectional because dural AVFs can present with thrombosis of the adjacent dural sinus or with partial thrombosis at the fistula site. Whether thrombosis adjacent to the fistulous site is related to flow conditions through the diseased vasculature or is the result of prior thrombosis that initially contributed to the fistula development is unknown.[2] In rodent models a causal relationship between venous hypertension and dural AVF genesis has been reproduced experimentally.[21] The authors demonstrated that with the production of venous hypertension in the absence of dural sinus thrombosis (creating carotid artery to

external jugular vein anastomosis) subsequent dural fistulas developed in 13 to 23% of animals. This experimental finding is best delineated clinically in a case report[24] describing sinus thrombosis with resultant venous hypertension initially angiographically negative for a dural fistula. This patient eventually developed a dural fistula proven on follow-up angiography (**Fig. 14–1**). Even though a correlation with dural sinus thrombosis and dural AVFs has been established a one to one relationship is not present. Other mechanisms for the development of dural AVFs must exist because most cases of dural thrombosis do not result in fistulae.[20] Regardless,

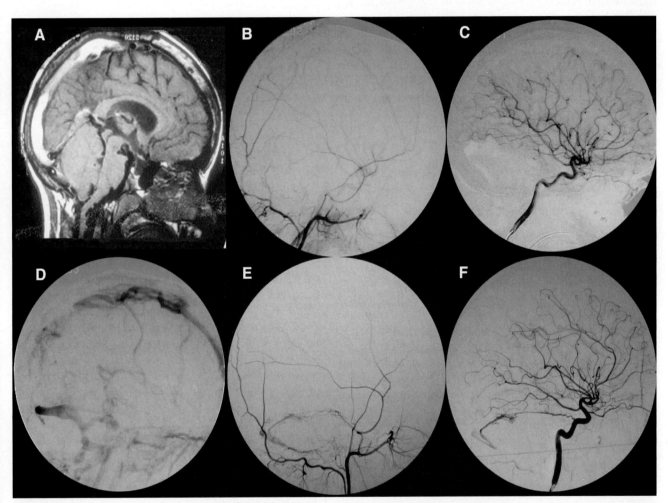

FIGURE 14–1 Acquired transverse-sigmoid dural arteriovenous fistula. A 12-year-old male with history of a fall from a tree presented with headache and pulsatile tinnitus and was worked up for a vascular anomaly. Initial magnetic resonance imaging (MRI) and angiogram demonstrated superior sagittal sinus thrombosis without evidence of a dural fistula. The patient returned 15 months later with acute onset of aphasia and hemiparesis. Repeat angiography demonstrated interval development of a transverse sigmoid dural arteriovenous fistula. **(A)** Sagittal T1-weighted MRI image of the head demonstrating T1 shortening (hyperintensity) involving the posterior aspect of the superior sagittal sinus consistent with acute thrombus.

(B) Initial angiogram demonstrating normal right external carotid angiographic anatomy. **(C)** Right internal carotid angiography (arterial phase) lateral projection was initially negative. **(D)** Right internal carotid angiography in lateral projection (venous phase) demonstrating thrombosis of the posterior aspect of the superior sagittal sinus. **(E)** Follow-up angiography 15 months later with right external carotid angiography demonstrating development of a transverse sigmoid dural arteriovenous fistula with supply via the posterior division of the middle meningeal artery. **(F)** Right internal carotid artery angiography on follow-up also revealed interval development of this fistula with additional supply from branches of the meningohypophyseal trunk.

patients with dural sinus thrombosis must be carefully followed clinically to exclude the possibility of the development of a dural fistula. A potential role of angiogenic growth factors has been postulated. In one study, basic fibroblast growth factor was shown to be present in surgical dural AVF specimens; however, it was absent in normal control patients.[25] This idea was expanded by Lawton et al in 1997[26] by measuring dural angiogenic activity in rodent models with iatrogenically induced fistulas. The findings suggest that the induction of venous hypertension or sinus thrombosis may alter the balance of angiogenic substances produced by the brain or dura. This alteration in angiogenic substances may be the causative final common pathway in the development of a fistula.[27,28]

In contrast to the acquired etiology, congenital causes to dural AVFs were proposed and theorized in the early literature.[29–31] The congenital theory resulted from several observations. These include reports of patients with dural fistulas with no prior development of sinus thrombosis or related dural insult and the presence of dural fistulas in neonates.[32] Opponents to the proposal of a congenital origin to dural AVFs state that most pediatric dural AVFs contain mature vasculature and are devoid of embryonic vascular patterns. Therefore some dural insult might have occurred in utero.[18,19] Currently, most feel dural AVFs are multifactorial in origin.

Pathological Findings

Only a relatively small number of detailed reports of the pathological findings associated with dural AVFs exist in the literature.[33–35] In one study, surgically excised specimens of dural AVFs demonstrated intimal thickening of the involved sinuses, arteries, and veins, with associated obliteration of the elastic lamina.[33] Stenosis of the sinus was more commonly the result of intimal thickening of the involved vasculature. Moreover, the site of the fistula involved the wall of the dural sinus and was not directly to the sinus itself.[2,33]

Clinical Presentation

The presenting symptoms of dural AVFs as well as their associated clinical signs are highly variable and depend upon several factors. The clinical presentation is heavily dependent on the location of the affected sinus and the pattern of venous drainage. Anterior cranial fossa and tentorial dural AVFs almost always drain into a cortical vein and are associated with a high degree of intracranial hemorrhage.[36,37] For example, in an adult, a transverse-sigmoid dural AVF with unobstructed venous flow usually presents with pulsatile tinnitus. When venous obstruction exists, patients can present with symptoms of venous infarction or intracranial hemorrhage due to impaired cortical venous drainage. Adults may present with other symptoms such as headache, impaired vision, mental deterioration, papilledema, and hemiparesis. In contrast, with regard to the pediatric population, the clinician must be keenly aware that a child may not complain of, nor view, pulsatile tinnitus as an abnormality because it may have been present since birth. A complete history and physical exam might elicit the findings by direct questioning in addition to auscultation around the location of the abnormality.

> **PEARL** Cardiac involvement, although essentially absent in adults, is more commonly seen in the pediatric age group and might be the sole presenting symptom of an intracranial AVF.

In children, clinical manifestations also vary by age as well as amount of the arteriovenous shunting. Cardiac involvement, although essentially absent in adults, is more commonly seen in the pediatric age group and might be the sole presenting symptom.[38] Furthermore, neonates usually demonstrate a larger degree of arteriovenous shunting and cardiac involvement when compared with their childhood and adult counterparts.[39] Neonates with dural fistulas can present in fulminant congestive heart failure whereas children with a lesser degree of shunting might only manifest with asymptomatic cardiomegaly found on a routine chest x-ray.[40] In general, neonates usually demonstrate systemic (cardiac) and cranial signs related to the shunt such as a heart murmur, heart failure, macrocephaly, and distended scalp veins whereas children may show neurological symptoms such as hydrocephalus and developmental delay.[5,39] Although exceedingly rare in children, a dural fistula occuring in the cavernous sinus presents with proptosis, chemosis, cranial bruit, increased intraocular pressure, diplopia, or diminished visual acuity.

Classification

Lasjaunias et al described a classification of dural fistulas based on age of presentation and severity of arteriovenous shunting.[5,39] The first group is a dural sinus malformation, usually presenting in the neonatal period with congestive heart failure. The second type is an infantile-type dural arteriovenous shunt, which more commonly presents in childhood. Third are the most common adult-type dural arteriovenous shunts.

The most common classification system used for dural AVFs involves a separation based on venous drainage away from the fistula. Djindjian et al[41] defined three types, with type 1 (low risk) draining via the ipsilateral sinus, type 2 (higher risk) draining toward the contralateral sinus, and type 3 (highest risk) draining via cortical veins. This classification system often allows one to predict the severity of presenting symptoms and risk of intraparenchymal hemorrhage. Type 1 patients usually present with headaches and bruits but rarely with neurological deficits or hemorrhage and are generally considered at low risk. Type 2 patients usually present with more severe symptoms, mostly related to increased intracranial pressure or papilledema. Type 3 patients are at greatest risk of intracranial hemorrhage or venous infarction. In one study, 44% of patients with dural AVFs and associated cortical venous drainage developed intracranial hemorrhage.[42] Some dural AVFs can spontaneously progress from a type 1 to either a type 2 or a type 3. The progression from thrombosis of venous drainage pathways can occur gradually or abruptly and is associated with a change in the patient's symptomatology. Close clinical follow-up is necessary and repeat angiography is essential if a patient with a known dural fistula develops new symptoms.

Location

At the authors' institution, one series[2,43] delineating the incidence of dural AVFs demonstrated the transverse and sigmoid sinus regions were the most common, representing 38% of the cases. The second most common site is the cavernous sinus region (34%). The remainder of locations include deep venous location (7%), superior petrosal sinus (5%), superior sagittal sinus (5%), ethmoidal sinus (4%), marginal sinus (4%), and inferior petrosal sinus (3%). Lesions affecting the occipital-suboccipital regions are reported to account for 50% of all dural AVFs.[44]

Radiological Evaluation

Pediatric dural AVFs are more commonly multifocal and generally demonstrate higher flow with larger connections when compared with adult dural AVFs.[7] Due to the bigger size of these arteriovenous shunts, the draining sinuses or veins are usually quite large and generally do not demonstrate cortical venous drainage. Sometimes the draining sinuses can be so massive they can be misinterpreted as extra-axial masses on imaging studies. In neonates with dural AVFs, classic signs of congestive heart failure might be present on a standard chest x-ray. These signs include cardiomegaly, pulmonary vascular congestion, and edema as well as cephalization of flow. Although not commonly performed for the evaluation of a dural fistula, plain film radiographs of the head might demonstrate widening of the middle meningeal grooves from high flow–induced arterial hypertrophy and enlargement of the sella secondary to elevated intracranial pressure.[45] If incidentally performed, Doppler ultrasound of the neck may demonstrate conversion from a normal high resistive pattern within the feeding external carotid system to a low resistive pattern normally observed in internal carotid circulation.

> **PEARL** Patients may develop irreversible brain injury when a dural fistula and resultant cerebral venous hypertension remain undiagnosed for a long period of time.

Radiological evaluation of the head in patients with dural AVFs tends to vary with age.[19] In adults with dural AVFs computed tomography (CT) of the head is frequently normal unless complicated by intracranial hemorrhage (intraparenchymal, subarachnoid, and, less commonly, subdural) or venous infarction. In neonates, an early presentation usually correlates with no radiographic or clinical brain injury. Therefore, the brain parenchyma is usually normal except for the enlarged venous structures (**Fig. 14–2**) related to the dural fistula, which can mimic an extra-axial mass and appear iso- to hyperdense. However, a higher percentage of patients develop irreversible brain injury when a dural fistula and resultant cerebral venous hypertension remain undiagnosed for a longer period of time. This irreversible brain injury manifests itself with dystrophic calcification in the brain parenchyma and white matter abnormalities such as thinning and demyelination.[19] Therefore, children with an undiagnosed long-standing dural fistula are more likely to present with signs and symptoms related to irreversible brain injury than neonates or recently diagnosed adults. Magnetic resonance imaging (MRI) in combination with ultrasound can reveal abnormally enlarged dural arteries, normal pial arteries, thrombosis of a dural sinus, and multiple serpentine vessels coursing through the brain parenchyma without a vascular nidus. MRI with its multiplanar capabilities can better delineate cerebellar tonsillar prolapse than CT. Cerebellar tonsillar prolapse, which has been described in children and neonates with dural fistulas, is usually the result of hydrovenous dysfunction of the posterior fossa and is reversible after therapy (**Fig. 14–1**). MRI is more sensitive for the evaluation of subtle white matter changes than CT. However, CT is better for the evaluation of parenchymal calcification and subarachnoid

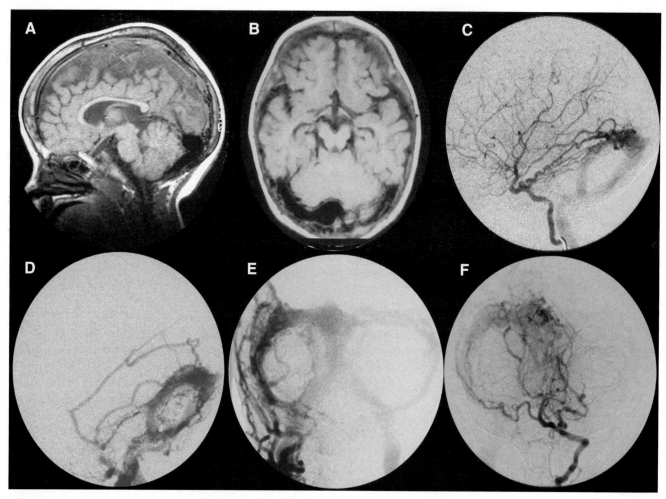

FIGURE 14–2 Childhood (congenital) transverse-sigmoid dural arteriovenous fistula. A 1-year-old female presented with increasing head circumference. The child was noted to have occipital scalp hemangioma and was neurologically normal. **(A)** Sagittal T1-weighted image demonstrates an enlarged and patent right transverse-sigmoid sinus with multiple serpentine flow voids surrounding this sinus. Structures at the foramen magnum are within normal limits without evidence of inferior tonsillar herniation. **(B)** Axial T1-weighted image through the posterior fossa also demonstrates the enlarged right transverse-sigmoid sinus with suggestion of arterial collaterals in this region. Note the prominent ventricles (dilatation of the temporal horns) and subarachnoid spaces more than likely the result of diminished cerebrospinal fluid resorption into the arterialized venous sinuses. **(C)** Right internal carotid angiogram (lateral projection) demonstrates enlarged meningohypophyseal trunk with supply to the fistula from the lateral (marginal) tentorial artery. Note the presence of an occipital sinus. **(D)** Right external carotid angiogram in the lateral projection also reveals abundant supply to the fistula from branches of the middle meningeal and occipital arteries. **(E)** Venous phase right external carotid angiogram demonstrates patent occipital sinus as well as both transverse-sigmoid sinuses. **(F)** Left vertebral artery injection (Towne's projection) shows supply from the posterior fossa through the posterior meningeal branches, both posterior inferior cerebellar arteries, and the right posterior cerebral artery.

hemorrhage. The evaluation of dural fistulas has broadened with improvements in magnetic resonance angiography (MRA) and magnetic resonance venography (MRV). MRA may demonstrate additional flow-related enhancement of serpentine vessels surrounding the site whereas MRV can evaluate for thrombosis of the recipient sinus. With regard to patient follow-up, MRI may serve as an adjunct when conventional angiography is not possible.

Conventional diagnostic cerebral angiography remains the gold standard and is mandatory for patients with suspected dural AVFs because MRI may be negative in some instances. A complete evaluation of the vasculature of the head and neck is required. This involves evaluation of common, internal, and external carotid systems as well as both vertebral arteries, including the extra- and intracranial segments. If necessary, injection

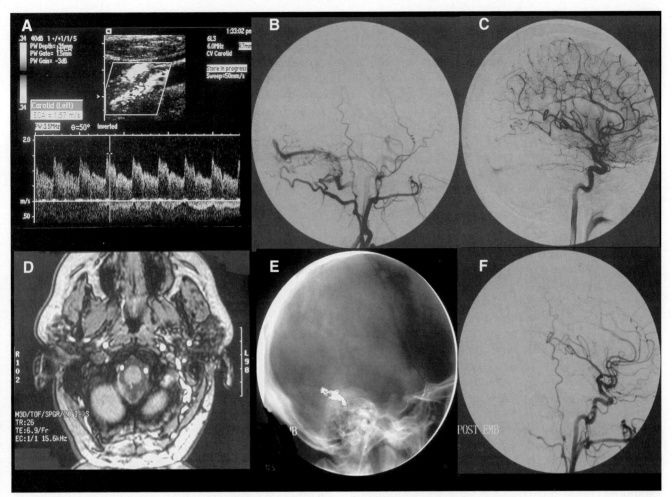

FIGURE 14–3 Transverse-sigmoid dural arteriovenous fistula. An 18-year-old female with a remote history of left occipital trauma presents with left-sided pulsatile tinnitus. **(A)** Doppler ultrasound of the left external carotid artery shows an abnormal low resistive waveform consistent with increased flow dynamics through this vessel. Note the external carotid waveform is typically a high-resistance pattern. **(B)** Lateral left external carotid angiogram (arterial phase) demonstrates a hypertrophied occipital artery, early arteriovenous shunting from transmastoid perforators of the occipital artery, as well as posterior division of the middle meningeal artery to a diseased segment of the sigmoid sinus. **(C)** Lateral projection left internal carotid arteriography reveals early arteriovenous shunting from tentorial arteries to the transverse-sigmoid sinus junction. **(B)** and **(C)** are consistent with a transverse-sigmoid dural arteriovenous fistula. **(D)** Partition image from a three-dimensional time-of-flight magnetic resonance angiogram demonstrates abnormal flow–related enhancement to the serpiginous vessels along the mastoid and occipital regions. **(E)** Scout film after transarterial (particulate agents) and later transvenous (fibered coils) embolization; platinum coils can be seen in the region of the diseased sigmoid sinus. **(F)** Postembolization left common carotid angiogram demonstrates no evidence of arteriovenous shunting consistent with thrombosis of the fistula. Patient after the procedure remained at neurological baseline and her tinnitus resolved.

of both thyrocervical or costocervical trunks might be indicated for evaluation of the neck or craniocervical junction.

Arterial Supply and Venous Drainage

Arterial supply and venous drainage patterns vary according to location of the fistula. Transverse sigmoid dural AVFs (**Fig. 14–3**) usually obtain their supply from the ipsilateral occipital artery (transmastoid perforators). Additional supply is via anterior and posterior divisions of the middle meningeal arteries, posterior auricular artery, neuromeningeal trunk of the ascending pharyngeal artery, posterior meningeal branches of the ipsilateral vertebral artery, as well as the meningohypophyseal trunk from the internal carotid artery. Venous drainage is variable and can be antegrade involving the ipsilateral sinus and depending upon the degree of sinus obstruction into the contralateral transverse sigmoid sinus or cortical veins. Arterial supply to superior sagittal sinus fistulas is via the coronal segments of either/both middle meningeal arteries or superficial temporal arteries. Additional supply can be via the anterior falcine artery of the ophthalmic artery and the posterior meningeal branch of the vertebral artery. Dural AVFs along the floor of the anterior cranial fossa (ethmoidal dural AVFs) achieve their blood supply from anterior and posterior ethmoidal branches of the ophthalmic artery and secondarily from the internal maxillary artery. Venous drainage from ethmoidal dural fistulas is usually through a pial vein commonly associated with a venous varix that is directed toward the superior sagittal sinus. Cavernous dural AVFs, although exceedingly rare in the pediatric population, can receive arterial supply from dural branches from the cavernous segment of the internal carotid artery (inferior lateral trunk, meningohypophyseal trunk) as well as distal internal maxillary artery branches, middle/accessory meningeal arteries, and distal branches of the ascending pharyngeal artery. Cavernous sinus dural fistulas drain into the superior ophthalmic vein, cavernous sinus, or cortical veins. Superior/inferior petrosal sinus dural fistulas and marginal sinus dural fistulas have variable supply from branches of the internal and external carotid arteries.

Treatment

In adults, therapeutic alternatives involving dural AVFs should be closely related to the patient's symptomatology, location of the fistula, pattern of venous drainage (high vs low risk), and benefits/risks of the treatment modality. With low-risk dural AVFs treatment is usually palliative, with the overall goal aimed at reduction in arteriovenous shunting. This is usually achieved by transarterial embolization with particulate agents. Treatment of high-risk dural AVFs, which can present with vision loss, hemorrhage, or infarction, should involve obliteration of the fistulous communication via endovascular or surgical routes. Most often some form of either definitive or adjunctive transvenous or transarterial endovascular therapy is utilized[46–48] (**Fig. 14–3**). Following preoperative embolization surgical obliteration could be required for definitive cure. Moreover, radiation therapy has been used in adults with localized slow flow lesions but should not be considered in children or neonates.[19,20]

In contrast with the adult population, therapy for dural AVFs in children must be performed with the understanding that these lesions are potentially life threatening because of their distinctive high-flow arteriovenous shunting.[5] The overall goal of therapy should be aimed at obliteration of the fistula. Several therapies exist and include endovascular treatment, surgical

resection, and compression therapy or a combination thereof. Compression therapy is usually reserved for highly motivated adult patients with low-risk dural fistulas located in the posterior fossa who have their primary arterial supply from the occipital artery. In one series at the authors' institution, compression therapy resulted in a reduction/thrombosis of the fistula in 27%.[49] The timing of therapy is also more critical in children and neonates when compared with adults, given the higher incidence of cardiac manifestations. For example, in a child with a large dural AVF who presents in congestive heart failure curative therapy might not be possible and therefore palliative embolization would be indicated. Palliative embolization may result in a reduction in congestive heart failure and allow for definitive embolization at a later date.

Endovascular alternatives, either as a definitive or an adjunctive treatment, are now largely used as the initial therapy.[2,19,45–49] However, in the pediatric population, appropriate medical management is necessary and often beneficial to the patient at the onset of cardiac manifestations.[19,40] Due to the persistence of a patent foramen ovale with some patients in the pediatric population, preembolization workup should include the need for right to left shunt studies. If a patient demonstrates a patent right to left shunt the chance of parodoxical embolus is a real consideration and can definitely change therapeutic alternatives. In the case of a persistent right to left shunt, embolization should be performed with coils rather than particulate agents (glue and polyvinyl alcohol) because coils have a diminished chance of delivery into the venous system, which could eventually reach the arterial system. Endovascular therapy should always be directed at the specific site of the lesion; more specifically, targeted toward the nidus if a cure is to be attained.[45] If a child has multiple fistulas endovascular therapy should be directed toward the site of the fistulous connection that correlates with the patient's symptoms.[19] Utilizing the endovascular technique, access to the nidus can be achieved from either a transarterial or a transvenous approach or both. Transarterial embolization is usually performed with particulate agents such as polyvinyl alcohol or a sclerosing agent such as absolute alcohol.[46] N-butyl cyanoacrylate liquid adhesive, a more permanent embolic, can also be used. If a more permanent agent is contemplated, care must be taken for embolization to occur at the fistulous site because proximal occlusion can be associated with a high rate of recurrence.[2,19,45,46] Transarterial embolization has been shown to be more effective in a focal fistula demonstrating reduced flow. Transvenous embolization with coils has proved to be more effective at closure of the fistula when the embolic agent is deposited at the fistula site. At our institution, transvenous embolization usually follows the transarterial approach. In some instances it may be

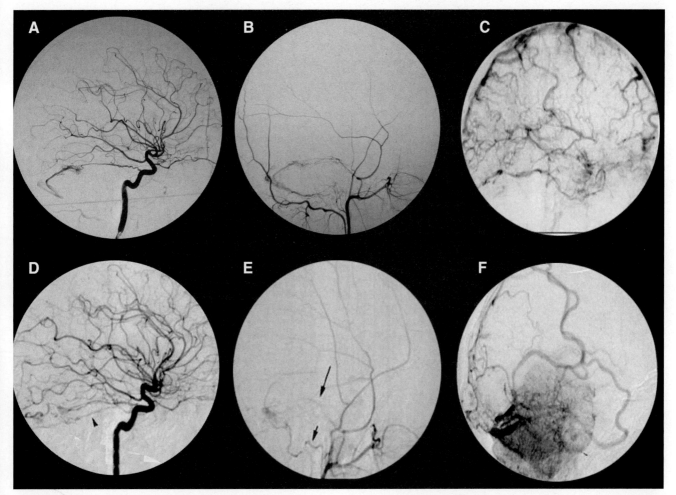

FIGURE 14–4 Endovascular recanalization with angioplasty and stenting for treatment of intracranial hypertension, Part 1. Same patient as Fig. 14–1. A 13-year-old male with history of a fall from a tree. The initial angiogram was negative when he presented with superior sagittal sinus thrombosis. The patient returned with aphasia and right hemiparesis and engorged scalp veins. Follow-up angiogram demonstrated a dural fistula involving each transverse sigmoid sinus. **(A)** Right internal carotid angiogram lateral projection demonstrates supply from the meningohypophyseal trunk. **(B)** Right external carotid angiogram shows supply to the fistula from the posterior division of the middle meningeal artery and neuromeningeal trunk of the ascending pharyngeal artery. **(C)** Right internal carotid angiogram (venous phase) in the lateral projection confirms venous sinus thrombosis in the posterior aspect of the superior sagittal sinus as well as both transverse sigmoid sinuses. Venous drainage is via cortical veins with diversion to the deep venous system and anteriorly into the cavernous sinus through transcortical pathways. **(D)** Left internal carotid digital subtraction angiography in the lateral projection shows supply to a left transverse sigmoid dural fistula from the meningohypophyseal trunk. **(E)** Left external carotid angiography reveals supply to the left-sided fistula from the posterior division of the middle meningeal artery and ascending pharyngeal artery (neuromeningeal trunk). **(F)** Left vertebral injection (venous phase–lateral projection) also better delineates the cortical as well as deep venous drainage.

necessary for complete closure of the involved recipient sinus; however, it is imperative not to secondarily occlude any cortical veins demonstrating a normal drainage pattern. In one case, angioplasty/stenting (**Figs. 14–4, 14–5,** and **14–6**) of a diseased sinus was performed for treatment of intracranial venous hypertension, which resulted in a reduction of shunting and improvement in symptoms.[24]

PEARL Transvenous embolization with coils has been shown to be more effective at closure of the fistula when the embolic agent is deposited at the fistula site.

Definitive cure can also be achieved by direct surgical resection. This is usually performed following transarterial

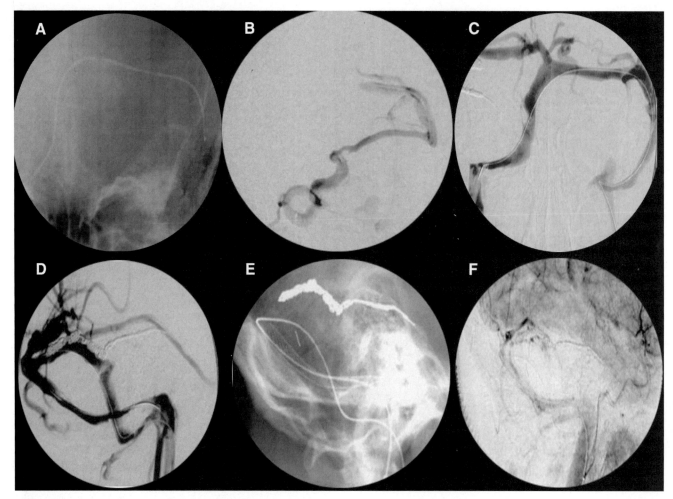

FIGURE 14–5 Endovascular recanalization with angioplasty and stenting for treatment of intracranial hypertension, Part 2. After transvenous and transarterial obliteration of the right-sided transverse-sigmoid dural fistula and angioplasty of the occipital and left transverse-sigmoid sinus (not shown) the patient was brought back to the neuroangiography operating room suite for worsening episodes of aphasia despite continued intravenous anticoagulation. Angiography (not shown) revealed reocclusion of the segments in which angioplasty had been performed. **(A)** Anteroposterior radiograph of the skull centered to the left demonstrates a microcatheter whose tip is located in the left transverse–sigmoid sinus junction. This microcatheter was from a transvenous femoral approach with a guiding catheter in the right jugular bulb and the microcatheter coursing from the occipital sinus through the torcular Herophili and into the diseased left transverse sinus. **(B)** Digital subtraction venography (Towne's projection) with distal injection of the microcatheter in the left transverse sinus revealing minimal flow through the largely thrombosed left transverse sinus. **(C,D)** Catheterization of the left internal jugular vein was performed utilizing a 300 cm exchange wire from a right internal jugular venous approach via the occipital sinus. Angioplasty of the occipital and left transverse-sigmoid sinus was subsequently performed over the guide wire. **(C)** Towne's and **(D)** lateral postangioplasty venography through the guiding catheter in the right internal jugular vein demonstrate significant improvement in venous outflow. **(E)** After angioplasty an 8 × 40 mm stent was deployed in the occipital sinus over the exchange wire. Lateral scout film demonstrating the stent in the occipital sinus. **(F)** Digital subtraction angiography of the left internal carotid artery (venous phase, lateral projection) demonstrates patency of the occipital sinus.

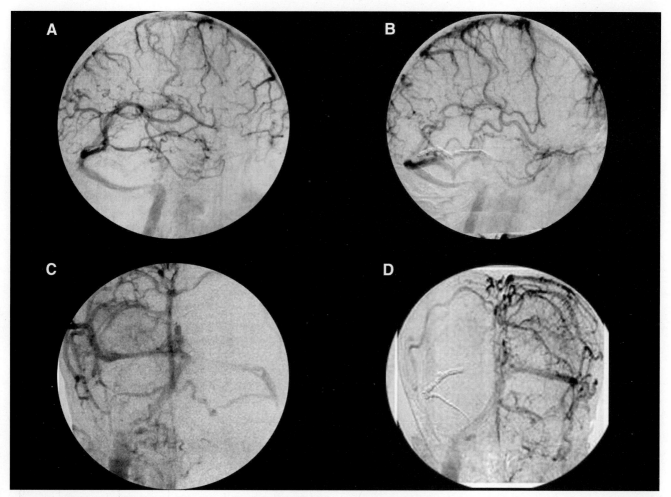

FIGURE 14–6 Endovascular recanalization with angioplasty and stenting for treatment of intracranial hypertension, Part 3. Follow-up digital subtraction angiography performed at 3 months after treatment. **(A)** Venous phase, right internal carotid angiography, lateral projection. **(B)** Venous phase, left internal carotid angiography, lateral projection. **(C)** Venous phase, right internal carotid angiography, anteroposterior (AP) projection. **(D)** Venous phase left internal carotid angiography, AP projection. These demonstrate continued patency of the stented occipital sinus, which constitutes the sole outflow among the major venous sinuses. Note that the left transverse sinus, which had previously undergone angioplasty, is now occluded.

embolization because surgical therapy without preoperative embolization is associated with a significant amount of blood loss. This operative blood loss is of particular concern to infants who are at more of a risk given their delicate volume status.[7,19] Various surgical techniques have been utilized and include ligation of feeding arteries, trapping/obliteration of the sinus, or excision/cauterization of the fistula.[5]

■ Carotid Cavernous Fistulas

Definition

A carotid cavernous fistula (CCF) is defined as a spontaneous or acquired abnormal arteriovenous communication between the cavernous segment of the internal carotid artery and the cavernous sinus. These can be further divided into direct or indirect fistulas. A direct CCF exists when the internal carotid artery communicates directly with the cavernous sinus and can be the result of trauma, ruptured cavernous artery aneurysm, collagen vascular anomalies, arterial dissection, or inadvertent surgical manipulation and is usually considered a high-flow lesion.[1,50–59] Indirect CCFs are low-flow lesions that consist of multiple dural arterial connections from the external and, to a lesser extent, internal carotid artery to the cavernous sinus. Several factors have been implicated in the development of indirect CCFs. Most are related to some degree of venous hypertension. Indirect (dural) CCFs are rare in children; therefore, the remainder of this section focuses on direct CCFs.

Pathophysiology

Direct CCFs are most commonly the result of trauma[50,54] and in children are usually caused by falls and penetrating injury.[60] Pathophysiologically, they occur when forces result in a laceration of the cavernous internal carotid artery with decompression of the high pressure arterial blood into the lower pressure cavernous sinus. This decompression with arterialization of the cavernous sinus can result in increased flow within surrounding venous structures, especially the superior ophthalmic vein. Clinically, this entity presents with pulsatile exophthalmos, bruit, headaches, and chemosis.[50,54,61] Diplopia can occur due to cranial nerve palsies or proptosis. Other less common presentations include intracranial hemorrhage, decreased visual acuity, blindness, epistaxis, progressive neurological deficits from cerebral steal, and hydrocephalus. The clinical signs and symptoms that characterize a hazardous CCF and represent an indication for urgent therapy include increased intracranial pressure, rapidly progressive proptosis, diminished visual acuity, hemorrhage, and transient ischemic attacks.[62]

Radiological Evaluation

Radiographic evaluation with CT and MRI in patients with CCFs usually demonstrates proptosis, engorgement of the ipsilateral cavernous sinus, and associated venous structures (superior ophthalmic vein and petrosal sinus). CT is more accurate in the assessment of surrounding bony structures if the condition is associated with trauma. MRI is more useful in evaluation of the surrounding brain parenchyma, optic nerves, and surrounding vasculature. Phase-contrast MRA may demonstrate reversal of flow away from the cavernous sinus on the affected side. High-resolution digital subtraction angiography can evaluate size, location, and number of fistulas; associated intracavernous aneurysms; patency of venous outflow pathways; associated risk factors (cortical venous drainage); and other vascular lesions. Angiography still remains the gold standard in evaluation of this condition.[1] Arterial phase of the cerebral angiogram usually demonstrates a high-flow fistula from the internal carotid artery to the cavernous sinus. The venous phase during cerebral angiography (**Fig. 14–7**) is excellent at establishing the pattern of venous drainage (ipsilateral or contralateral superior ophthalmic vein, superior or inferior petrosal sinus, and sphenoparietal sinus).

Treatment

Therapeutic alternatives for treatment of direct CCFs should involve obliteration of the arteriovenous fistulous site. Previous attempts at surgical ligation of the internal carotid artery were ineffective because of their inability to permanently close the arteriovenous communication. In one series, 67% of patients with direct CCFs treated with surgical ligation of the internal carotid artery failed to demonstrate improvement in cranial neuropathy.[63] Currently, direct neurosurgical therapy for this entity has largely been replaced by newer endovascular techniques.[63,64] These techniques generally involve closure of the fistula through a transarterial or transvenous approach. Transarterial balloon embolization is the preferred therapeutic treatment of choice and is curative in 90% of cases (**Fig. 14–7**). However, when the balloon cannot be manipulated into the necessary position transvenous or transarterial coil embolization might be utilized as adjunctive or curative therapy. The balloon can be filled with contrast that has the same osmolarity as blood or with a more permanent solidifying agent such as 2-hydroxyethyl methacrylate.[65] During embolization, preservation of the parent carotid artery is paramount. It is rarely necessary to occlude the internal carotid artery during therapy. However, if occlusion is necessary then temporary balloon test occlusion should be performed with provocative hypotensive neurological testing. If the endovascular approach is not feasible, surgical exposure of the cavernous sinus and packing with an embolic agent have been shown to be an effective alternative.[66] Carotid/jugular vein neck compressive therapy has been shown to be effective in treatment of smaller CCFs.[67] After endovascular therapy, some patients might develop worsening of presenting symptoms, which will generally resolve over several months.

■ Vertebral Arteriovenous Fistulas

Definition

Defined as an abnormal arteriovenous communication between the vertebral artery and the surrounding paravertebral venous plexus these are most commonly the result of trauma but congenital fistulas have been reported.[68–73] Additionally, some disease states such as neurofibromatosis type 1 may predispose patients to development of vertebral arteriovenous fistulas. Patients with vertebral AVFs can present with neck pain, a bruit, or posterior fossa transient ischemic episodes (secondary to vascular steal). Myelopathic or radiculopathic symptoms, if present, are usually the result of either mass effect from dilated venous structures compressing the cord and/or nerve roots, venous congestion or progressive arterial steal from the spinal column. Although uncommon, a patient with this condition might present with subarachnoid hemorrhage if rupture of a dilated medullary venous structure occurs. As with dural arteriovenous fistulas the pediatric patients may not complain of symptoms if the bruit has been present for a long time.

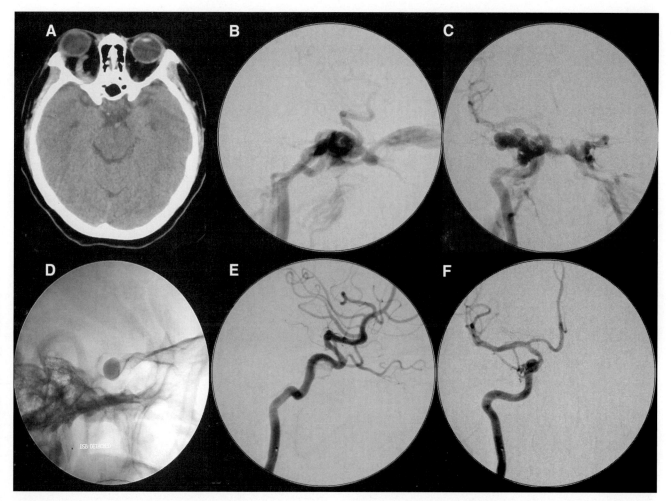

FIGURE 14–7 Direct carotid–cavernous fistula. A 17-year-old boy status post–motorcycle accident with multiple facial fractures developed worsening proptosis and chemosis. On physical exam an intracranial bruit could be auscultated. **(A)** Axial nonenhanced computed tomographic scan of the brain at the level of the cavernous sinus demonstrates right-sided proptosis as well as dilatation of the right superior ophthalmic vein (SOV). **(B)** Lateral image from right internal carotid injection shows antegrade flow within the carotid artery, filling of a direct right carotid cavernous fistula with subsequent retrograde filling of a dilated ipsilateral SOV, and antegrade filling of the ipsilateral inferior petrosal sinus, then into the internal jugular vein. **(C)** Anteroposterior (AP) digital subtraction angiogram from right internal carotid injection additionally demonstrates filling of the contralateral dilated inferior petrosal sinus, cavernous sinus, and dilated left SOV. **(D)** Scout film in the lateral projection after transarterial deployment of a detachable silicone balloon. **(E)** Right lateral internal carotid injection following embolization, and **(F)** AP internal carotid injection demonstrates eradication of the fistula.

Radiological Evaluation

Although the presence of a vertebral AVF might be detected with contrast-enhanced CT/CT angiography versus MRI/MRA of the neck, definitive diagnosis is only completely assessed with conventional angiography. CT/MR is best at the delineation of dilated vascular structures and their relationship to the surrounding soft tissues and spinal canal as well as assessment of the possibility of stroke involving the posterior fossa. In the evaluation of vertebral AVF a complete cerebral angiogram is warranted. The angiographic study should include evaluation of both internal and external carotid circulation in addition to close examination of the vertebral arteries in their intracranial and extracranial extent. The information provided via a complete cerebral angiogram will give the clinician a better understanding of the collateral circulation present and the exact location of the fistula and will enhance the ability to differentiate between a vertebral AVF with or without the presence of vertebral artery transection.

Treatment

If the patient is shown to harbor a single AVF without vertebral artery transection the therapeutic objective

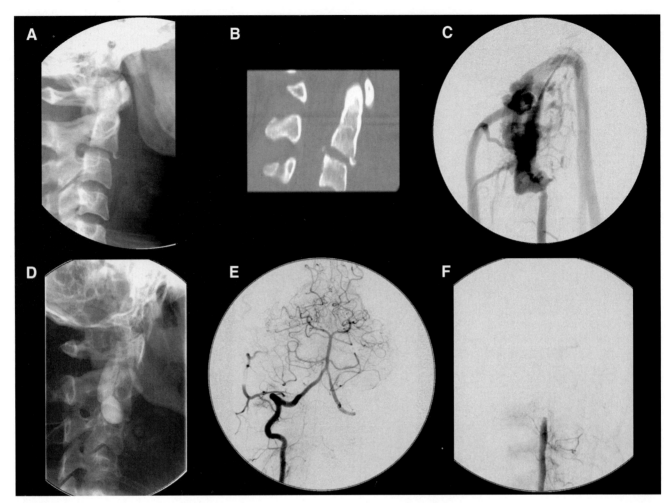

FIGURE 14–8 Posttraumatic vertebral arteriovenous fistula. A 16-year-old male involved in a high-speed motor vehicle accident presenting with an audible bruit. **(A)** Lateral radiograph of the cervical spine demonstrating fracture of the anterior inferior aspect of C2 with anterior subluxation of C2 on C3 worrisome for posterior column instability. **(B)** Three-dimensional reconstructed image in the sagittal plane from a computed tomographic scan of the cervical spine additionally reveals a fracture of the posterior inferior corner of the C2 vertebral body. **(C)** Digital subtraction angiography of the left vertebral artery (lateral projection) centered over the neck demonstrates antegrade flow in the cervical segment of the left vertebral artery, filling of a large venous pouch, and filling of the paravertebral plexus in the neck in a caudal direction consistent with a vertebral arteriovenous fistula. Note there is no antegrade filling of the vertebral artery distal to the fistula. **(D)** Lateral radiograph of the neck after embolization of the fistula and deconstructive occlusion of the vertebral artery with two detachable silicone balloons filled with contrast. Note the balloons' location at the C2/C3 level. **(E)** Postembolization angiogram of the right vertebral artery demonstrating patency of the vertebrobasilar system, no major branch occlusions, and retrograde filling of the left vertebral artery to the level of the occlusion. **(F)** Postembolization angiography of the left vertebral artery in the lateral projection demonstrating absence of filling of the fistula with collateralization of the distal left vertebral artery cephalad to the fistulous site via muscular collaterals.

should include closure of the fistula with preservation of the parent artery. This can be achieved though endovascular techniques utilizing placement of a detachable silicone balloon at the fistula site. Less commonly used embolization materials include coils or n-butyl cyanoacrylate liquid adhesive. Postprocedure care for these patients, especially those with long-standing fistulas, should include close monitoring of blood pressure to avoid normal perfusion pressure breakthrough.[70] If vertebral artery transection is present with the fistula (**Fig. 14–8**), therapeutic intervention should involve trapping of the fistula with deconstructive occlusion of the artery. This can be accomplished via an endovascular approach. Care must be taken to occlude the fistula at its proximal and distal aspect and not to proximally occlude the vertebral artery. If proximal occlusion is performed without closure of the fistula, the arteriovenous shunt will continue to remain patent and receive arterial supply from retrograde flow through the cephalad extent of the transected artery via the contralateral vertebral artery, making further attempts at embolization more difficult.

REFERENCES

1. Connors JJWJ III. Interventional Neuroradiology: Strategies and Practical Techniques. Philadelphia: WB Saunders; 1999
2. Malek AM, Halbach VV, Higashida RT, Phatouros CC, Meyers PM, Dowd CF. Treatment of dural arteriovenous malformations and fistulas. Neurosurg Clin N Am 2000;11:147–166
3. Chaudhary MY, Sachdev VP, Cho SH, Weitzner I Jr, Puljic S, Huang YP. Dural arteriovenous malformation of the major venous sinuses: an acquired lesion. AJNR Am J Neuroradiol 1982;3:13–19
4. Vanderwerf AJ. Sur un cas d'aneurymme arterio-veineux intradural bilateral de la fosse posterieur chez un enfant [On a case of bilateral intradural arteriovenous aneurysm of the posterior fossa in a child]. Neurochirurgie 1964;10:140–144
5. Rosenbloom S, Edwards MH. Dural arteriovenous malformations. In: Edwards MH, ed. Cerebral Vascular Disease in Children and Adolescents. Baltimore: Williams & Wilkins; 1989:343–365
6. Al-Mefty O, Jinkins JR, Fox JL. Extensive dural arteriovenous malformation: case report. J Neurosurg 1986;65:417–420
7. Albright AL, Latchaw RE, Price RA. Posterior dural arteriovenous malformations in infancy. Neurosurgery 1983;13:129–135
8. Chan ST, Weeks RD. Dural arteriovenous malformation presenting as cardiac failure in a neonate. Acta Neurochir (Wien) 1988;91:134–138
9. Debrun G, Chartres A. Infra and supratentorial arteriovenous malformations, a general review: about 2 cases of spontaneous supratentorial arteriovenous malformation of the dura. Neuroradiology 1972;3:184–192
10. Epstein B, Platt N. Visualization of an intracranial arteriovenous fistula during angiocardiography in an infant with congestive heart failure. Radiology 1962;79:629–627
11. Gordon IJ, Shah BL, Hardman DR, Chameides L. Giant dural supratentorial arteriovenous malformation. AJR Am J Roentgenol 1977;129:734–736
12. Konishi Y, Hieshima GB, Hara M, Yoshino K, Yano K, Takeuchi K. Congenital fistula of the dural carotid-cavernous sinus: case report and review of the literature. Neurosurgery 1990;27:120–126
13. Newton T, Hoyt W. Spontaneous arteriovenous fistula between dural branches of the internal maxillary artery and the posterior cavernous sinus. Radiology 1968;91:1147–1150
14. Robinson JL, Sedzimir CB. External carotid-transverse sinus fistula: case report. J Neurosurg 1970;33:718–720
15. Ross DA, Walker J, Edwards MS. Unusual posterior fossa dural arteriovenous malformation in a neonate: case report. Neurosurgery 1986;19:1021–1024
16. Sundt TM Jr, Piepgras DG. The surgical approach to arteriovenous malformations of the lateral and sigmoid dural sinuses. J Neurosurg 1983;59:32–39
17. Tsugane R, Sato O, Watabe T. Noncommunicating hydrocephalus caused by dural arteriovenous malformation. Surg Neurol 1979;12:393–396
18. Garcia-Monaco R, Rodesch G, TerBrugge K, Burrows P, Lasjaunias P. Multifocal dural arteriovenous shunts in children. Childs Nerv Syst 1991;7:425–431
19. Kincaid PK, Duckwiler GR, Gobin YP, Vinuela F. Dural arteriovenous fistula in children: endovascular treatment and outcomes in seven cases. AJNR Am J Neuroradiol 2001;22:1217–1225
20. Berenstein A, Lasjaunias P. Surgical Neuroangiography. Berlin: Springer-Verlag; 1992
21. Terada T, Higashida RT, Halbach VV, et al. Development of acquired arteriovenous fistulas in rats due to venous hypertension. J Neurosurg 1994;80:884–889
22. Picard L, Bracard S, Mallet J, et al. Spontaneous dural arteriovenous fistulas. Semin Intervent Radiol 1987;4:219–240
23. Houser OW, Campbell JK, Campbell RJ, Sundt TM Jr. Arteriovenous malformation affecting the transverse dural venous sinus: an acquired lesion. Mayo Clin Proc 1979;54:651–661
24. Malek AM, Higashida RT, Balousek PA, et al. Endovascular recanalization with balloon angioplasty and stenting of an occluded occipital sinus for treatment of intracranial venous hypertension: technical case report. Neurosurgery 1999;44:896–901
25. Terada T, Tsuura M, Komai N, et al. The role of angiogenic factor in bFGF in the development of dural AVFs. Acta Neurochir (Wien) 1996;138:877–883
26. Lawton MT, Jacobowitz R, Spetzler RF. Redefined role of angiogenesis in the pathogenesis of dural arteriovenous malformation. J Neurosurg 1997;87:267–274
27. Folkman J, D'Amore PA. Blood vessel formation: what is its molecular basis? [comment] Cell 1996;87:1153–1155
28. Folkman J. Clinical applications of research on angiogenesis [see comments]. N Engl J Med 1995;333:1757–1763
29. Aminoff M. Vascular anomalies in the intracranial dura mater. Brain 1973;96:601–612
30. Newton T, Greitz T. Arteriovenous communication between the occipital artery and the transverse sinus. Radiology 1966;87:824–828
31. Takekawa S, Holman C. Roentgenologic diagnosis of anomalous communications between the external carotid artery and intracranial veins. Am J Roentgenol Radium Ther Nucl Med 1965;95:822–825
32. Vanderwerf AJ. Sur un cas d'aneurymme arterio-veineux intradural bilateral de la fosse posterieur chez un enfant [On a case of bilateral intradural arteriovenous aneurysm of the posterior fossa in a child]. Neurochirurgie 1964;10:140–144
33. Nishijima M, Takaku A, Endo S, et al. Etiological evaluation of dural arteriovenous malformation of the lateral and sigmoid sinuses based on histopathological examinations. J Neurosurg 1992;76:600–606
34. Findlay JM, Mielke BW. Fatal rebleeding from a dural arteriovenous malformation of the posterior fossa: case report with pathological examination. Can J Neurol Sci 1994;21:67–71
35. Graeb DA, Dolman CL. Radiological and pathological aspects of dural arteriovenous fistulas. J Neurosurg 1986;64:962–967
36. Ito J, Imamura H, Kobayashi K, et al. Dural arteriovenous malformations of the base of the anterior cranial fossa. Neuroradiology 1983;24:149–154
37. Hunt WE. Dural arteriovenous malformations. In: Wilson CB, Stein BM, eds. Intracranial Arteriovenous Malformations. Baltimore: Williams & Wilkins; 1984:222–233
38. Hook O, Werko L, Ohrberg G. Intracranial arteriovenous aneurysms: a study of their effect on the cardiovascular system. AMA Arch Neurol Psychiatry 1958;79:622–632
39. Lasjaunias P, Magufis A, Goulao R, Suthipongchai S, Rodesch R, Alvarez H. Anatomoclinical aspects of dural arteriovenous shunts in children. Intervent Neuroradiol 1996;2:179–191
40. Garcia-Monaco R, De Victor D, Mann C, Hannedouche A, Terbrugge K, Lasjaunias P. Congestive cardiac manifestations from cerebrocranial arteriovenous shunts: endovascular management in 30 children. Childs Nerv Syst 1991;7:48–52
41. Djindjian R, Cophignon J, Theron J. Embolization by superselective arteriography from the femoral route in neuroradiology: review of 60 cases, technique, indications, complications. Neuroradiology 1973;6:20–26
42. Castaigne P, Bories J, Brunet P, Cassan JL, Meninger V, Merland JJ. Fistules arterio-veineuses de la dure-mere. Ann Med Interne (Paris) 1975;126:813–817
43. McDougall CG, Halbach VV, Higashida RT, et al. Treatment of dural arteriovenous fistulas. Neurosurg Q 1997;7:110–134
44. Ushikoshi S, Kikuchi Y, Miyasaka K. Multiple dural arteriovenous shunts in a 5-year-old boy. AJNR Am J Neuroradiol 1999;20:728–730
45. Malek AM, Halbach VV, Dowd CF, Higashida RT. Diagnosis and treatment of dural arteriovenous fistulas. Neuroimaging Clin N Am 1998;8:445–468

46. Halbach V, Higashida R, Dowd C, Barnwell S, Hieshima G. Treament of dural arteriovenous fistulas involving the transverse and sigmoid sinuses by transvenous embolization: results in 20 patients. Neuroradiology 1991;33(Suppl):550–552

47. Barnwell SL, Halbach VV, Dowd CF, Higashida RT, Hieshima GB. Dural arteriovenous fistulas involving the inferior petrosal sinus: angiographic findings in six patients. AJNR Am J Neuroradiol 1990;11:511–516

48. Barnwell SL, Halbach VV, Dowd CF, Higashida RT, Hieshima GB, Wilson CB. A variant of arteriovenous fistulas within the wall of dural sinuses: results of combined surgical and endovascular therapy. J Neurosurg 1991;74:199–204

49. Halbach VV, Higashida RT, Hieshima GB, Goto K, Norman D, Newton TH. Dural fistulas involving the transverse and sigmoid sinuses: results of treatment in 28 patients. Radiology 1987;163:443–447

50. Dandy W. Carotid-cavernous aneurysms (pulsatile exophthalmos). Zentralbl Neurochir 1937;2:77–113

51. Dany F, Fraysse A, Priollet P, et al. Dysmorphic syndrome and vascular dysplasia: an atypical form of type IV Ehlers-Danlos syndrome [in French]. J Mal Vasc 1986;11:263–269

52. Eggers F, Lukin R, Chambers AA, Tomsick TA, Sawaya R. Iatrogenic carotid-cavernous fistula following Fogarty catheter thromboendarterectomy: case report. J Neurosurg 1979;51:543–545

53. Fischbein NJ, Dillon WP, Barkovich AJ. Teaching Atlas of Brain Imaging. New York: Thieme; 2000

54. Hamby WB. Carotid Cavernous Fistula. Springfield: Charles C Thomas; 1966

55. Lister JR, Sypert GW. Traumatic false aneurysm and carotid-cavernous fistula: a complication of sphenoidotomy. Neurosurgery 1979;5:473–475

56. Motarjeme A, Keifer JW. Carotid-cavernous sinus fistula as a complication of carotid endarterectomy: a case report. Radiology 1973;108:83–84

57. Pedersen RA, Troost BT, Schramm VL. Carotid-cavernous sinus fistula after external ethmoid-sphenoid surgery: clinical course and management. Arch Otolaryngol 1981;107:307–309

58. Song IC, Bromberg BE. Carotid-cavernous sinus fistula occurring after a rhinoplasty: case report. Plast Reconstr Surg 1975;55:92–96

59. Takahashi M, Killeffer F, Wilson G. Iatrogenic carotid cavernous fistula: case report. J Neurosurg 1969;30:498–500

60. Kupersmith MJ, Berenstein A. Neurovascular Neuro-ophthalmology. Berlin: Springer-Verlag; 1993:70–108

61. Sattler CH. Pulsierender Exophthalmus: Handbuch der gesamten Augenheikunde. Berlin: Springer; 1920

62. Halbach VV, Hieshima GB, Higashida RT, Reicher M. Carotid cavernous fistula: indication for urgent therapy. AJR Roentgenol 1987;149:587–593

63. Debrun GB, Lacour P, Vinuela F, et al. Treatment of 54 traumatic carotid cavernous fistulas. J Neurosurg 1981;55:678–692

64. Norman D, Newton TH, Edwards MJ. Carotid cavernous fistula: closure with detachable silicone balloon. Radiology 1983;149: 149–159

65. Goto K, Halbach VV, Hardin CW, Higashida RT, Hieshima GB. Permanent inflation of detachable balloons with a low-viscosity, hydrophilic polymerizing system. Radiology 1988;169: 787–790

66. Batjer HH, Purdy PD, Neiman M, Samson DS. Subtemporal transdural use of detachable balloons for traumatic CCF. Neurosurgery 1988;22:290–296

67. Higashida RT, Hieshima GB, Halbach VV, Bentson JR, Goto K. Closure of carotid cavernous sinus fistulae by external compression of the carotid artery and jugular vein. Acta Radiol 1986;369(Suppl):580–583

68. Meyers P, Halbach V, Barkovich A. Anomalies of cerebral vasculature: diagnostic and endovascular considerations. In: Barkovich A, ed. Pediatric Neuroimaging. Philadelphia: Lippincott Williams & Wilkins; 2000:771–814

69. Hayes P, Gerlock J, AJ, Cobb CA. Cervical spine trauma: a cause of vertebral artery injury. J Trauma 1980;20:904–905

70. Halbach VV, Higashida RT, Hieshima GB, Norman D. Normal perfusion pressure breakthrough occurring during treatment of carotid and vertebral fistulas. AJNR Am J Neuroradiol 1987;8: 751–756

71. Halbach VV, Higashida RT, Heishima GB. Treatment of vertebral arteriovenous fistulas. AJR Am J Roentgenol; 22:297–300

72. Matas R. Traumatisms and traumatic aneurysms of the vertebral artery and their surgical treatment with the report of a cured case. Ann Surg 1893;18:477–521.

73. Weinberg PE, Flom RA. Traumatic vertebral arteriovenous fistula. Surg Neurol 1973;1:162–167

15

Endovascular Treatment of Cerebral Arteriovenous Malformations in Children

OSAMA O. ZAIDAT AND MICHAEL J. ALEXANDER

In children who are diagnosed with cerebral pial arteriovenous malformations (AVMs), several treatment strategies are available depending on the size, location, and angioarchitectural features of the AVM and the patient's age and size in addition to other factors. For patients who have not had previous hemorrhage from their AVM, therapeutic approaches of surgical excision, endovascular embolization, stereotactic radiosurgery or radiotherapy, multimodal treatment, and conservative expectant therapy are options.[1,2] However, patients presenting with cerebral hemorrhage may require more expedient treatment, and the surgical and endovascular options become more important.[1–3] This chapter discusses the endovascular treatment for nondurally based intracranial AVMs in the pediatric age group.

Several aspects differentiate pediatric from adult AVMs. The Spetzler-Martin scale, devised for assessing the outcome of AVM resection with respect to neurological morbidity and mortality, was developed using primarily adult data.[4] The elements of eloquence and venous drainage are important factors in pediatric AVMs; however, the size criteria of the Spetzler-Martin grading system cannot be directly correlated. The size of the AVM nidus must be adjusted to the size of the infant or pediatric brain, which may affect the length and duration of the surgical excision or endovascular intervention. Moreover, the remote effects of an AVM in children may challenge the idea of eloquence in the Spetzler-Martin scale. In neonates it is more common to present with hemodynamic and systemic manifestations rather than local mass effect or ischemia from steal. Finally, the plasticity of the young brain will also affect the outcome following endovascular or surgical intervention.

The goal of endovascular AVM treatment in children is similar to that for adults—attempted complete obliteration of the AVM nidus. The exception is in the neonatal and infant age group where immediate and urgent partial intervention may be a goal in itself, with reduction in arteriovenous shunting to prevent further medical or neurological deterioration. This chapter first discusses the embryology, epidemiology, and clinical presentation of pediatric AVMs, followed by the management approach, functional testing, principles of endovascular approach, embolization materials, technical considerations, and complications.

■ Embryology and Pathology

Cerebral AVMs have long been thought of as congenital vascular anomalies. The congenital theory proposes the persistence of primitive arteriovenous connections or the development of these connections prior to delivery.[1,2] In the late 1980s, a second theory explained the AVM as a "proliferative capillaropathy" arising from the fact that the AVM is a constantly changing lesion rather than an abnormal static connection. This theory was supported by the inability to diagnose these lesions perinatally and the argument that AVMs are dynamic, rather than static, vascular lesions.[1–3] A third theory in the 1990s was based on genetic aberration in the development of AVMs and proposed dysfunctional biological vascular remodeling, secondary to genetic errors and mutations in the genes controlling angiogenesis. The growth of an AVM in the genetic theory is explained by hemodynamic stress factors and secondary angiopathy or angiogenesis after ischemia or hemorrhage.[1–3]

■ Epidemiology

The incidence of cerebral AVMs in general population studies has been reported to be 1.34 per 100,000 person-years (95% CI, 1.18 to 1.49), and in the pediatric population it is 0.014 to 0.028%.[1–3,5,6] However, cerebral AVMs are 10 times more frequent in children than saccular aneurysms, with pediatric AVMs constituting 10 to 26% of all diagnosed AVMs. In general, 10% of the AVMs are diagnosed before the age of 10 and 16% between 10 and 19.9 years.[1–3,5,6] Although many continue to believe that cerebral AVMs are congenital in origin, it is clear that only a small number are diagnosed in the first 2 decades of life. The theory behind later presentation in life is related to the proposed progressive vascular changes over time, leading to excessive thinning of the vascular wall and bleeding. Stimulation of vascular growth by blood shunting is another theory, which has been thought to explain this regrowth. De novo cerebral AVMs have been reported, and it is speculated that localized angiogenic cytokines may be responsible for their development.[7]

■ Clinical Presentation

In children, one third of the patients present acutely. In the general pediatrics group (those <20 years of age), a total of 65 to 80% present with intracerebral hemorrhage (ICH), 36% with seizure and hydrocephalus, and 18% with congestive heart failure.[1–3] In neonates, 50% present with congestive heart failure and systemic presentation, and 25% with neurocognitive decline. In infants, the ICH presentation predominates again.[1–3]

Compared with those in adults, pediatric AVMs more frequently present with spontaneous intracranial hemorrhage, with an average presentation of 75 to 80% in the child versus 50% in the adult. The annual rate of bleeding is also higher in children (5 to 6%) than in adults (2 to 4%).[3,5,6,8,9]

Progressive brain injury from cerebral arteriovenous shunting has been well described by Lasjaunias and others.[3] Melting-brain syndrome is rapid brain destruction, usually of the white matter, with ventriculomegaly. This syndrome occurs in all types of vascular malformations with arteriovenous shunting during the neonatal and early infancy period, but in cerebral AVMs it usually occurs between 7 and 8 months of age due to progressive spontaneous thrombosis of the venous drainage with absent alternate venous pathways.[3] Patients usually have symmetrical white matter signs with increased tone, spasticity, and hyperreflexia.[3]

> ***PEARL*** Risks of embolization and surgery may not be additive because a thorough embolization can actually reduce the risk of surgery.

■ Endovascular Management

Surgical excision is the standard treatment of choice and allows removal and obliteration of the AVM in selective cases. The complication rate in AVM resection can be predicted by the factors of the Spetzler-Martin grade. AVM embolization can be implemented prior to surgery or radiosurgery and is occasionally used as the sole modality of treatment. Despite the poor prognosis and increased mortality of pediatric AVMs, 10 to 40% of pediatric patients may not be treated due to the large size of the AVM, a deeply located lesion, or poor vascular access.[8,9] Risks of embolization and surgery may not be additive because a thorough embolization can actually reduce the risk of surgery.

General Principles of Cerebral Arteriovenous Malformation Embolization

There are several technical considerations for pediatric cerebral AVM embolization. We must carefully monitor the amount of contrast administration over a given period of time per the patient's weight, the amount of radiation exposure during therapy by both fluoroscopy and angiographic runs, arterial access issues, intravenous fluid volume administration, and general anesthetic issues.[10,11]

We prefer to perform all pediatric cerebral AVM embolization under general anesthesia. An experienced pediatric anesthesia team is essential in performing these sometimes complex procedures. Following embolization, the patient may be kept sedated with normal pressure overnight in the intensive care unit or a monitored bed.[12]

Micropuncture access to the femoral artery is preferred and we will typically use a 5 French guide catheter for the largest share of transarterial pediatric embolization. For pediatric cerebral AVM embolization, we usually perform a diagnostic cerebral angiogram to plan embolization of separate pedicles in advance. In most cases, even high-quality magnetic resonance angiography or computed tomographic angiography is not sufficient for this type of planning. Performing the cerebral angiogram prior to the date of embolization allows for more latitude with contrast administration and radiation dosage.

In infants and pediatric patients less than 1 year of age, a 4 or 5 French sheath and guide catheter may be occlusive in the artery, which requires careful monitoring to assess skin color and capillary refill in the lower extremities.

Likewise, if repeated procedures are necessary, with repeated access in the same artery, fibrosis and scarring may occur, which may limit access for future procedures.

Follow-up angiography may be performed 3 to 6 months postembolization; if no neovascularization and recruitment are found no further angiograms are needed. Imaging follow-up may be obtained with other noninvasive tests.

Imaging Preplanning and Functional Testing

Functional testing is controversial, but because pediatric AVM embolization is usually performed under general anesthesia, functional imaging would be useful prior to embolization.[1-3,13] Functional magnetic resonance imaging (fMRI) may delineate the functional topography of the brain areas in the vicinity of the AVM.[14] Some studies have observed reorganization of the cortex secondary to the AVM using a combination of blood oxygen–dependent contrast with the spatial resolution of MRI. The eloquence of the surrounding cortex of the AVM may be determined prior to endovascular intervention (**Fig. 15–1**). Sensory and language function can also be localized using sensory positron emission tomography, but it is less readily available than fMRI. In older children, where the endovascular embolization may be performed under sedation, the superselective Wada test, performed by injecting sodium amytal, with neurological assessment may be helpful prior to the embolization of arterial feeders in eloquent regions. Electroencephalographic recording with a four- to eight-lead electroencephalogram or somatosensory evoked potential may be used and can aid with safe embolization in conjunction with Wada's test in those who are undergoing endovascular AVM embolization under general anesthesia.[13]

Recently developed computer-assisted MRA techniques may improve the safety of preembolization planning. The segmentation and interconnectedness of extraction techniques can accurately depict the blood vessels and their branching pattern, increasing the precision and consistency of planning for the interventional procedure. The hypothesized treatment plan may be tested by experimental software to simulate the passage of the microcatheter, rendering only the distal vasculature. Interactive visualization reflects the important functional information needed to test the embolization theory.[15]

Approach to Endovascular Treatment

The goals of endovascular treatment in children may share some similarities with those for adults, but there are some differences.[16-18] In children, complete obliteration of the AVM may not mean cure, and recanalization has been reported following complete exclusion of the AVM with endovascular and surgical excision.[19] However, partial treatment may lead to progressive thrombosis and subsequent cure, and spontaneous thrombosis and occlusion of the AVM following ICH have been reported. Diagnostic angiography prior to embolization is recommended to assess the number of feeders to be embolized and whether to use complete or staged embolization.[1-3,16-19] **Figure 15–2** shows an example of a gadolinium-enhanced MRI scan and diagnostic cerebral angiography depicting the pertinent AVM anatomy.

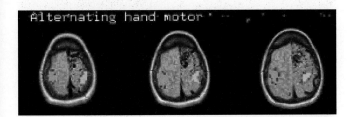

FIGURE 15–1 Functional magnetic resonance imaging (fMRI) helps to localize functional regions such as motor and speech areas with respect to the arteriovenous malformation (AVM) nidus. Here the fMRI demonstrates this paracentral left frontal AVM nidus to be at least one gyrus anterior to the primary motor cortex activation for hand movement (see Color Plate 15–1).

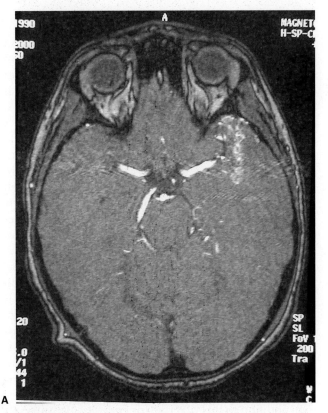

A

FIGURE 15–2 (A) Axial magnetic resonance imaging scan with gadolinium demonstrating a 3 cm left temporal lobe arteriovenous malformation (AVM) in a 10-year-old boy who presented with a new onset of generalized seizures.

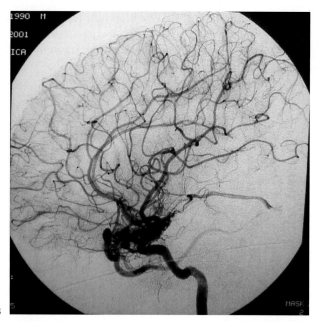

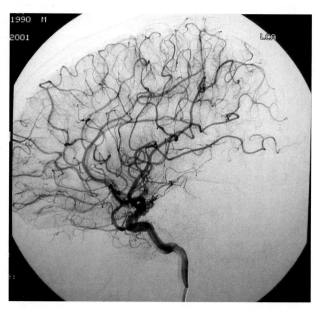

FIGURE 15–2 (*Continued*) **(B)** Lateral angiogram demonstrating the elongated temporal AVM nidus, which was fed primarily by the anterior temporal artery, and drains via superficial and deep venous pathways. **(C)** Lateral angiogram following n-butyl-2-cyanoacrylate embolization of four separate middle cerebral artery feeder artery pedicles. A very small residual nidus remains for surgical excision. Note there is still early filling of the venous drainage to the superior petrosal sinus.

Particularly in large AVMs, complete embolization in one session carries a higher risk of embolization-related hemorrhage. In these situations, a staged embolization is recommend. Staged endovascular treatment, although controversial in adults, has been recommended in neonates and infants less than 1 year old, particularly in large AVMs by some.[1,3] Timing of the intervention is another vital aspect of endovascular embolization of the cerebral AVM in infants and neonates.[1,3] This age group commonly presents with progressive neurocognitive decline secondary to atrophy, leukomalacia, hydrocephaly, and macrocephaly. Leukomalacia and atrophy may occur rapidly and is specific for this age group. Untreated patients usually have a poor prognosis, and an endovascular approach would be preferred sooner rather than later. When targeted at the points of angioarchitectural weakness, embolization contributes to stabilizing the vascular lesion.[1,3] It should be undertaken rapidly to avoid loss of brain substance secondary to hemorrhage, atrophy, or leukomalacia, and to allow neurocognitive recovery and normal brain maturation. The AVMs in this group are the most aggressive ones for the maturing brain and the most difficult to approach technically, but they merit the risk of early intervention.[1,3]

In addition to this vital role for endovascular intervention in neonates and infants, currently the endovascular role in managing cerebral AVMs is similar to that for adults and may be divided into presurgical, or preradiosurgical, palliative, curative, and partial (**Table 15–1**).

TABLE 15–1 Approach to Endovascular Arteriovenous Malformation Management in Children

Age Group	Recommendations
Neonates and infants	Urgent, but elective endovascular treatment for the main feeding artery feeding artery to halt progression of neurological decline
1–15 years of age	Endovascular therapy prior to surgery or radiosurgery, small AVM with <3 cm, and fewer than four feeders may be cured
>15 years of age	Similar to adults: Adjunctive role prior to surgery or radiosurgery; Partial embolization for seizure or progressive neurological deficit; Palliative embolization, and rarely curative
All age groups	Functional testing: MRI, PET, and superselective Wada test with neurological exam, EEG, or somatosensory evoked potentials; Pretreatment diagnostic angiogram; Embolization under general anesthesia; Staged embolization versus complete one; Postembolization: overnight sedation and normotensive in neurointensive care unit; Follow-up angiogram in 3–6 months

AVM, arteriovenous malformation; EEG, electroencephalography; MRI, magnetic resonance imaging; PET, positron emission tomography.

Partial obliteration of AVMs in the pediatric population can be attained in 54 to 90% of cases.[1–3,16–18] In children, this has been recommended to be performed prior to surgery or radiosurgery and also to control refractory seizures and progressing neurological deficits.[1–3,16–18]

Embolization cure rates of cerebral AVMs ranging from 5 to 16.6% have been reported.[1–3,16–18] Some authors attributed the low cure rate in the endovascular literature to the referral bias of large AVM size, with multiple and deep perforating feeders. The rate of complete cure is indeed affected by the size of the AVM and the number of arterial feeders. The rate of complete obliteration is inversely related to the AVM nidus size (<3 cm) and the number of arterial feeders (fewer than four feeders). **Figure 15–3** depicts a 15-year-old girl who underwent endovascular embolization of a cerebral AVM with complete angiographic cure after one session.

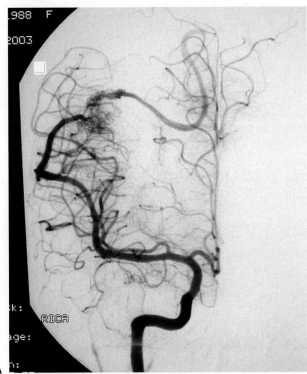

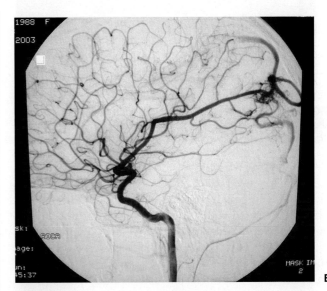

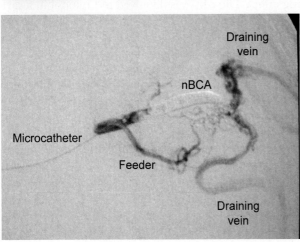

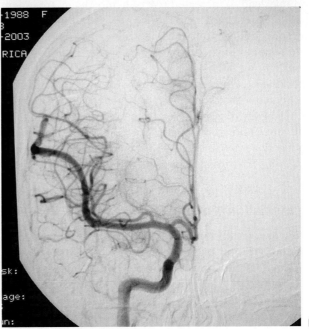

FIGURE 15–3 (A) Anteroposterior (AP) and **(B)** lateral cerebral angiogram of a 15-year-old girl who presented with subarachnoid hemorrhage demonstrating a small right parietal arteriovenous malformation (AVM) nidus, which is not compact. **(C)** Microcatheter angiography after the embolization of one pedicle of the AVM with n-butyl-2-cyanoacrylate (nBCA) shows one remaining feeder to the diffuse AVM and two remaining draining veins. **(D)** AP and **(E)** lateral angiograms show no residual filling of the AVM and no early venous drainage after a two-pedicle embolization with nBCA.

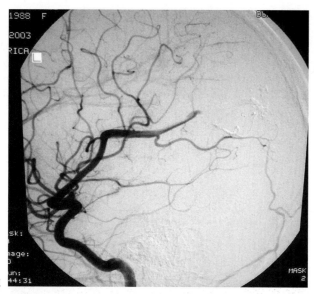

FIGURE 15–3 (*Continued*) **(D)** AP and **(E)** lateral angiograms show no residual filling of the AVM and no early venous drainage after a two-pedicle embolization with nBCA.

TABLE 15–2 Cerebral Arteriovenous Malformation Embolization Agents, Pros and Cons

Embolic Agents	Comments
• nBCA	Immediate solidification, risk of escape of the embolic agent, and microcatheter adhesions; microcatheter can be used once; pre-radiotherapy.
• Ethibloc	Slow solidification, microcatheter can be used up to four times; risk of rupture of the microcatheter (1.8F)
• PVA	Several particle sizes 150–1000 μ, temporary occlusion, mainly used preoperatively
• Embospheres, Onyx, GDC, Gelfoam, Silastic or latex balloon, fibrin silicon, hydrogel glue, calcium alginate, silk thread, and others	

AVM, arteriovenous malformation; nBCA, n-butyl-2-cyanoacrylate; PVA, polyvinyl alcohol particles; GDC, Guglielmi detachable coils.

The adjunctive role of endovascular therapy in combination with surgery is usually more successful. In patients who were treated with one-stage embolization followed by surgery a cure rate of more than 95% has been reported.[17,18] The association between cerebral AVMs and aneurysmal formation has been estimated at 5 to 15%.[20] Because it has been postulated that such an association may lead to increased risk of hemorrhage, treatment of these aneurysms may reduce this risk. Endovascular therapy is used to treat feeding arteries and intranidal or venous aneurysms, either as a palliative therapy, prior to surgery or radiosurgery, or during curative or partial embolization. Proximal aneurysms on the feeding artery are treated with coil embolization, with considerations to the tortuosity of the arteries, the fragility of the aneurysm wall, and the high-flow pattern. Intranidal or distal feeding artery aneurysms may be treated with glue embolization using flow-directed or flow-assisted microcatheters.

Embolization Materials and Technical Notes

There are several types of materials that may be used in the embolization of pediatric cerebral AVMs. They are mainly classified as solid versus liquid materials and are summarized in **Table 15–2**. The solid materials may include polyvinyl alcohol (PVA) particles, silicone spheres, microhydrogel spheres, calcium alginate, Silastic or latex balloon, Gelfoam particles, surgical silk threads, and platinum or polymer-coated coils.[1,14] The liquid materials may include n-butyl-2-cyanoacrylate (nBCA) (TruFill, Cordis Neurovascular, Miami Lakes, FL), 100% ethanol, ethylene vinyl alcohol copolymer (Onyx, Micro

Therapeutics, Inc., Irvine, CA), fibrin glue, cellulose, and Ethibloc.

> **PEARL** In high-flow fistulas, the largest fistula should be occluded first to prevent early reflux around the catheter by arterial steal if a less important feeder has been chosen.

The most commonly used embolic agent is nBCA, which solidifies immediately upon contact with the free hydrogen ion in the blood, creating a permanent casting effect. The nBCA is dissolved in Lipiodol in a variety of concentrations, and injected via the flow-directed or flow-assisted microcatheter. Pure glue injection (100%) may be performed in high-flow fistulas, and the largest fistula should be occluded first to prevent early reflux around the catheter by arterial steal if a less important feeder has been chosen. Injection against the wall will reduce the risk of glue migration. Loops from the microcatheter should be removed before injecting the glue to assure immediate response upon pulling the catheter. Injecting pure glue into the nidus or high-flow fistula requires extra caution and years of experience.

The risk with nBCA includes escape of the agent to the venous side or normal arteries, subsequently leading to cerebral infarction. Another potential risk is adhesion of the catheter to the wall of the blood vessel due to the reflux of nBCA around the microcatheter tip. Consequently, each microcatheter can be used only once and should be withdrawn immediately upon completion of the injection.

TABLE 15–3 Potential Complications following Endovascular Arteriovenous Malformation Embolization

Complications	Comments
Angiography related:	
• Contrast allergy	Weight-based contrast dose (5 mL/kg)
• Contrast-induced renal injury	Mucomyst, hydration
• Radiation injury	Limit fluoroscopy time and angiographic runs
• Arterial scarring and stenosis	Secondary to multiple femoral punctures
• Arterial vasospasm	Intra-arterial Nitroglycerin administration
• Groin and retroperitoneal hematoma	Expectant management/vascular surgery consult
• Vessel perforation	Very rare and <0.5%
Embolization related:	
• Minor stroke/no disability	Related to normal arterial glue embolization 8%
• Moderate stroke with minor disability	Related to normal arterial glue embolization 4%
• Death	Secondary to ICH and edema, related to venous occlusion and hypertension 1%
• Pulmonary embolism	Small emboli typically asymptomatic
• Peripheral vascular occlusion	May require embolectomy
• Consumption coagulopathy	FFP, factor replacement

FFP, fresh frozen plasma; ICH, intracerebral hemorrhage.

Ethibloc is a solution of ethanol and the corn protein zein (210 mg/mL of ethanol). In an aqueous solution such as blood, the ethanol dissolves and the zein precipitates. Ethibloc provides an advantage over nBCA by being less adhesive to the microcatheter, which allows reuse of the flow-directed micro-catheters. Unfortunately, it has to be infused via a microcatheter with an outer diameter of 1.8 French or it will lead to rupture of the microcatheter. Both ethibloc and nBCA are to be mixed with lipid-based oil before injection. Other agents are also used, including PVA of different particle sizes: small (45 to 150 μm), medium (250 to 450 μm), and large (500 to 750 μm) and macrospheres or embospheres with sizes between 750 and 2000 μm.

These materials are chosen based on the goal of the embolization. For example, if the embolization is presurgical, then solid polymer embolization using platinum or polymer-coated coils or PVA particles may be considered. However, in cases where surgical excision is not planned in the near future, we typically avoid PVA particles as an embolization material, primarily because the recanalization rate is higher than with other materials (40 to 80% at 1 month postembolization with PVA).[1,14]

PEARL In cases where surgical excision is not planned in the near future, we typically avoid PVA particles because the recanalization rate is higher than with other materials.

In cases in which we plan postembolization radio-therapy or staged embolization over a longer period of time, we prefer the use of liquid polymer such as nBCA or Onyx. Platinum coils are typically used when there is a significant arteriovenous fistula component to the AVM.

■ Complications of Endovascular Therapy

The clinical complications following endovascular intervention may be correlated with clinical and angioarchitectural features (**Table 15–3**). The Spetzler-Martin grading scale was originally devised to predict outcome following surgical intervention in adults; however, it has been applied prior to endovascular intervention. Hartmann et al have performed one of the largest AVM embolization studies, with 233 patients in all age groups undergoing 545 embolization procedures.[21] Some assessed neurological deficit occurred in 14% of their patients. Of those, 2% (five patients) had permanent neurological disability, with a modified Rankin scale of ≤2, and death secondary to ICH occurred in two patients (1%). The complications were more frequent with increased patient age (OR 1.04, 1.01 to 1.08), number of embolizations (mean of 3.5 procedures, OR 1.41, 1.16 to 1.70), and absence of pretreatment neurological deficit (OR 4.55, 1.03 to 20.0).[22] Rebleeding between sessions of embolization may occur, but it is very low, and in children, the risk of complete aggressive embolization may outweigh the risk of rebleeding between sessions.[1]

Hemorrhage and stroke are the most important complications related to cerebral AVM embolization; however, there are other potential risks to be aware of. During cerebral AVM embolization, the fluoroscopy and angiography run time is longer, with more radiation exposure and more contrast dose. The lower weight of pediatric patients requires more judicious use of contrast administration, particularly in long, complex embolizations. The recommended dosage of contrast may be estimated by patient weight using the following formula: weight (kg) × 5/serum creatinine (mg/dL), or 5 to 6 mL per kg with normal kidney function. This is a conservative formula, and 10 to 20% additional contrast volume may be administered in the long and complicated endovascular procedure. Diluting the contrast to a ratio of 70/30 is advised during long interventional procedures, particularly with newer and higher-quality digital subtraction angiography machines. Radiation-induced skin eruption and hair loss may occur with prolonged radiation exposure. The rapidly growing tissue of pediatric patients may be more susceptible to radiation injury in dose-related (deterministic, such as skin ulceration, erythema, and hair loss) or not dose-related effect (stochastic, such as neoplasm). Use of filters and limiting time on the fluoroscopy pedal are the main effective measures in reducing radiation exposure.

In children, in addition to the potential for contrast and radiation injury, fluid administration may lead to volume overload. In general 1 to 2 mL/kg of isotonic fluids is adequate for a maintenance volume. Other complications related to embolization may include groin or retroperitoneal hematoma. Blood loss in the pediatric age group can be detrimental and a small hematoma may lead to hemodynamic compromise and require blood transfusion. Arterial vasospasm is common in children and may lead to limb ischemia if it happens at the common femoral or iliac arteries.

During the interventional procedure itself and while advancing the flow-guided or flow-assisted microcatheter over the micro–guide wire, a vessel perforation may occur, and contrast extravasation may be seen. Vessel perforation and bleeding may occur and may lead to increased intracranial pressure and death. This occurs in less than 0.5% of cases with the transarterial approach and is more common during the transvenous and transtorcular approach in up to 10%.[1] Treatment would entail continuing embolization if feasible, followed by immediate imaging to assess the extent of ICH secondary to the vessel perforation and the need for possible hematoma evacuation.

Additional complications may be related to the glue and particles embolization. Glue embolization to an arterial branch feeding normal brain tissue can cause stroke; across the AVM, may lead to occlusion of the draining vein and sinuses causing venous hypertension, infarction, and hemorrhage; or to the lung can cause pulmonary embolism. If the cerebral venous occlusion is partial, the patient may be started on heparin for anticoagulation.[1] Caution with removal of the flow-directed microcatheter should be taken because a drop of glue in the pediatric population with small vessel calibers may lead to occlusion of any branch on the way out, such as the aorta or internal iliac or radicular arteries. Partial occlusion may resolve spontaneously, and complete occlusion will require an immediate vascular surgery consult.[1]

> **PEARL** Polymer embolization across the AVM may lead to occlusion of the draining vein, potentially leading to hemorrhage.

Care must be taken not to allow reflux of the nBCA polymer back around the flow-guided microcatheter. If the microcatheter is glued in place, it could be cut as proximal as possible to the arterial wall under tension and allowed to retract to the aortic lumen, or it can be secured to the subcutaneous tissue. In either case the microcatheter will be pushed to the side and will be incorporated into the arterial wall.

■ Summary and Conclusions

In children, cerebral AVM presentation, endovascular management, and complications share some similarities with adults, but there are significant differences.

The mortality and morbidity from AVM hemorrhage in the pediatric age group are higher than in adults (5 to 15% for supratentorial AVMs and 40 to 50% for infratentorial AVMs), which warrants aggressive treatment and less expectant therapy. Moreover, the longer life expectancy of children justifies the interest in early treatment. Pediatric cerebral AVMs constitute a heterogeneous group and management should be tailored according to the location as well as the size and age of the patients. More urgent therapy is preferred in neonates and infants, and usually with an endovascular approach to halt the progression of irreversible neurocognitive decline and melting-brain syndrome. In those older than 1 year of age, the role of endovascular therapy remains an integral portion of multimodality AVM therapy and the sole therapy in ~10% of cases with a small AVM nidus and few feeding arteries. Moreover, partial AVM embolization may lead to complete occlusion, and complete occlusion may recanalize later on.

The complications following an endovascular approach include those related to the contrast and radiation exposure and to glue embolization and vessel thrombosis. Recanalization or recurrence can occur after complete angiographic cure with endovascular, surgical, or radiotherapy techniques more frequently than in adult AVMs.

REFERENCES

1. Lasjaunias P. Vascular Diseases in Neonates, Infants and Children: Interventional Neuroradiology Management. 1st ed. Berlin: Springer-Verlag; 1997
2. Lasjaunias P, Hui F, Zerah M, et al. Cerebral arteriovenous malformations in children: management of 179 consecutive cases and review of the literature. Childs Nerv Syst 1995;11:66–79

3. Rodesch G, Malherbe V, Alvarez H, Zerah M, Devictor D, Lasjaunias P. Nongalenic cerebral arteriovenous malformations in neonates and infants: review of 26 consecutive cases (1982–1992). Childs Nerv Syst 1995;11:231–241

4. Spetzler RF, Martin NA. A proposed grading system for arteriovenous malformations. J Neurosurg 1986;65:476–483

5. Hofmeister C, Stapf C, Hartmann A, et al. Demographic, morphological, and clinical characteristics of 1289 patients with brain arteriovenous malformation. Stroke 2000;31:1307–1310

6. The Arteriovenous Malformation Study Group. Arteriovenous malformations of the brain in adults. N Engl J Med 1999;340:1812–1818

7. Bulsara KR, Alexander MJ, Villavicencio AT, Graffagnino C. De novo cerebral arteriovenous malformation: case report. Neurosurgery 2002;50:1137–1141

8. Hladky JP, Lejeune JP, Blond S, Pruvo JP, Dhellemmes P. Cerebral arteriovenous malformations in children: report on 62 cases. Childs Nerv Syst 1994;10:328–333

9. Ciricillo SF, Cogen PH, Edwards MS. Pediatric cryptic vascular malformations: presentation, diagnosis and treatment. Pediatr Neurosurg 1994;20:137–147

10. Armstrong DC, ter Brugge K. Selected interventional procedures for pediatric head and neck vascular lesions. Neuroimaging Clin N Am 2000;10:271–292

11. terBrugge KG. Neurointerventional procedures in the pediatric age group. Childs Nerv Syst 1999;15:751–754

12. Newfield P, Hamid RK. Pediatric neuroanesthesia: arteriovenous malformations. Anesthesiol Clin North America 2001; 19:229–235

13. Paulsen RD, Steinberg GK, Norbash AM, Marcellus ML, Lopez JR, Marks MP. Embolization of rolandic cortex arteriovenous malformations. Neurosurgery 1999;44:479–484; discussion 484–486

14. Fleetwood IG, Steinberg GK. Arteriovenous malformation. Lancet 2002;359:863–873

15. Bullitt E, Aylward S, Bernard EJ, Gerig G. Computer-assisted visualization of arteriovenous malformation on the home personal computer. Neurosurgery 2001;48:576–583

16. Perini S, Zampieri P, Rosta L, et al. Endovascular treatment of pial AVMs: technical options, indications and limits in pediatric age patients. J Neurosurg Sci 1997;41:325–330

17. Humphreys RP, Hoffman HJ, Drake JM, Rutka JT. Choices in the 1990s for the management of pediatric cerebral arteriovenous malformations. Pediatr Neurosurg 1996;25:277–285

18. Hoh BL, Ogilvy CS, Butler WE, Loeffler JS, Putman CM, Chapman PH. Multimodality treatment of nongalenic arteriovenous malformations in pediatric patients. Neurosurgery 2000;47:346–357; discussion 357–358

19. Ali MJ, Bendok BR, Rosenblatt S, Rose JE, Getch CC, Batjer HH. Recurrence of pediatric cerebral arteriovenous malformations after angiographically documented resection. Pediatr Neurosurg 2003;39:32–38

20. Meisel HJ, Mansmann U, Alvarez H, Rodesch G, Brock M, Lasjaunias P. Cerebral arteriovenous malformations and associated aneurysms: analysis of 305 cases from a series of 662 patients. Neurosurgery 2000;46:793–800; discussion 800–802

21. Hartmann A, Pile-Spellman J, Stapf C, et al. Risk of endovascular treatment of brain arteriovenous malformations. Stroke 2002;33:1816–1820

16

Endovascular Treatment of Vein of Galen Malformations in Children

KAREL G. TERBRUGGE

Vein of Galen arteriovenous malformations (VGAMs) reflect a choroidal arteriovenous disease and may be the only embryonic vascular malformations. Unlike pial arteriovenous malformations (AVMs), the actual shunt lies in the subarachnoid space. Raybaud et al first recognized that the ectatic vein in a VGAM is, in fact, the median vein of prosencephalon, the embryonic precursor of the vein of Galen itself.[1] Additionally, alternative routes for deep venous drainage persist, most often the choroidal vein and the thalamostriate vein do not drain into the vein of Galen.[2] The clinical presentation of VGAMs and their natural history vary significantly from that of pial AVMs. The management options, timing of intervention, and potential complication make it imperative that this condition be recognized precisely and accurately and managed at an experienced center at the optimal time to ensure that a child develops normally.

■ Angioarchitecture of Vein of Galen Arteriovenous Malformations

It is possible to distinguish the angioarchitectural differences between an AVM involving the vein of Galen forerunner; that is, the median vein of prosencephalon (VGAM) and an AVM with venous drainage into a dilated vein of Galen, which has been called a vein of Galen aneurysmal dilatation (VGAD) by Lasjaunias.[3] VGAMs involve the choroidal fissure and extend from the interventricular foramen rostrally to the atrium laterally.[3] The arterial supply usually involves all choroidal arteries, including subfornical and anterior choroidal contributions. It also may receive significant contributions from

the subependymal network from the posterior circle of Willis. Involvement of transmesencephalic arteries, which are easily identified on magnetic resonance imaging (MRI), excludes the diagnosis of VGAM. Subependymal and transcerebral contributions appear accessory in the supply to the shunt and are possibly created by the venous-sump effect.[3] Their spontaneous disappearance after appropriate treatment of the major supply to the shunt supports this hypothesis. The limbic arterial arch that bridges the cortical branch of the anterior choroidal artery with the posterior cerebral artery secondarily with the pericallosal artery is often seen. The nidus of the lesion is usually located in the midline and usually receives a bilateral and symmetrical blood supply.

Dural contributions to a VGAM are possible and may be located remote from the choroidal fissure. They represent secondary arteriovenous (AV) shunts after sinus thrombosis or are a consequence of the sump effect. Rarely, an arterial disposition resembles a moyamoya pattern and usually reflects irreversible damage to the brain. It is associated with a very poor prognosis.

Lasjaunias broadly divided VGAMs into two types on the basis of their angioarchitecture: choroidal and mural.[3] The choroidal types (**Figs. 16–1A** and **16–2D**, pages 177 and 180) correspond to a primitive condition. They receive a contribution from all the choroidal arteries, and an interposed network is present before opening into the large venous pouch. It is mostly encountered in neonates with poor clinical scores. In contrast, mural types of VGAMs (**Fig. 16–3B**, page 182) represent direct AV fistulas within the wall of the median vein of prosencephalon. These fistulas can be single or multiple. They can converge into a single venous chamber or into multiple venous lobulations located

176

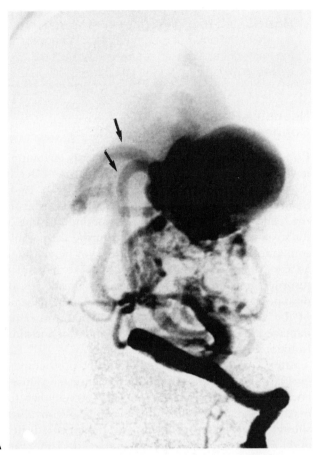

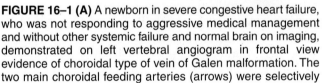

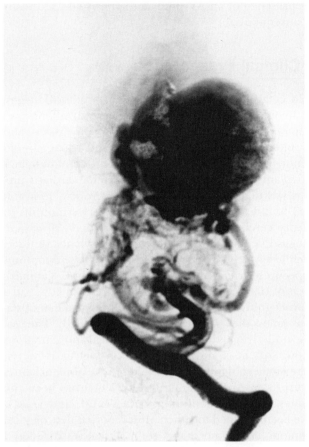

A   B

FIGURE 16–1 (A) A newborn in severe congestive heart failure, who was not responding to aggressive medical management and without other systemic failure and normal brain on imaging, demonstrated on left vertebral angiogram in frontal view evidence of choroidal type of vein of Galen malformation. The two main choroidal feeding arteries (arrows) were selectively catheterized and embolized with pure glue. **(B)** The immediate postembolization left vertebral angiogram in frontal view demonstrates significantly decreased flow through the lesion, which resulted in dramatic clinical improvement and extubation of the neonate in 36 hours and discharge on cardiac medication 8 days later.

along the anterior aspect of the pouch or along the anterior choroidal veins of the fissure. Mural VGAMs tend to occur in infants with higher clinical scores.

By definition, venous drainage is toward the dilated median vein of prosencephalon, and no communication exists with the deep venous system of the brain. Thalamostriate veins open into the posterior and inferior thalamic veins, which occurs normally during the third month in utero. They secondarily join either the anterior confluence or a subtemporal vein, demonstrating a typical epsilon shape on lateral angiography. Because the choroidal veins are the embryonic tributaries of the median vein, potentially fistulous communications may exist some distance from the pouch. In older children, the choroidal veins opening into the VGAM may become visible if the skull base outlet has been restricted. The remainder of the venous drainage is variable, with the straight sinus being absent in almost all cases.

VGAD, a major differential diagnosis, is a pial AVM draining into the deep venous system with an acquired dilatation of the vein of Galen confluence either caused by stenosis at the venodural junction or thrombosis of the straight sinus. The dilated vein drains the normal brain in addition to the malformation. The presence of a primary opening of the shunt into a nonchoroidal vein or demonstration of reflux into normal cerebral venous tributaries that open into the venous pouch confirms the diagnosis of VGAD. Typically these lesions are found in older children with clinical presentations that resemble other pial AVMs. Characteristic symptoms are progressive neurological deficits associated with a mass effect and/or retrograde venous congestion, and hemorrhage of a venous origin. When present, dural AV shunts are usually secondary lesions caused by a sump effect and thrombosis of the outflow sinuses. Vein of Galen varices rarely are seen without the presence of an AV shunt and are usually clinically inconsequential.

■ Clinical Presentation

Gold et al described three consecutive clinical stages: (1) neonates with cardiac insufficiency, (2) infants and young children with hydrocephaly and convulsions, and (3) older children with headaches and subarachnoid hemorrhage.[4] Subsequently, a fourth group of neonates and infants with macrocephaly and minimal cardiac symptoms was described.[5] In an exhaustive review, Johnston et al found the following as the primary symptoms in infants: cerebrospinal fluid (CSF) disorders, 70%; neurological deficits, 31%; and neurocognitve delays, 12%. In children between ages 1 and 5 years, these symptoms respectively occurred in 61, 33, and 5%.[6] In Lasjaunias's series of 109 neonates and infants, more than 50% had a neurocognitive delay. None had neurological manifestations unless they had been previously shunted.[3] The reason underlying these variable clinical presentations among patients and different series is unclear. However, there has been significant confusion in the nomenclature. A pial brain AVM draining into a VGAD has been the greatest source of confusion: both VGAMs and VGADs have been grouped together. Most reported neurological symptoms and hemorrhages are in mistakenly diagnosed VGAMs or are the result of changes in angioarchitecture. Only recently has the negative effect of ventricular drainage on the neurological evaluation of these patients been recognized.

On the basis of the literature the natural history of these lesions is unclear. The primary reasons are the relative rarity of the lesion and the confusing nomenclature. Lasjaunias have proposed a logical sequence in the natural history of this disease that not only improves understanding of the disease and its pathophysiology but also helps in choosing the appropriate timing of intervention.[3]

■ Angioarchitecture and Clinical Symptomatology: Implications and Indications for Treatment

The clinical manifestations of VGAMs are broadly classified into three groups: (1) neonates with congestive cardiac failure, (2) infants with hydrocephalus and hydrovenous disorder, and (3) children with neurocognitive delay. The appropriate management for each stage differs and is considered individually. These scenarios overlap considerably when decision making is based on the underlying pathophysiology. Emergency management should be limited to specific situations.

> **PEARL** Angiography in the neonatal workup is not indicated and not recommended. In neonates, the immediate goal is to restore a satisfactory systemic physiology and to gain time.

Neonates Presenting with Congestive Cardiac Failure

Congestive cardiac failure (CCF) is mainly encountered in choroidal forms of VGAM, which are the most frequent AV shunts diagnosed in that age group (**Fig. 16–1A**). Severe forms of CCF are associated with persistence of the fetal type of circulation. Septal communications and ductus arteriosus are often noted during cardiac ultrasonography. These structures should not be considered as associated cardiac malformations. Like most of the disorders encountered under these circumstances, they disappear spontaneously after endovascular management of the vein of Galen shunts itself. Renal and hepatic damage may further aggravate CCF, and liver and kidney function may be impaired transiently.

After a VGAM is suspected clinically, pretherapeutic evaluations should be obtained. Clinical evaluation and documentation of all possible events that have occurred since birth, including presence of convulsions, should be evaluated clinically and documented. Renal and liver function should be evaluated. Transcranial ultrasonography is needed to evaluate the patient for encephalomalacia. Cardiac ultrasonography should be performed to assess cardiac tolerance and to diagnose associated conditions. A good-quality MRI examination is necessary to provide morphological information about the lesion and to evaluate the status of myelinization. Finally, if the child is in the intensive care unit, electroencephalography should be performed.

Angiography is neither indicated nor recommended for the evaluation of neonates. In neonates, the immediate goal is to restore a satisfactory systemic physiology and to gain time. The first few months of clinical assessment are crucial to be able to prognose the child's future neurological state. The goal is to deliver a baby who is stable on medication for cardiac insufficiency and to gain time for easier technical management. It is important to recognize the presence of a significant developmental delay as well as early features of hydrocephalus and macrocrania. In our experience the presence of encephalomalacia and moyamoya pattern predicts poor clinical outcomes. A decrease in head circumference is probably the worst finding because it indicates loss of brain substance and early fusion of suture.

We follow a scoring system proposed by Lasjaunias to decide the timing of intervention.[3] It is also extremely helpful in maintaining a consistent management strategy and for comparing results. A poor score mandates against intervention. Emergency management in neonates should be restricted to specific situations. In the scoring system proposed by Lasjaunias, a score between 8 and 12 entails emergency endovascular management.[3] The emergency procedure partially reduces the degree of shunting to eliminate CCF. We usually embolize one or two major pedicles. At this stage, the aim of management is not necessarily to obliterate the shunt completely.

The management team also should direct its attention to the management of CCF. There are two strategies: to reduce oxygen consumption and to improve oxygen delivery. These goals can be achieved by tracheal intubation, mechanical ventilation, and drug therapy (e.g., administering a diuretic) in conjunction with expert advice from a pediatric cardiologist.

In summary, time is gained by managing the CCF, recognizing and excluding neonates where irreversible brain damage has already occurred, and partially embolizing to reduce the degree of AV shunting in a select group of patients.

Ventricular Enlargement and Increasing Head Size

Unlike CCFs, disorders of CSF circulation manifest at any age: in utero, in neonates, and in infants. Choroidal and mural VGAMs also give rise to these manifestations (**Figs. 16–2A–C, 16–3A**, pages 180 and 182), which result from the abnormal hemodynamic condition in the torcular venous sinus confluence, the posterior conversion of the venous drainage of the brain, and the immaturity of the pacchionian granulation system. Compression of the aqueduct by the dilated vein is rarely a contributing factor[7,8] as evidenced by demonstrations of patency of the aqueduct itself and by the presence of prominent CSF spaces in relation to the cerebral sulci. An enlarging head can stabilize spontaneously and the ventricles can dilate with cavernous sinus capture of the sylvian veins. A new low-pressure venous system then offers an alternative pathway for water resorption, and the hydration status of the cerebral tissue improves.

Ventricular shunting in a VGAM carries an additional risk of complications (**Fig. 16–3D**, page 182). It does not deal with the problem created by the hydrodynamic disorders and only transiently and incompletely resolves the emergency situation at the ventricular level. Various series have consistently reported poor clinical outcomes in shunted infants.[6,8,9] The deficits, seizures, and hemorrhage that follow ventricular shunting are so well accepted that they have even been considered as part of the natural history of VGAMs. Endovascular management in the same situation stops the progression of these disorders (**Fig. 16–2C,G**). Complete obliteration of the fistula is seldom necessary, and even partial embolization often rapidly reverses the overhydration of brain tissue. If the head circumference appears to increase too rapidly, if there is preclinical MRI evidence of intraventricular hyperpressure, or if clinical follow-up demonstrates a significant developmental delay, urgent embolization should be performed. Ventricular shunting should be avoided unless pressure within the ventricles is increased despite an adequate attempt at embolization.

> **PEARL** The presence of venous infarcts or calcifications as well as encephalomalacia would suggest irreversible brain damage, whereas hydrovenous disorders and hydrocephalus are potentially treatable conditions.

Developmental Delay

Developmental delay is part of the natural history of an untreated VGAM. Careful evaluations of neurocognitive performances show that most children with increasing head size exhibit some degree of mental retardation. During infancy, assessment of neurocognitive delay is challenging and requires collaboration with a specialist. Consistent and uniform well-established grading scales should be used. The major aim of such testing is not to compare children but to follow a child's ongoing development. From the perspective of management, it is important to recognize irreversible brain damage and potentially treatable or preventable situations. The presence of venous infarcts or calcifications and encephalomalacia suggests irreversible brain damage. Hydrovenous disorders and hydrocephalus are potentially treatable conditions (**Fig. 16–2C,G**, pages 180 and 181). Again, hydrovenous disorders should be treated by eradicating the fistula, rather than by shunting the patient. As head size increases, obstruction of venous outflow related to narrowing of the jugular veins at the level of the jugular bulb tends to become apparent.

■ Chronic Vein of Galen Aneurysm Malformation with Patent Sinuses

Patients who do not undergo decompensation from CCF or CSF hydrodynamic disorders enter a stage of chronicity. Clinical manifestations and the prognosis primarily depend on the patency of the draining dural sinuses. If the draining sinuses are patent, the prognosis tends to be good. Seizures and mental retardation are the major symptoms if AV shunt is not corrected in time. Some unusual endocrine manifestations, such as precocious puberty and failure to thrive, have been reported.

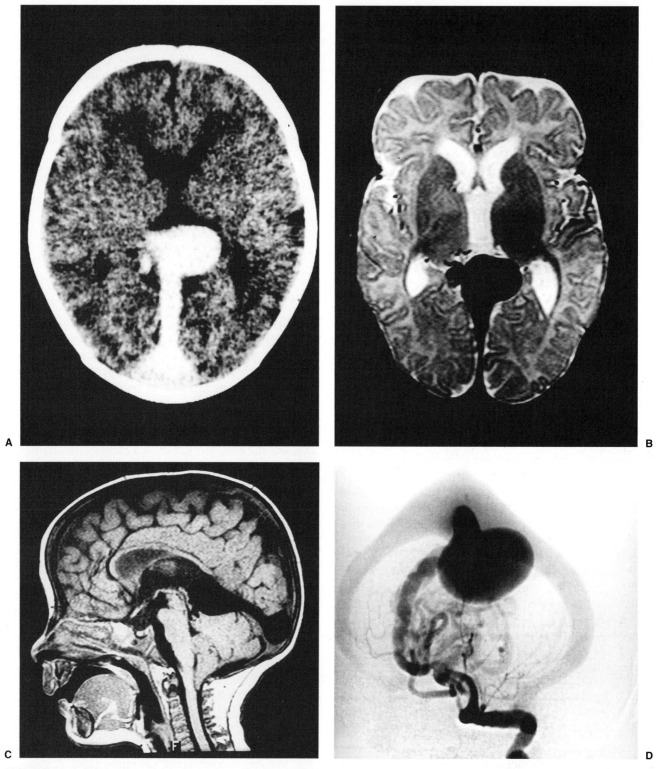

FIGURE 16–2 (A) A neonate was born in moderate congestive heart failure that could be managed with medical therapy, showed on enhanced computed tomography evidence of vein of Galen malformation and normal-sized ventricles. **(B)** Follow-up magnetic resonance imaging (MRI) examination at 5 months of age demonstrated on axial and **(C)** sagittal views evidence of progressive ventricular enlargement as well as cerebellar tonsillar prolapse. **(D)** Left vertebral angiogram in frontal view performed at 5.5 months of age demonstrates choroidal type of vein of Galen malformation.

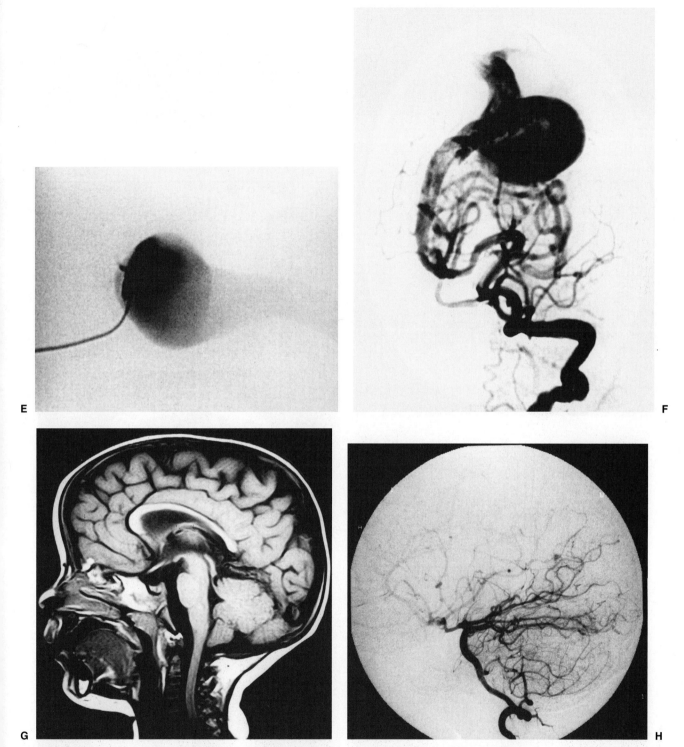

FIGURE 16–2 (*Continued*) **(E)** Selective catheterization of the main feeding artery was achieved and embolization with pure glue performed resulting in **(F)** significant reduction in the flow through the lesion as shown on the immediate postembolization left vertebral angiogram in frontal view. **(G)** MRI in sagittal view obtained 3 months later demonstrated a normal position of the cerebellar tonsils and normal-sized ventricles. **(H)** Delayed vertebral angiogram in lateral view 18 months after the partial embolization with glue demonstrated progressive complete obliteration of the vein of Galen malformation. The child developed normally with normal neurological function at 5 years follow-up.

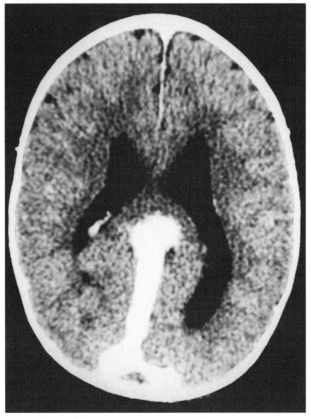

A

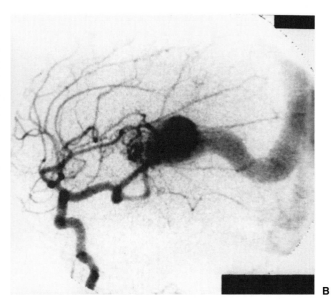

B

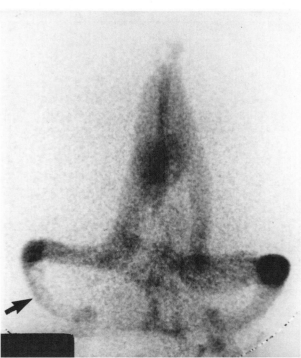

C

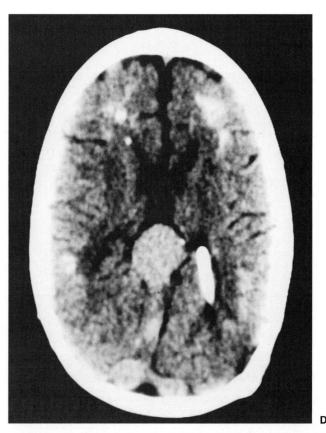

D

FIGURE 16–3 (A) An infant born with mild congestive heart failure and diagnosed with vein of Galen malformation developed progressive increasing head circumference at age 6 months and showed on enhanced computed tomographic (CT) examination evidence of vein of Galen malformation associated with ventricular enlargement. **(B)** Left internal carotid angiogram in lateral view performed at the age of 1 month had shown a mural type of vein of Galen malformation and **(C)** patency of the dural sinuses (arrow) on the venous phase of the vertebral angiogram frontal view. **(D)** Ventricular shunting was performed at age 7 months and unenhanced CT scan at 12 months of age demonstrated smaller-sized ventricles but a slight increase in the size of the vein of Galen malformation and significant subcortical calcifications.

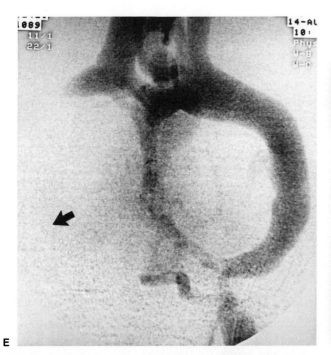

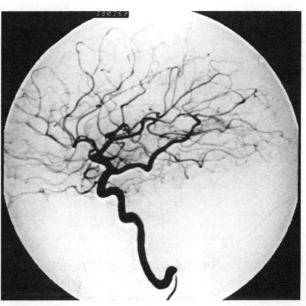

E   F

FIGURE 16–3 (*Continued*) **(E)** The venous phase of the vertebral angiogram in frontal view at 13 months of age showed there was no longer patency of the right transverse sinus (arrow). **(F)** Transarterial embolization with pure glue was performed at that time and resulted in good angiographic outcome with immediate obliteration of the malformation, as shown on the left internal carotid angiogram in lateral view, but unfortunately the developmental delay that occurred after ventricular shunting was not reversible and resulted in permanent mental retardation.

Morphological sequelae express themselves in the form of calcifications, subependymal atrophies, and eventually the stigmata of previous acute accidents with cortical and subcortical atrophy. Because there is no pial or subpial reflux in a classic VGAM, focal venous infarcts or parenchymal hemorrhages are unusual.

The insult to the brain is slow and permanent and usually manifests in the form of calcifications and atrophy. There are three types of calcifications in the vein of Galen.[3] The first type is mural related to partial or complete thrombosis of the lesion. The second type is subcortical in the white matter. These calcifications reflect the failure of the deep hydrovenous watershed when the compliance of the medullary veins began to lose its ventriculocortical gradient. These calcifications are usually bilateral and symmetrically located, preferentially in the frontal region. The third type of calcification is located in the striatum, particularly in the caudate and putamen bilaterally. These calcifications are an expression of the subacute ischemia in the region of the prominent collateral circulation system after the cortical veins are unable to drain the cerebral white substance, or when the persisting thalamic pathways are overloaded by the drainage of the parietal-occipital regions. The calcifications are not produced by arterial steal.[10]

Therefore, the timing of intervention is important. Most of these sequelae can be prevented by early occlusion of the shunt. However, the clinical outcomes of children with patent sinuses are relatively good compared with those with secondarily occluded sinuses.

■ Dural Sinus Occlusion and Supratentorial Congestion and Reflux

This evolution of VGAMs is common (**Fig. 16–3C,E**). The cause of the dural sinus thrombosis is unknown. It may be influenced by abnormal skull base growth and maturation caused by increased head size. Although hypothesized, the role of venous high angiopathy is unclear. Thrombosis is a hallmark of brain AVMs in children compared with those in adults. It is usually progressive and may develop slowly without symptoms over a long period. The development of jugular bulb stenosis protects the heart; however, it exposes the brain to congestion, venous infarcts, and hemorrhagic manifestations. The capture of the sylvian veins by the cavernous sinus would significantly influence the overall course of events.[3] Impending occlusion of jugular veins with rerouting of blood flow of the brain and possibly of the malformation toward the cavernous sinuses and finally the facial venous system is an emergency situation. As stressed earlier, shunting the ventricles is not the solution to this problem. Emergency endovascular management may be warranted to reduce blood flow across the AV shunt to allow easier drainage of the brain.

Another potential complication of thrombosis and occlusion of the dural sinuses is the development of dural AV shunts. Although these shunts seldom cause specific clinical symptoms and disappear after complete obliteration of the VGAM, they can complicate the interpretation of diagnostic angiography.

Overall, the cause of occlusion of the dural sinuses is understood poorly. Neither has it been possible to predict precisely the patients who will evolve toward this occlusive phenomenon. After occlusion, the overall prognosis remains guarded and little can be done in terms of management. Hence, identification of the therapeutic window before the onset of this occlusive phenomenon is important.

The infratentorial consequence of the dural sinus occlusion is tonsillar prolapse. The prolapse is caused by posterior fossa venous congestion and usually disappears when the AV shunt is corrected. Syringomyelia also has been described as a consequence of this tonsillar prolapse.[11]

Spontaneous Thrombosis

Spontaneous thrombosis of a VGAM is rare. In the series by Lasjaunias, five of 120 (4%) patients developed spontaneous thrombosis, but only two were normal neurologically.[3] Compression of the arterial feeders by the tentorial edge, combined with secondary intraluminal thrombosis and stenosed draining veins, might favor the development of spontaneous thrombosis. In any event, this thrombosis tends to occur after cerebral damage is already irreversible. Spontaneous thrombosis should not be considered a favorable outcome. Waiting for spontaneous thrombosis to occur does not represent an appropriate therapeutic strategy and, in our opinion, constitutes an unacceptable choice.

■ Endovascular Management

Goals

In our experience endovascular management of VGAMs is clearly superior to other forms of treatment. Like Lasjaunias, we use a transarterial approach and n-butyl-2-cyanoacrylate (nBCA) as the embolic agent (**Figs. 16–1A,B; 16–2D–F,H; and 16–3B,F**).[3] There are a few case reports of using a transvenous approach to reach the dilated sac. Conceptually, the aim of treatment is to exclude the malformation from the circulation. Theoretically, whether an arterial or venous route is used, the result should be similar. However, interventional experience with the venous route is limited[12–16] and the

lack of published outcome analyses does not seem to support the venous route. We therefore continue to believe that the best outcomes are obtained with the transarterial route.

Possible reasons for the poor outcomes associated with the venous approach may be related to interventional practitioners' limited overall understanding of the anatomy and pathophysiology of the lesion they think they are treating. In a mural type of VGAM with a single hole, excellent outcomes should be possible by either of the two routes. However, if reflux into any of the fistulas from the arteries of the brain parenchyma is possible as a consequence of the sump effect, the venous approach may lead to complications such as hemorrhage. We also strongly believe that for the choroidal types of VGAMs, the venous approach would be unsuitable.

> **PEARL**   Multiple, staged arterial embolizations aimed at slowly reducing the flow across the AV fistula are recommended in vein of Galen malformations.

Identification of irreversible brain damage is exceedingly important (**Fig. 16–3D**). MRI features of myelomalacia, extensive venous infarction, occlusion of the venous outlet, and the presence of moyamoya phenomenon should mitigate against any kind of management. Emergency management should be limited to a few situations, such as nonresolving CCF, increasing head circumference due to altered CSF hydrodynamics, and impending occlusion of the jugular veins with rerouting of blood to the facial venous system. Our approach has been to perform multiple-staged arterial embolizations aimed at slowly reducing the blood flow across the AV fistula.

■ Results

Lasjaunias have reported the largest experience with treating of VGAMs.[3] They used a consistent and reproducible set of management principles, embolization techniques, and patient follow-up. They divided their results into four groups: fetus, neonates, infants (up to 2 years old), and children.

Of the fetuses antenatally diagnosed with VGAMs, five had irreversible brain damage at the time of their initial presentation and were not treated. Of the 14 patients treated, 12 have had excellent neurological outcomes. About a third of the neonatal group had irreversible brain damage at the time of their initial presentation. No one in this group was neurologically normal at their first presentation. The incidence of permanent neurological deficit despite treatment was 50%. The difference in outcomes between the antenatal and neonatal groups suggests that the latter group had a more severe condition than the former. The antenatal group reflects an unselected population and thus probably better reflects the true aggressiveness of this malformation. In the infant group, Lasjaunias included children up to the age of 2 years, which they thought represented a good cutoff point from the perspective of brain maturation and the development of pacchionian granulations.[3] Most of these patients were embolized and 22 of 26 patients had a good neurological outcome. The predominant presenting symptom in this group was macrocrania.

Relatively few patients become symptomatic at an older age. Lasjaunias managed 12 children who were symptom free in the first few years of their life. Of these, 75% underwent embolization.[3] Each child who presented with neurological symptoms had a malformation in which the venous drainage of the AV shunt was modified spontaneously, resulting in reflux to the pial veins.

Limited information is available on long-term results of alternative treatment modalities for VGAMs, including a venous approach to endovascular treatment, surgery, and radiation therapy. Based on these limited reports and compared with the large reported experience with arterial embolization of VGAMs, it seems that arterial embolization by an experienced team is currently the treatment of choice.

■ Complications

Nonneurological complications related to embolization and the technical difficulties of injecting glue are rare.[3] Lasjaunias found a 4% complication rate, which was related to glue causing an asymptomatic occlusion of the internal iliac artery or to the microcatheter getting glued in place. Our experience is similar with an exceedingly low nonneurological complication rate. Repeated punctures of the femoral artery do not seem to cause significant problems.

The risk of venous passage of glue is obvious, especially in inexperienced hands. The malformations are typically high flow, and we usually use a high concentration of glue during embolization in these patients (2.5 mL nBCA and 0.5 mL Lipiodol). Tantulum powder is added to the mixture to increase opacification. The injection is made under induced hypotension. Venous infarction as a consequence of venous passage of glue is rare (4% in our personal series of 25 embolized VGAMs). The phenomenon of perfusion breakthrough has not occurred in our experience nor in that of Lasjaunias.[3] Acute closure of these high-flow fistulas does not seem to cause problems if performed by arterial embolization. In our experience and in that of Lasjaunias consumption coagulopathy has not been observed.[3] Overall, arterial embolizations can be performed with a low complication rate in experienced hands using a staged procedure approach to VGAMs.

The stenosis of the jugular foramina and the timing of capture of the cavernous sinus affect overall prognosis. At present, these cannot be predicted. Stenosis of the jugular foramina after capture of the cavernous sinuses allows an alternative route of drainage for the brain. However, if it occurs before capture of the cavernous sinuses, outcomes are uniformly dismal.

■ Conclusion

In the past 15 years major progress has been made in understanding and managing neonates, infants, and children with VGAMs. The apparent dismal prognosis of these patients ~20 years ago has now become a more optimistic outlook. Although significant challenges in the management of patients with VGAMs continue to exist, their predictability and response to endovascular treatment are now widely recognized.

Patient selection and the timing of treatment are essential in the decision-making process. When done properly by an experienced team, favorable outcomes and a normally developing child can be expected. We recommend the arterial approach as the method of choice for embolization therapy because its published results compare favorably with those of the venous approach and surgical intervention. Ventricular shunting should be avoided because it negatively affects VGAMs and, unlike arterial embolization, it does not reduce the venous hyperpressure phenomenon responsible for most of the clinical symptomatology. The management of patients with VGAMs more than any other vascular disorder affecting the central nervous system depends on the presence and coordination of a multidisciplinary treatment team, which must consist of an experienced interventionalist, pediatric interventionalist, neurosurgeon with pediatric expertise, neuroradiologist, and development assessment teams. If such a team is unavailable, patients with this disorder should be sent to a specialized treatment center to ensure optimum decision making and care.

REFERENCES

1. Raybaud CA, Strother CM, Hald JK. Aneurysms of the vein of Galen: embryonic considerations and anatomical features relating to the pathogenesis of the malformation. Neuroradiology 1989;31: 109–128
2. Lasjaunias P, Garcia-Monaco R, Rodesch G, TerBrugge K. Deep venous drainage in great cerebral vein (vein of Galen) absence and malformations. Neuroradiology 1991a;33:234–242
3. Lasjaunias P. Vein of Galen aneurysmal malformation. In: Lasjaunias P. Vascular Diseases in Neonates, Infants and Children. Berlin: Springer-Verlag; 1997:67–202

4. Gold AP, Ransohoff J, Carter S. Vein of Galen malformation. Acta Neurol Scand 1964;11:5–31

5. Amacher AL, Shillito J Jr. The syndromes and surgical treatment of aneurysms of the great vein of Galen. J Neurosurg 1973;39:89–98

6. Johnston IH, Whittle I, Besser M, Morgan MK. Vein of Galen malformation: diagnosis and management. Neurosurgery 1987;20:747–757

7. Diebler C, Dulac O, Renier D, Ernest C, Lalande G. Aneurysms of the vein of Galen in infants aged 2 to 15 months: diagnosis and natural evolution. Neuroradiology 1981;21:185–197

8. Zerah M, Garcio-Monaco R, Rodesch G, et al. Hydrodynamics in vein of Galen malformation in 43 cases. Childs Nerv Syst 1992;8:111–117

9. Quisling RG, Mickle JP. Venous pressure measurements in vein of Galen aneurysms. AJNR Am J Neuroradiol 1989;10:411–417

10. Yu YL, Chiu EKW, Woo E, et al. Dystrophic intracranial calcification: CT evidence of "cerebral steal" from arteriovenous malformation. Neuroradiology 1987;29:519–522

11. Apsimon HT, Ives FJ, Khangure MS. Cranial dural arteriovenous malformation and fistula: radiological diagnosis and management: review of thirty-four patients. Australas Radiol 1993;37:2–25

12. Halbach VV, Down CF, Higashida T, Balousek PA, Ciricillo SF, Edwards MSB. Endovascular treatment of mural-type vein of Galen malformations. J Neurosurg 1998;89:74–80

13. Casasco A, Lylyk P, Hodes JE, Kohan G, Aymard A, Merland JJ. Percutaneous transvenous catheterization and embolization of vein of Galen aneurysms. Neurosurgery 1991;28:260–266

14. Mickle JP, Quisling RG. The transtorcular embolization of vein of Galen aneurysms. J Neurosurg 1986;64:731–735

15. Dowd CF, Halbach VV, Barnwell SL, et al. Transfemoral venous embolization of vein of Galen malformations. AJNR Am J Neuroradiol 1990;11:643–648

16. Lylyk P, Vinuela F, Dion JE, et al. Therapeutic alternatives for vein of Galen vascular malformations. J Neurosurg 1993;78:438–445

17

Endovascular Treatment of Spinal Vascular Malformations in Children

OSAMA O. ZAIDAT AND MICHAEL J. ALEXANDER

■ Epidemiology of Spinal Vascular Malformations

Spinal vascular malformations are a rare heterogeneous group of pathologies that constitute a small proportion of all vascular malformations. The exact prevalence of vascular spinal malformations in children is unknown and is not well defined, but it may represent less than 5 to 10% of all arteriovenous malformations (AVMs) in all age groups. There is a clear male predominance in these lesions.[1] The topographical classifications of intradural, extradural, and dural spinal vascular lesions have been well described.[2] Dural spinal fistulas and slow-flow lesions are rarely encountered in young patients and will not be discussed in this chapter. The intradural spinal vascular lesions that are commonly diagnosed in children are thought to be congenital in origin, whereas the dural late-onset spinal vascular lesions are thought to be acquired lesions following prior recognized or unrecognized trauma.

The topographical classification and underlying pathophysiology of spinal vascular malformations play a pivotal role in deciding the best treatment approach. Hemorrhage, venous hypertension or congestion, or venous steal phenomena are some of the clinical presentations that may require a targeted therapeutic approach to eliminate patient symptoms or reduce the future risk of rebleeding.

■ Pertinent Spinal Cord Vascular Anatomy

The key to successful spinal cord AVM (SCAVM) endovascular intervention, or surgical resection, is a knowledge of the normal spinal cord vascular anatomy.

This knowledge provides a basis for understanding the aberrant anatomy of the SCAVM and helps in formulating the surgical or endovascular treatment plan.

The spinal cord receives blood supply from three longitudinal channels, one midline anterior spinal artery and two dorsolateral posterior spinal arteries (**Fig. 17–1A,B**). Spinal arteries branch off segmental arteries entering the neural foramen where they form radicular arteries supplying the nerve roots or medullary arteries supplying the spinal cord. On average, there are seven to eight medullary arteries supplying the anterior spinal artery. The posterior spinal arteries are more variable in location, and the number of posterior medullary arteries tributaries is less predictable compared to the arterior vasculature.[3]

The midthoracic region has the most tenuous arterial blood supply. The artery of Adamkiewicz supplies the thoracolumbar spinal cord area below T9, entering between T5 and L2 in 85% of cases and from left side in 80% of cases.[3] The spinal cord venous drainage is via radial veins, which drain into the coronal venous plexus, and longitudinal spinal veins on the cord surface (**Fig. 17–1B**). **Figure 17–2** shows a left T9 segmental artery angiogram, which demonstrates both the artery of Adamkiewicz and a posterior spinal artery contribution.

■ Classification of Spinal Cord Arteriovenous Malformations

SCAVMs are most commonly encountered in the midthoracic region (22%), followed by the cervical spine region (14%), and the rest in the lower thoracic, lumbar, and sacral areas.[1,2] A few classification schemes have been developed for the SCAVM.[2,4–7]

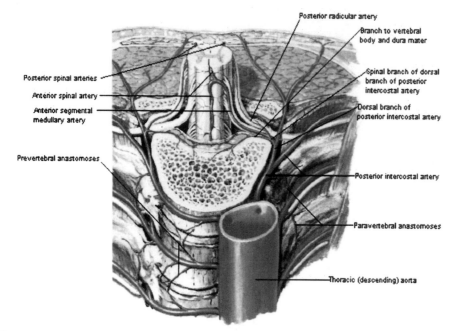

A

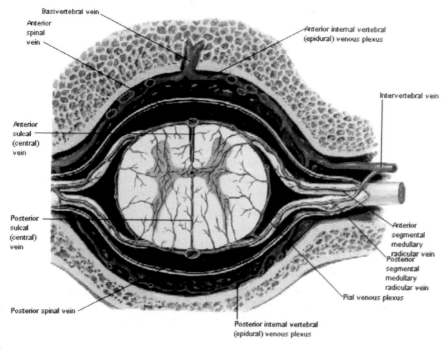

B

FIGURE 17–1 (A) Axial illustration at the thoracic aorta level illustrates the arterial supply to the spinal cord and the origin of the intercostal arteries left and right from the aorta. Note the supply to the anterior spinal artery. **(B)** The venous drainage from the spinal cord in an axial cross section (see Color Plate 17–1).

The traditional classification of the SCAVM has been based on the axial location in relation to the spinal cord parenchyma and its meninges (perimedullary and peridural), angioarchitectural features (niduses versus shunt), arterial supply, and venous drainage, which is usually via radicular, subpial coronal venous plexus, or subarachnoid venous channels.

The most commonly used topographical classification divides the spinal vascular malformation into four subtypes; type I or dural, which is further subdivided into IA with single arterial feeder and IB with multiple feeders. This type is not present in children. Type II is common in children and includes the intramedullary glomus or juvenile SCAVM. Type III is intramedullary

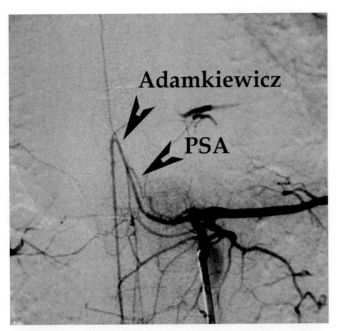

FIGURE 17–2 Anterior view left T9 segmental artery angiogram showing the artery of Adamkiewicz and a posterior spinal artery (PSA) contribution.

with extension to the extramedullary space, with complex multiple feeders. This type may be encountered in children, but less often than type II or IV. Type IV is an intradural-perimedullary SCAVM (**Table 17–1**).

A modified classification has been proposed by Spetzler et al[2] (**Table 17–1**). In this scheme, the spinal cord vascular lesions are divided into three broad categories: vascular neoplasms, aneurysms, and arteriovenous lesions. The vascular neoplastic lesions include hemangioblastoma and cavernous malformation. Spinal aneurysms may be related to dissection or blood flow

TABLE 17–1 Classification of Spinal Vascular Lesions

Traditional Classification

Type IA: dural SCAVMs (TLS, single feeding artery)
Type IB: dural SCAVM (two or more arterial feeders)
Type II: intramedullary SCAVM with compact nidus (glomus). Rapid flow, with feeders from the anterior spinal artery
Type III: intra- and extramedullary, large, complex AVM, with multiple feeders from multiple levels
Type IV: intradural-perimedullary

Modified Classification

Neoplastic vascular lesion: hemangioblastoma and cavernous malformation
Spinal aneurysm
Arteriovenous fistulas: extradural and intradural (dorsal and ventral)
AVMs: extradural-intradural, intradural (intramedullary, compact, diffuse, conus medullaris)

AVM, arteriovenous malformation; SCAVM, spinal cord arteriovenous malformation; TLS, thoraco-lumbar-sacral.

hemodynamics and are rarely encountered in pediatric population. The third category is divided into spinal cord arteriovenous fistulas and SCAVMs. Spinal arteriovenous fistulas are further subdivided into intradural and extradural; small-, medium-, or large-shunts; single or multiple feeders; and ventral or dorsal location. The spinal vascular fistulas are not usually seen in children.

The SCAVMs are further subdivided into extradural-intradural and intradural. The intradural SCAVMs are further subdivided into intramedullary, intramedullary-extramedullary, and conus medullaris. The traditional and the modified classifications are summarized in **Table 17–1**.

SCAVMs can be associated with metameric AVMs (Cobb's syndrome) and fistulas can be associated with Rendu-Osler-Weber syndrome. Other syndromes and vascular lesions that may be encountered with spinal vascular lesions are cerebral aneurysms, Klippel-Trénaunay-Weber syndrome, neurofibromatosis, and Parkes-Weber syndrome.

■ Clinical Features

The SCAVMs become clinically overt between 10 and 30 years of age; they are rarely diagnosed before the age of 10.[8] Cervical SCAVMs tend to become clinically evident earlier than SCAVMs elsewhere in the spinal cord. Various modes of clinical presentation may occur. In the pediatric population, presentation varies according to the age group.[9] Fourteen percent of SCAVMs present and are diagnosed in the pediatric age group. An additional 16% are diagnosed in adults who, in retrospect, had symptoms beginning in childhood.[9]

The underlying mechanisms for various clinical presentations are thought to be related to venous hypertension with venous congestion and ischemia, subarachnoid or intramedullary hemorrhage, mass effect by enlarged and arterialized veins, venous thrombosis, and vascular steal syndrome leading to spinal cord infarction.[10–13]

The majority of patients will present with motor or sensory symptoms as mono- or paraparesis or anesthesia (80%) and ~10% will have sphincteric involvement.[14]

> **PEARL** An acute onset of neurological deficit is the most common clinical presentation of SCAVM in children

Sudden acute onset of neurological deficit is the most common clinical presentation of SCAVM in children and occurs in 50 to 70% of cases, due to subarachnoid

- Venous hypertension related: progressive myelopathy
- Arterial steal phenomenon: spinal cord ischemia/infarction
- Venous arterialization: mass effect from venous varix
- Subarachnoid hemorrhage and hematomyelia: acute presentation, severe low back pain with para- or quadriparesis
- Cobb's syndrome: metameric involvement of the skin, vertebral body, and spinal cord at the same segment
- Rendu-Osler-Weber syndrome in 9% of the cases, with high-flow fistula
- Klippel-Trénaunay-Weber syndrome in 5% of the cases

hemorrhage (SAH) in 50% of cases and hematomyelia with or without SAH in the remaining cases. Hemorrhagic presentation reveals itself with acute severe back pain with paraplegia, with or without sphincteric dysfunction.[14] A progressive neurological deficit is a less common presentation, but it may occur in 9% cases with arterial steal syndrome and venous hypertension or slowly enlarging mass due to venous congestion.[9,14]

Other, less typical, clinical presentations include mass effect with scoliosis and other musculoskeletal abnormalities, radicular pain, abnormal gait, asymptomatic bruit, hemodynamic shunts with congestive heart failure, and cutaneous angioma or discoloration that can be enhanced by Valsalva's maneuver.[9–14] Bouts of abdominal pain may occur due to the sympathetic tract involvement in the intramedullary lesions.[15] Spinal vascular lesions can also be diagnosed incidentally in 6% of the pediatric cases with no neurological symptoms.[8]

Overall, the SCAVM is usually a single entity, but it may be associated with other vascular dysplasia, as mentioned earlier, such as Cobb's syndrome, Rendu-Osler-Weber syndrome (hereditary hemorrhagic telangiectasia), and Klippel-Trénaunay-Weber syndrome. The following conditions may mimic SCAVM: transverse myelitis, spondylosis, motor neuron disease, Devic's disease, syringomyelia, and spinal abscess or arachnoiditis.[14] **Table 17–2** summarizes the clinical findings in SCAVM.

■ Radiological Evaluation

With the advent of magnetic resonance imaging (MRI), the tradition of obtaining plain films, computed tomographic myelography, or intravenous contrast-enhanced spine tomography as an initial workup for SCAVM has been abandoned. Multifocal SCAVMs are infrequent but may occur, and this further supports the use of MRI for SCAVM screening. The MRI findings consist of heterogeneous and serpiginous signal voids with enlarged spinal canal on T1- and T2-weighted MRI sequences localized to the involved spinal cord segments. Recent advances in MRI technology have

made the diagnosis of SCAVM readily attainable.[16,17] Magnetic resonance angiography (MRA) with and without gadolinium administration provides valuable information pre- and postendovascular intervention and surgical resection. Mascalchi and coworkers studied 34 patients who underwent endovascular and surgical treatment of their spinal vascular malformation, and MRA was found to be very sensitive in detecting new residual or recanalization in their SCAVMs.[18]

Spinal digital subtraction angiography is the current standard for diagnosing SCAVMs. Spinal angiography shows details of the arterial feeders, the nidus, and the venous drainage pattern. In addition to its diagnostic value, spinal angiography is vital for surgical and endovascular treatment planning. The arterial phase of the angiogram should show good filling of the spinal arteries, which have a more tortuous course in the pediatric population than in adults and should not be mistaken for abnormal vessels. The venous phase should show good opacification of the venous drainage to allow complete assessment of the SCAVM. On spinal angiography, SCAVMs appear as compacted nidus-type malformations in 88% of the lesions, whereas the remaining may appear as fistula-type malformations. The fistula type is usually associated with Rendu-Osler-Weber syndrome. AVM-associated aneurysms are very infrequent in SCAVMs. These could be related to different hemodynamic patterns between spinal and cerebral AVMs with different endothelial responses to such shear forces. When seen, these aneurysms are usually associated with thrombosed venous outflow and hematomyelia, and are more commonly found in thoracic spinal AVMs. Venous ectasia and outflow venous stenosis are frequently seen in SCAVMs during spinal angiography.

More recently, three-dimensional (3D) volume-averaged angiography based on the digital subtraction spine angiography has been employed during the workup for SCAVM. The 3D spinal angiography may better delineate the lesions associated with SCAVM, such as intranidal or venous aneurysms and vein varicosities, and may better define the topographical localization of the SCAVM and its feeders.[19] Currently, this technique for SCAVM assessment has the limitations of increased contrast load and prolonged procedure time but may prove to be beneficial in the future as further advancements in the technique and more complex software become available.

■ Diagnosis and Treatment

Spinal Angiography

The diagnosis and management plan for SCAVM depend on high-quality digital subtraction spinal angiography. The development of refined angiographic

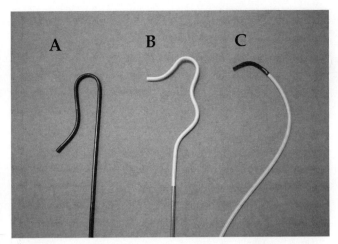

FIGURE 17–3 The primary catheters for diagnostic spinal angiography and embolization. **(A)** Simmons catheter; **(B)** Mikaelsson catheter; **(C)** Cobra catheter.

and endovascular tools in addition to the newer angiographic suites and radiographic software has improved the quality of images and roadmap fluoroscopy and has improved the diagnostic and interventional capabilities during embolization in the SCAVM.

We prefer to perform the diagnostic spinal angiography with the child under general anesthesia. This allows us to obtain the best-quality angiogram with no respiration artifact, and to better plan the interventional procedure sessions. For lesions below the thoracic spine, some authors recommend using glucagon (0.5 mg IV) prior to performing the run to suppress the bowel movement; however, we do not find this necessary. To help restrict the contrast load, the diagnostic angiogram and the procedure should be performed on different days.

Spinal angiography may be performed utilizing diagnostic catheters ranging in size from 4 to 5 French. We primarily use the Cobra (AngioDynamics, Inc., Queensbury, NY) and Mikaelsson (Merit Medical Systems, Inc., South Jordan, UT), as well as Simmons catheters (Boston Scientific, Natick, MA) (**Fig. 17–3**) introduced via 4 to 5 French introducer sheath. The choice of catheter depends on the angle of the segmental arteries with respect to the aorta.

A complete spinal angiogram is recommended to look for SCAVM. Segmental arteries are selected sequentially by rotating the catheter 30 to 45 degrees to the left and right. Cervical and upper thoracic radiculomedullary and radiculopial arteries may be studied by selectively catheterizing the bilateral vertebral, costocervical, and thyrocervical arteries. Selecting the lower lumbar and sacral segmental arteries requires injecting the common and internal iliac arteries, which can be selected using Mikaelsson or Simmons-I catheters. Occasionally, external carotid arteries may be required to assess the contribution of ascending pharyngeal and occipital arteries to the

cervical spine AVM, which may provide an excellent indirect alternative for AVM embolization.

Obtaining images in the frontal projection is satisfactory in most cases, but occasionally lateral, oblique, or 3D projections may be needed to better delineate the angioarchitectural characteristics of the SCAVM. Several anatomical variations in children can be encountered, including normal increase in spinal artery tortuosity in comparison to adults, lower segmental arteries originating at acute angles and with an oblique, rostrally oriented course, one segmental spinal medullary artery supplying multiple levels, a segmental artery from the sacrococcygeal area supplying the anterior or posterior spinal arteries, unilateral origin of segmental arteries, and the bidirectionality of the spinal artery flow within the same level.

Endovascular Therapy

General Considerations

We perform all of our pediatric spinal vascular malformation embolization procedures under general anesthesia. Premedication with anxiolytics and steroids may be administered, and we routinely administer dexamethasone 2 to 6 mg every 6 hours for 24 to 48 hours following the procedure. Patients may be discharged on a 2-week prednisone taper. Patients are usually admitted to the neurointensive care unit following the procedure, their blood pressure is maintained within 20% of their baseline mean arterial blood pressure, and isotonic saline is administered to keep them euvolemic. If a large fistula is embolized, heparin anticoagulation is administered overnight to prevent extension of venous thrombosis.

Indications and Limitations

Embolization is considered the first choice of treatment in medullary and perimedullary AVMs or multifocal SCAVMs and may be considered in all other types of SCAVM as a palliative treatment or in combination with surgical resection. Some cases are excluded from the endovascular therapy based on the preprocedure diagnostic spinal angiography. Technical limitations that preclude endovascular therapy include inaccessible arterial feeders, inaccessible nidus, and potential increased risk of spinal cord infarction when the feeder is jointly supplying the AVM and normal spinal cord region. When embolic material has to travel more than three to four vertebral body segments, the likelihood of spinal cord infarction increases.

> **PEARL** When embolic material has to travel more than three to four vertebral body segments, the likelihood of spinal cord infarction increases.

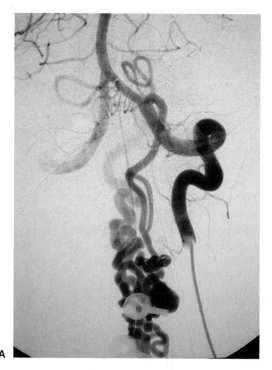 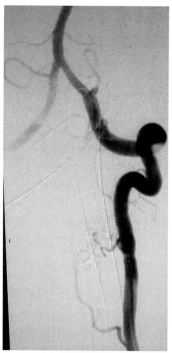

FIGURE 17–4 Selective left vertebral artery angiography in a 14-year-old girl with subarachnoid hemorrhage secondary to a ruptured cervical spinal cord arteriovenous malformation **(A)** prior to and **(B)** following embolization with n-butyl cyanoacrylate.

In summary, the technical feasibility of endovascular embolization of SCAVMs is limited by the ability to safely reach and withdraw from a safe embolization position. These limitations vary among interventionalists based on individual experience and interpretation of the SCAVM angioarchitecture. The embolization can be performed acutely in cases with high risk of rebleeding such as outflow obstruction, stenosis, or associated aneurysm. However, a delay of 1 to 2 months is usually recommended following the acute incidence to allow for hematoma and edema resolution prior to endovascular therapy.

Embolic Material

Two embolic materials are commonly used in the endovascular treatment of SCAVM: polyvinyl alcohol (PVA) particles for preoperative embolization and n-butyl cyanoacrylate (nBCA) permanent glue for curative or palliative embolization (**Fig. 17–4**). PVA has a more graduated delivery but is associated with an increased rate of recanalization and is more time-consuming. It is provided in particle sizes ranging from small (50 μ) to large (1000 μ).[20–23] The nBCA glue is provided in 1 mg tubes that need to be mixed with lipophilic oil to obtain various dilutions and concentrations, and is sometimes mixed with tantalum powder for improved radiopacity, particularly when the Lipiodol concentration falls below 50%. The glue seems to be well tolerated, and the long-term effect appears to be very safe with no delayed consequences on children. It is less likely to recanalize than

PVA and polymerization is assumed to be permanent.[20–23] Dimethyl sulfoxide (Onyx liquid embolic system, Micro Therapeutics, Inc., Irvine, CA) has been reported in a few cases of SCAVM treatment with good results, and appears to be more promising with potentially predictable use than currently available liquid embolic materials.[24] Other materials, including Gelfoam, fat particles, Ethibloc, balloons, silks, and liquid coils are not frequently used in spinal cord vascular malformation.

Spinal Cord Arteriovenous Malformation Embolization Technique

The introducer sheath is inserted in the common femoral artery via the micropuncture technique in all pediatric cases using a 4 or 5 French sheath according to the patient's weight. The flow-directed microcatheter, 1.5 and 1.8 French, is usually used to select the arterial feeder, and the microcatheter is positioned as close as possible to the SCAVM nidus (**Fig. 17–5**). We use an Elite flow-directed microcatheter (Boston Scientific–Neurovascular, Fremont, CA) for SCAVM embolization, and we occasionally use an Excelsior-SL-10 microcatheter (Boston Scientific–Neurovascular, Fremont, CA) for the larger feeders. The microcatheter is advanced over 0.008 in. microwire. We use Mirage 0.008 in. (Micro Therapeutics, Inc., Irvine, CA), which has better compatibility with the flow-directed microcatheters than the 0.010 in. wires.

A preembolization superselective angiogram is routinely performed via the microcatheter to obtain

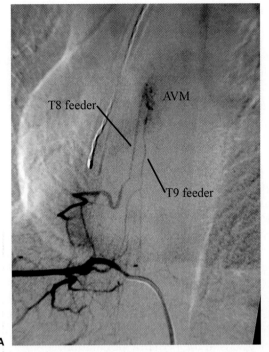

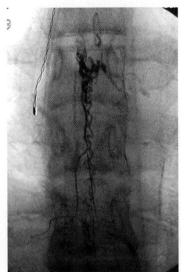

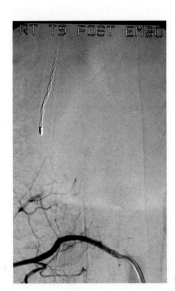

A   **B**   **C**

FIGURE 17–5 Selective right T9 injection spinal angiogram with a Cobra diagnostic catheter in a 17-year-old girl who presented with lower extremity numbness. **(A)** A T6–7–level spinal cord arteriovenous malformation (SCAVM) is fed by right T8 and T9 feeders. **(B)** A 1.5 French Elite catheter is used to superselectively enter the T9 feeder. **(C)** Following n-butyl cyanoacrylate embolization, there is no further filling of the SCAVM from the right T9 injection.

an improved baseline image of the SCAVM angioarchitecture. This allows the interventionalist to ascertain the amount of pressure needed to inject the polymer into the SCAVM nidus. An additional benefit of using general anesthesia for these cases is that the anesthesiologist may suspend respirations during the injection to yield higher-quality images. The glue injection is performed under a blank roadmap. Flow control prior to embolization, with microcatheter wedging, allows low-pressure glue injection. Glue mixtures may vary between 5 and 100%, depending on the flow rate in the spinal vascular shunt. The addition of glacial acetic acid may also allow for a slower delivery due to increased polymerization times. The microcatheter should be flushed with 5% dextrose prior to glue injection, and the microcatheter should be pulled immediately after the injection.

Intraprocedural Monitoring

In intramedullary or perimedullary lesions physiological and functional evaluation prior to embolization of particular arterial feeder is recommended. Provocative physiological testing under general anesthesia for evaluation of the potential arterial feeder contribution to the particular spinal cord functional segment is usually recommended. We routinely perform SCAVM embolization under general anesthesia, and do not

recommend an intervention in young children with conscious sedation.

> **PEARL** Evoked potential monitoring during SCAVM embolization is critical to reduce the risk of complications.

In most SCAVM embolizations, we perform provocative testing by administering 20 to 40 mg of sodium amytal superselectively as already described, while continuously monitoring the evoked potentials (e.g., somatosensory or motor). Berenstein and his group have reported a 97% negative predictive value of provocative amytal testing using evoked potential monitoring in SCAVM embolization.[25] Despite the lack of supportive data and randomized studies, we believe that neurophysiological evoked potential monitoring during the embolization is critical to reduce the risk of complications, particularly in intra- and perimedullary SCAVMs.[26]

Complications

The risks of endovascular intervention may be divided into those related to the diagnostic procedure and those related to the interventional procedure. The complications related to the diagnostic procedure are universal to angiography and include vessel injury, dissection, pseudoaneurysm, bleeding and hematoma, infection, allergic reaction to the ionic-based x-ray contrast agent, contrast load–related nephropathy, and fluid overload. Complications related to the interventional procedure may include inadvertently occluding a feeder to the SCAVM that supplies normal spinal cord leading to ischemic infarction, or early occlusion of the main venous drainage with outflow obstruction and hemorrhage, or feeding vessel perforation and bleeding, arterial spasm, and inadvertent microcatheter adherence to the glue cast. Pulmonary embolization of the glue material in SCAVM embolization is rarely encountered, and it does not lead to respiratory compromise. Inadvertent glue leak via the diagnostic catheter may lead to acute arterial occlusion and ischemia to the affected territory, which may require immediate vascular surgery for glue cast removal.

Alopecia and skin desquamation may occur in prolonged radiation exposure due to repeated embolization sessions that may be required in children. To eliminate the contrast overload in children, we use a 70:30 concentration ratio of the nonionic contrast dilution, and we monitor the total volume administered during the procedure so as not to exceed 5 mL/kg per session.

Prognosis and Outcome

The natural history of untreated SCAVMs is not well-established[27] because few of the discovered cases go untreated. Vodoff et al reported a case of cervical intramedullary SCAVM in a 9-year-old child treated with steroids who had spontaneous regression within 2 weeks. This may have been related to hemorrhage and spontaneous thrombosis.[28] Moreover, reports of long-term outcome and prognosis following SCAVM treatment are scarce and limited to case series of patients of various ages with different types of SCAVM types that were treated with various approaches of surgical, interventional, and combined therapies.

The intramedullary and perimedullary spinal vascular malformations are associated with early and rapid deterioration secondary to hemodynamic or hemorrhagic complications.[11] However, dural, extradural, and extra- or perimedullary SCAVMs are usually associated with better prognosis than intramedullary or dorsal SCAVMs. The outcome with endovascular treatment in children is not clearly documented. Lasjaunias has reported one of the largest SCAVM series with clinical outcome. In one review of 69 patients with SCAVM who were treated, 20 were children.[29] Good clinical outcomes, assessed by Karnofsky scale score, were obtained in 83% of the patients, with 4% permanent severe complications (Karnofsky scale score ≤70), and 9% mild worsening (Karnofsky scale score, 80).[5,29]

■ Summary

Pediatric SCAVMs are less common than those in adults and they present clinically between 10 to 20 years of age. SCAVMs in neonates and infants have been reported, however. Association with other metameric syndromes may occur.[30,31] Most of the cases are intra- and perimedullary in location, with a compact nidus on angiography, which makes the endovascular approach a safe and attractive alternative to open surgical resection. SCAVMs in children frequently present with acute onset of hemorrhagic complications, SAH, or hematomyelia, resulting in severe acute back pain with or without paresis and sphincteric dysfunction. The outcome following endovascular therapy using nBCA glue seems to be favorable, with a 4% rate of permanent neurological deficit or disability, and >80% of the cases having 50% or more of their arteriovenous shunting reduced.

Future advances in imaging, interventional devices, and embolic materials technologies will only improve the safety and efficacy of endovascular interventions in treating SCAVMs in the pediatric population.

REFERENCES

1. Cogen P, Stein BM. Spinal cord arteriovenous malformations with intramedullary components. J Neurosurg 1983;59:471–478
2. Spetzler RF, Detwiler PW, Riina HA, Porter RW. Modified classification of spinal cord vascular lesions. J Neurosurg 2002;96(Suppl 2): 145–156
3. Krauss WE. Vascular anatomy of the spinal cord. Neurosurg Clin N Am 1999;10:9–15
4. Lasjaunias P. Spinal cord vascular lesions. J Neurosurg 2003; 98(Suppl 1):117–119
5. Rodesch G, Hurth M, Alvarez H, Tadie M, Lasjaunias P. Classification of spinal cord arteriovenous shunts: proposal for a reappraisal: the Bicetre experience with 155 consecutive patients treated between 1981 and 1999. Neurosurgery 2002;51:374–379; discussion 379–380
6. Bao YH, Ling F. Classification and therapeutic modalities of spinal vascular malformations in 80 patients. Neurosurgery 1997;40:75–81
7. Anson JA, Spetzler RF. Classification of spinal arteriovenous malformations and implications for treatment. BNI Q 1992;8:2
8. Berenstein A, Lasjaunias P. Spinal cord arteriovenous malformations. In: Berenstein A, Lasjaunias P, eds. Endovascular Treatment of Spine and Spinal Cord Lesions. New York: Springer-Verlag; 1994:24–109. Berenstein A, Lasjaunias P, eds. Surgical Neuroangiography; vol 5
9. Rodesch G, Lasjaunias P, Berenstein A. Embolization of arteriovenous malformations of the spinal cord. In: Valavanis A, ed. Interventional Neuroradiology. New York: Springer-Verlag; 1993:135–150
10. Detweiler PW, Porter RW, Spetzler RF. Spinal arteriovenous malformations. Neurosurg Clin N Am 1999;10:89–100
11. Grote EH, Voigt K. Clinical syndromes, natural history, and pathophysiology of vascular lesions of the spinal cord. Neurosurg Clin N Am 1999;10:17–45
12. Bandyopadhyay S, Sheth RD. Acute spinal cord infarction: vascular steal in arteriovenous malformation. J Child Neurol 1999;14: 685–687
13. Riche MC, Modenesi-Freitas J, Djindjian M, Merland JJ. Arteriovenous malformation of the spinal cord in children: a review of 38 cases. Neuroradiology 1982;22:171–180

14. Rosenblum B, Oldfield EH, Doppman JL, Di Chiro G. Spinal arteri-ovenous malformations: a comparison of dural arteriovenous fistulas and intradural AVMs in 81 patients. J Neurosurg 1987;67:795–802

15. Bjork A, Eeg-Olofsson O, Svendsen P, Mostrom U, Pellettieri L. Endovascular treatment of a spinal arteriovenous malformation in a 21-month-old boy. Acta Paediatr 1994;83:1326–1331

16. Binkert CA, Kollias SS, Valavanis A. Spinal cord vascular disease: characterization with fast three-dimensional contrast-enhanced mr angiography. AJNR Am J Neuroradiol 1999;20:1785–1793

17. Mascalchi M, Quilici N, Ferrito G, et al. Identification of the feeding arteries of spinal vascular lesions via phase-contrast MR angiography with three-dimensional acquisition and phase display. AJNR Am J Neuroradiol 1997;18:351–358

18. Mascalchi M, Ferrito G, Quilici N, et al. Spinal vascular malforma-tion: MR angiography after treatment. Radiology 2001;219:346–353

19. Prestigiacomo CJ, Niimi Y, Setton A, Bernestein A. Three-dimensional rotational spinal angiography in the evaluation and treatment of vascular malformation. AJNR Am J Neuroradiol 2003;24:1429–1435

20. Biondi A, Merland JJ, Reizine D, et al. Embolization with particles in thoracic intramedullary arteriovenous malformations: long-term angiographic and clinical results. Radiology 1990;177:651–658

21. Hall WA, Oldfield EH, Doppman JL. Recanalization of spinal arte-riovenous malformations following embolization. J Neurosurg 1989;70:714–720

22. Rodesch G, Hurth M, Alvarez H, Lasjaunias P. Embolization of spinal cord arteriovenous malformations (SCAVMs) with glue through the anterior spinal axis: review of 20 cases. Interv Neuro-radiol 1997;3:131–143

23. Kahara VJ, Seppanen SK, Kuurne T, Laasonen EM. Diagnosis and embolizing of spinal arteriovenous malformations. Ann Med 1997;29:377–382

24. Molyneux AJ, Coley SC. Embolization of spinal cord arteriovenous malformations with ethylene vinyl alcohol copolymer dissolved in dimethyl sulfoxide (Onyx liquid embolic system): report of two cases. J Neurosurg 2000;93(Suppl 2):304–308

25. Niimi Y, Sala F, Deletis V, Setton A, Bueno de Camargo A, Berenstein A. Neurophysiologic monitoring and pharmacologic provocative testing for embolization of spinal cord arteriovenous malformations. AJNR Am J Neuroradiol 2004;25:1131–1138

26. Sala F, Niimi Y, Krzan MJ, Berenstein A, Deletis V. Embolization of a spinal arteriovenous malformation: correlation between motor evoked potentials and angiographic findings: technical case report. Neurosurgery 1999;45:932–938

27. Aminoff MJ, Logue V. The prognosis of patients with spinal vascular malformations. Brain 1974;97:211–218

28. Vodoff MV, Gilbert B, Le Breton F, et al. Paraplegia and medullary arteriovenous malformation: role of surgery, corticosteroids, and embolization. Arch Pediatr 2001;8:608–610

29. Rodesch G, Hurth M, Alvarez H, David P, Tadie M, Lasjaunias P. Embolization of spinal cord arteriovenous shunts: morphological and clinical follow-up and results–review of 69 consecutive cases. Neurosurgery 2003;53:40–49; discussion 49–50

30. Meisel HJ, Lasjaunias P, Brock M. Multiple arteriovenous malfor-mations of the spinal cord in an adolescent: case report. Neuro-radiology 1996;38:490–493

31. Matsumaru Y, Pongpech S, Laothamas J, Alvarez H, Rodesch G, Lasjaunias P. Multifocal and metameric spinal cord arteriovenous malformations: review of 19 cases. Interv Neuroradiol 1999;5:27–34

18

Thrombolysis in Children

FELIPE C. ALBUQUERQUE AND CAMERON G. McDOUGALL

In contrast to strokes in adults, which typically result from the sequelae of atherosclerosis and hypertension, a variety of pathological conditions can incite stroke in the pediatric population: congenital heart diseases, genetic disorders, systemic and cerebral infections, blood dyscrasias and coagulopathies, neoplasia, and adverse reactions to medications. As in the adult population, endovascular techniques in the pediatric population are tailored toward revascularization through mechanical and pharmaceutical means. These techniques are best assessed by qualifying the disease process as arterial or venous.

■ Arterial Pediatric Strokes

Epidemiology

The prevalence of stroke in children ranges from 2.5 to 3.3 per 100,000.[1–6] Despite the relative rarity of stroke in this population, outcomes are decidedly poor: 50 to 90% of patients sustain adverse neurological outcomes.[1–6] Mortality rates are higher in males than in females and in blacks than in whites.[1–6] The cause of almost a third of childhood strokes remains unknown.[1–6] The other cases have several etiologies.[1–6] Although infection, particularly from *Hemophilus influenza*, was once a common cause of stroke in this population, advances in antimicrobial therapy have altered this relationship.[1–6] Now, congenital heart diseases, sickle cell anemia, coagulation disorders, and traumatic injuries are the most prevalent underlying causes.[1–7]

> **PEARL** In some series, cardiac diseases have accounted for as many as 50% of cases of childhood stroke.

Heart diseases, both congenital and acquired, trigger strokes in children through thromboembolism.[1,2,4–6] This mechanism produces either watershed infarction or focal cortical injury, depending on the site and extent of the embolus.[1,4–6] In some series, cardiac diseases have accounted for as many as 50% of cases of childhood stroke.[1,4–6] Offending lesions include intracardiac anomalies such as an atrial septal defect and patent foramen ovale as well as complex congenital malformations such as tetralogy of Fallot and coarctation of the aorta.[1,4–6] Less frequently, acquired cardiac diseases such as rheumatic fever, bacterial endocarditis, and atrial myxoma cause pediatric arterial infarcts.[1,4–6]

Sickle cell disease causes strokes in both children and adults.[1,8] In this setting, arterial infarcts result from either small vessel hypoperfusion or large, proximal vessel stenosis or occlusion.[1,8] Within this subset of patients, the incidence of clinically apparent infarcts is 9% whereas silent strokes may affect as many as 13%.[1,8] The annual risk of stroke for these patients has been estimated at 0.7% per year whereas the rate of subsequent stroke ranges from 50 to 75% among untreated (e.g., not transfused) patients.[1,8] Overall, a child with sickle cell anemia is 200 to 400 times more likely to suffer a stroke than a healthy child.[1,8] Sickle cell disease is the most common cause of stroke among black children. Moreover, stroke related to sickle cell disease is most prevalent in less developed nations.[1,8] Although infection and aplastic crisis are known to precipitate stroke in patients with sickle cell disease, few cases manifest such antecedent events.[1,8]

Several genetic coagulopathies are associated with pediatric stroke: deficiencies of protein C, S, and antithrombin III as well as mutations of the factor V Leiden and prothrombin genes.[5,6,9] Other congenital diseases are known risk factors for pediatric stroke.[5,6,9] Of these, homocystinuria, Fabry's disease, fibromuscular dysplasia, and neurofibromatosis type 1 are the most common.[6,9]

The pathophysiological mechanisms underlying these diseases are distinct and complex, but all predispose individuals to arterial thromboses.[9] In addition, acquired hypercoagulation states can be precipitated by medications, hepatorenal disease, and infection.[6,9]

Infections of varying etiology are involved in pediatric arterial strokes in as many as a third of the cases.[1,5,6] In this subgroup, bacterial meningitis is the most common inciting factor.[1,5,6] The intracranial vasculitis that ensues from this disease produces arterial thromboses, intraparenchymal and subarachnoid hemorrhage, and sinovenous occlusion.[1,5,6] Other bacterial, infectious causes of pediatric stroke include rheumatic heart disease, other endocarditides,[1,5,6] as well as systemic infections such as bacterial and viral pneumonias (**Fig. 18–1**). Tuberculous meningitis predisposes individuals to basal ganglia

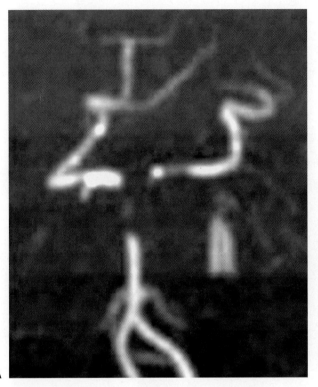

A

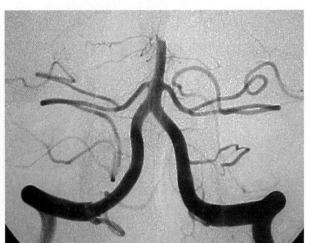

B

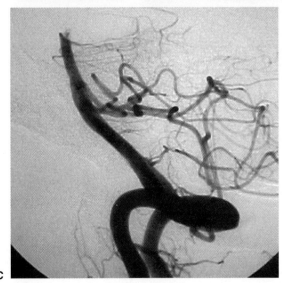

C

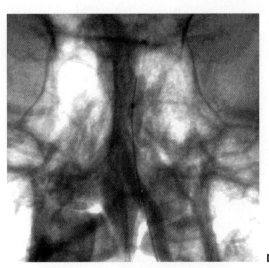

D

FIGURE 18–1 (A) Magnetic resonance angiography demonstrating thrombosis of the distal basilar artery. This 15-year-old girl presented with a 1-week history of bacterial pneumonia as well as patent foramen ovale. She rapidly progressed to quadriparesis and lethargy. **(B)** Left vertebral artery digital subtraction angiogram (DSA) demonstrating thrombotic occlusion of the distal basilar artery (posteroanterior projection). **(C)** Lateral projection. **(D)** Unsubtracted skull film demonstrating an angioplasty balloon in the distal basilar artery. Arrow demarcates proximal balloon marker.

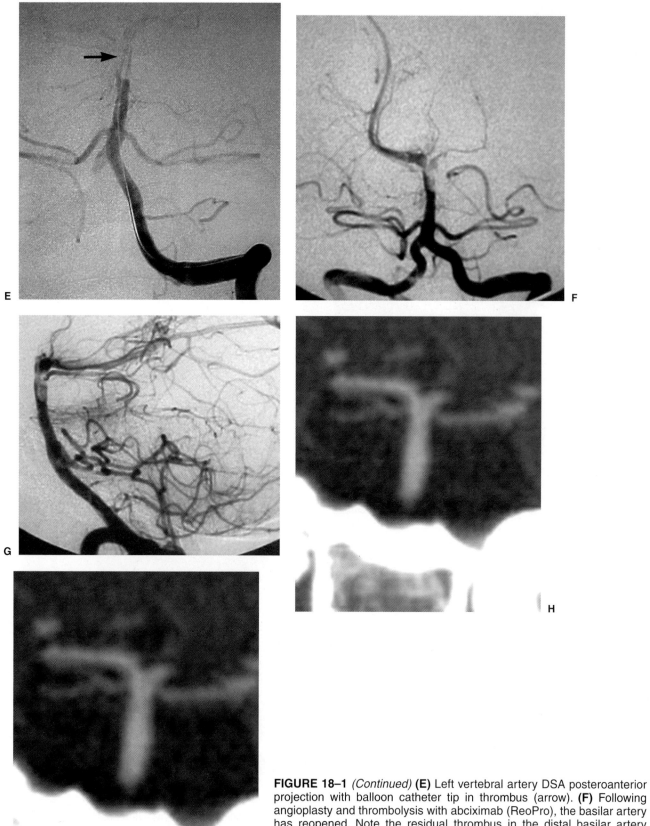

FIGURE 18–1 *(Continued)* **(E)** Left vertebral artery DSA posteroanterior projection with balloon catheter tip in thrombus (arrow). **(F)** Following angioplasty and thrombolysis with abciximab (ReoPro), the basilar artery has reopened. Note the residual thrombus in the distal basilar artery (posteroanterior projection). **(G)** Lateral projection of the left vertebral artery DSA. **(H,I)** Computed tomography angiograms obtained 6 months after thrombolysis demonstrate normal patency of the distal basilar artery.

infarctions and is more likely to produce this sequela in infected children than in adults.[1,5,6]

An apparent association also exists between antecedent varicella-zoster infection and ischemic infarction in children.[10] This association is thought to be related to the development of postvaricella angiopathy, which often persists for 9 months after infection and is characterized by distal cervical and proximal intracranial carotid stenoses.[10] As in cases of tuberculous meningitis, infarctions from varicella infection typically involve the basal ganglia.[10] Infection-related pediatric strokes are also regional. Examples include borreliosis in Scandinavia and malaria in endemic regions of Africa and Asia.[6] Finally, the human immunodeficiency virus predisposes both children and adults to several pathogens that cause stroke, including viral and fungal vectors.[6]

Cervical and cranial traumatic injuries can cause stroke in children through the sequelae of arterial dissection and thromboembolism.[1,2,7,11] Such infarctions can occur when the artery is injured or in a delayed fashion. Recurrent ischemic events after traumatic injuries to the head or neck should prompt diagnostic evaluation of the brachiocephalic vessels. The cervical and proximal intracranial carotid arteries are more often affected than the vertebral arteries.[1,2,7,11] In children, intracranial dissections are as common as those affecting the cervical vessels. Dissections can also occur spontaneously and manifest much like their traumatic counterparts.[1,2,7] In cases of dissection and distal thromboembolism, endovascular techniques are geared toward reestablishing the patency of both the proximal and the distal affected arterial segments. To do so may necessitate angioplasty and stenting of the dissection before the embolus is addressed by either mechanical or pharmaceutical thrombolytic techniques. Penetrating injuries to the vertebral and carotid arteries also may require a variety of surgical and endovascular techniques as precursors to managing the thromboembolic sequelae.

> **PEARL** Angioplasty and stenting of some dissections may be necessary to properly treat the associated distal embolus.

Neoplastic diseases, particularly acute leukemia, predispose children to both ischemic and hemorrhagic arterial strokes.[12] Embolic or thrombotic stroke (either arterial or venous) occurs in 3% of cases of noncentral nervous system primary malignancies.[12] Such cases may be triggered by these patients' predisposition to intracranial infections but are more often the result of adverse reactions to chemotherapeutic agents. Causative agents include L-asparaginase, which is known to create a hypercoagulable condition, methotrexate, and many platinum-based chemotherapeutic agents.[12]

In addition to the chemotherapeutic agents already discussed, oral contraceptive pills are also associated with a higher likelihood of thromboembolic infarction— a risk factor that may be further enhanced by cigarette smoking.[2] Although this scenario is most common in women, cases involving teenage girls have become more prevalent.[2] Other causes of pediatric stroke related to cancer include disease-related coagulation disorders, arterial injury from radiation, and metastases to the calvarium.[12]

Finally, the inflammatory vasculopathy, moyamoya disease, is another cause of arterial infarctions in the young.[1,13] Once considered a heritable disease prevalent in Japan, moyamoya disease has gained further recognition in the West as diagnostic strides have been made.[1,13] This occlusive disease affects the distal internal carotid artery and circle of Willis and typically manifests with stuttering neurological deterioration as a result of progressive infarction.[1,13] Patients usually become symptomatic within the first to fourth decades of life.[1,13] The disease has been associated with other pathological conditions such as Down syndrome, neurofibromatosis, and sickle cell disease.[1,13] The surgical management of moyamoya disease consists of a variety of bypass techniques.[1,13] Endovascular therapy, primarily angioplasty or thrombolysis, is seldom involved in the management of these patients.

Endovascular Management: Medical and Mechanical Thrombolysis

The use of intra-arterial thrombolytic medications to treat acute thromboembolic stroke is an established practice in adults. Debate over dosage and safety, coupled with the relative infrequency of pediatric strokes, has rendered this practice controversial in children.[14–18] Moreover, in younger children, lower functional plasminogen levels and higher concentrations of plasmin inhibitor may make thrombolysis more difficult.[15–17] Reports of intra-arterial thrombolysis in children are few, and little can be said with certainty regarding the efficacy of and potential complications associated with this therapy.[15–18] Nonetheless, this technique and the various agents employed offer a practical alternative to more accepted and less invasive treatment modalities. The practice of microcatheterization of the intracranial vasculature is straightforward and varies little from adults to children, but the pharmacology of the various thrombolytic agents is complex.

> **PEARL** In younger children, lower functional plasminogen levels and higher concentrations of plasmin inhibitor may make thrombolysis more difficult.

Tissue plasminogen activator (t-PA) is a serine protease glycoprotein that exists in two recombinant forms: a single chain (alteplase) and a double chain (duteplase) molecule.[19] t-PA catalyzes the conversion of plasminogen to plasmin but does so preferentially when bound to fibrin.[19] This mechanism selectively promotes the conversion of plasminogen to plasmin at the site of thrombosis. Alteplase is synthesized by inserting complementary human deoxyribose nucleic acid from a melanoma cell line into a hamster ovarian cell line.[19] Because metabolism of the agent is hepatic, variability in its efficacy may be related to blood flow through the liver.[19] The typical half-life of alteplase is 2 to 5 minutes.[19]

In contrast to t-PA, streptokinase and urokinase are nonspecific, allowing plasminogen to be converted to plasmin throughout the circulation.[19] Streptokinase, one of the earliest thrombolytic agents used, is a protein by-product of β-hemolytic streptococci.[19] It does not trigger the conversion of plasminogen directly.[19] Rather, it binds to plasminogen, creating a protein complex that activates the conversion of other plasminogen molecules to plasmin.[19] However, in human studies the bacterial nature of the drug rarely induced antibody formation and subsequent toxic reactions such as anaphylaxis.[19] This discovery prompted the discontinuation of streptokinase use.[19]

Systemic intravenous administration of t-PA in children has been reported in several small-scale analyses.[20-23] Reports have detailed systemic thrombolytic therapy for a variety of arterial and venous thrombotic conditions, including postcardiac catheterization thromboses, brachial artery thromboses, and thromboses of the inferior vena cava and renal veins.[20-23] These studies document a reasonable recanalization rate (as high as 65%).[20-23] However, the risk of complications, including hemorrhagic complications at the intravenous puncture site and mucosal and internal bleeding, is high (40% in one study).[24] Complications are most common in small patients, in those who have lengthy infusions, and in those experiencing a large decline in fibrinogen levels after receiving t-PA.[20-24] Neonates receiving intravenous t-PA also may have a disproportionately high risk of spontaneous intracerebral hemorrhage.[20-24]

Although intravenous t-PA is seldom used in children, its intracranial intra-arterial use is even more rare.[16,17] Most reports have involved only a single case.[16,17] In a review of a case of pediatric cardioembolic stroke, Gruber et al[16] used an intra-arterial dose of recombinant t-PA of 0.11 mg/kg body weight to treat acute thrombosis of the right middle cerebral artery in a 6-year-old child. The authors argued that this dose corresponded to the approximate amount of the drug that would enter the carotid circulation had it been given intravenously according to the standard established by the National Institute of Neurological Disorders and Stroke trial.[16,25] In this case,

local thrombolysis resulted in recanalization of the vessel.[16] The authors contend that intra-arterial delivery of this medication may reduce the risk of systemic hemorrhagic complications often associated with the intravenous administration of t-PA.

Other intravenous and potentially intra-arterial agents include the glycoprotein IIb/IIIa inhibitors (GPIIb/IIIa).[19] These agents preferentially block the GPIIb/IIIa receptor, thereby inhibiting platelet aggregation.[19] The safety of these agents, which include abciximab (ReoPro) and eptifibatide (Integrilin), has been established by several large, prospective, randomized trials of patients undergoing endovascular treatment for coronary atherosclerotic disease.[19] This work established that such medications reduced the risks of death, myocardial infarction, and myocardial ischemia by 35 to 50%.[19] Nonetheless, the efficacy and safety of intracranial intra-arterial use have not been established in either adult or pediatric populations.

As in the intra-arterial treatment of adult strokes, microcatheterization of the thrombosed arterial segment is the desired endovascular goal. t-PA can thereby be administered directly into the clot, likely increasing the rate of recanalization. Other techniques such as percutaneous transluminal angioplasty, which mechanically disrupts a thrombus, may improve the efficacy of t-PA when it is delivered secondarily. Cognard et al[15] treated an 8-year-old child with basilar artery occlusion in this fashion. The child deteriorated to the point of losing consciousness and extensor posturing and was treated 36 hours after the onset of symptoms.[15] The authors argued that angioplasty serves two roles: It reestablishes blood flow beyond the thrombosed segment and increases surface area of clot exposed to the subsequent administration of thrombolytic agents.[15] This technique also may be reserved for patients in whom the direct intra-arterial administration of thrombolytic agents fails to produce recanalization. Several different snare devices can be used to disrupt clots mechanically.[26] These techniques, angioplasty and snaring, are usually associated with a low rate of complications.[26] However, their safety and efficacy have not been evaluated in children.

The success of such agents and techniques in children is predicated on the successful management of the primary disease process that produced the original thromboembolic event. Such treatment includes the repair or medical management of an underlying cardiac anomaly, transfusion and medical therapy of sickle cell anemia, and chemotherapy of congenital coagulation disorders and infections. If a patient has had previous cardiac surgery, local intra-arterial treatment may actually be preferred to systemic treatment, which may increase the risk of hemorrhage at the thoracic operative site. Cases involving traumatic dissections of the brachiocephalic and intracranial circulation are managed on an individual basis. The goal of preventing thromboembolic complications may necessitate endovascular stent repair or anticoagulant or antiplatelet therapy. These techniques and agents are beyond the scope of this review. Nonetheless, the endovascular management of procedural thromboembolic complications related to angioplasty and stenting of these injuries is the same as already discussed. Similarly, management of complications associated with the treatment of other pediatric lesions, such as aneurysms or arteriovenous malformations, may necessitate such techniques.

■ Venous Pediatric Strokes

Epidemiology

Once considered rare, venous sinus thrombosis in children is now diagnosed more frequently for two reasons.[27–30] Superior imaging techniques have improved our ability to make the diagnosis, and children with diseases that predispose to such thromboses are surviving longer.[27–30] The incidence of pediatric venous sinus thrombosis has been estimated at 0.29 to 0.67 per 100,000 per year and accounts for 25% of cases of pediatric cerebrovascular ischemia.[27–30] Risk factors for venous sinus thrombosis are myriad: infectious disorders of the head and neck, acute systemic illnesses such as perinatal complications and dehydration, traumatic injuries of the head and neck, neoplastic diseases such as leukemia and lymphoma, and prothrombic conditions like the presence of anticardiolipin antibody.[27–30] These risk factors differ substantially from those in adults where pregnancy, cancer, and oral contraceptive use are the predominant causes.[27–30]

Risk factors and presenting symptoms may be further stratified by age within the pediatric population. Neonates are most likely to develop sinus thromboses as a result of perinatal complications and most often become symptomatic with seizures and focal neurological deficits.[27–30] Infectious diseases of the head and neck such as mastoiditis and meningitis are the most frequent causes of sinus thrombosis in preschoolers, whereas chronic diseases such as neoplasia and coagulation disorders are more common predisposing conditions in older children.[27–30] This older group of children is most likely to present with signs of intracranial hypertension such as obtundation, headache, and cranial neuropathy.[27–30]

Congenital coagulation disorders, including deficiencies of antithrombin III, protein C, and protein S as well the presence of factor V Leiden, are important causes of both primary and recurrent sinovenous thrombosis in children, especially in those who have other predisposing factors such as prior surgery, trauma, or infection.[27,28,30] Screening the patient and family members is mandatory to initiate prophylactic therapy to protect against recurrent

thrombosis.[27,28,30] In adults with sinus thrombosis, the frequency of such prothrombic conditions ranges from 15 to 21%, but as many as 50% of affected children manifest such diseases.[27,28,30]

The prognosis for pediatric patients with sinus thrombosis is related to the extent of sinus involvement and the presence of cerebral infarction.[27,28,30] Mortality rates may approach 16% whereas the rate of serious permanent neurological injury is almost 22%.[27,28,30] Overall, neonates appear to fare more favorably than nonneonates.[27,28,30] In one study, 77% of this affected group was neurologically normal 2.1 years later compared with 52% of the nonneonates.[27] These figures may vary with longer follow-up because signs of neurological injury sustained during the neonatal period often manifest in a delayed fashion. Regardless, the presence of multiple sinus involvement is predictive of developmental delay in almost 100% of neonatal cases.[27,28,30] The coexistence of ischemic or hemorrhagic infarctions is also predictive of negative outcomes and is frequently associated with a more virulent presentation and disease course.[27,28,30]

Management: Medical Therapy and Endovascular Techniques

The variety of causes of sinus thrombosis has produced several therapeutic options. Treatments include aggressive rehydration, antibiotics, steroids, antiplatelet agents, systemic anticoagulation, transvenous thrombolysis, and mechanical clot disruption.[27,28,30] Rehydration remains the first-line therapeutic maneuver whereas antibiotic administration combined with surgical debridement is critical in the management of cases related to paranasal sinus infection and mastoiditis (**Fig. 18–2**).[27,28,30] Anticonvulsants play an obvious beneficial role in the management of secondary seizures. Although potentially life-saving in cases of refractory intracranial hypertension, the use of diuretic agents also may exacerbate thrombosis by further depleting intravascular volume.[27,28,30] Steroids may be used in cases of cerebral edema or as the primary management of select prothrombic conditions such as systemic lupus erythematosus.[27,28,30] These agents inhibit fibrinolysis and can promote further thrombosis.[27,28,30]

The role of systemic anticoagulation, specifically intravenous heparin, has been widely debated. Results in adults have been variable. One prospective trial documented a complete recovery rate of 80% in patients treated with heparin compared with 10% in those treated with placebo.[31] Results from subsequent retrospective studies have been inconsistent.[28–30,32,33] The unpredictability of the success of heparinization may reflect the heterogeneous nature of the disease, including factors such as the rate of thrombus development, the extent of clot, and the predisposing comorbid conditions.[28–33] In reviews of pediatric sinus

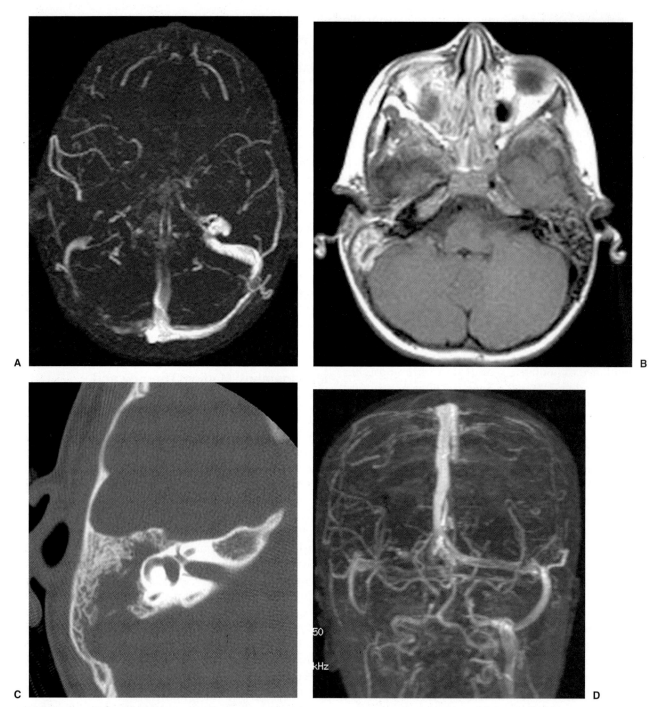

FIGURE 18–2 (A) Magnetic resonance (MR) venography in this 5-year-old girl with fever and mastoiditis demonstrates partial thrombosis of the right transverse sinus. **(B)** MR imaging with gadolinium demonstrates inflammation within the right mastoid process. **(C)** Temporal bone computed tomography demonstrates erosion of the mastoid air cells consistent with mastoiditis. **(D)** Coronal MR venography 6 months after conservative treatment with antibiotics demonstrates partial reopening of the right transverse and sigmoid sinuses. The patient remains neurologically intact and without complaints.

thrombosis, Barron et al,[34] Medlock et al,[35] and Reddingius et al[36] have reported resolution of thromboses without the use of systemic anticoagulation.[34–36] Although the dosage for administration has been extrapolated from adult cases, neither the duration of therapy nor the incidence of hemorrhagic complications has been analyzed prospectively in the pediatric population. Consequently, this therapy has primarily been used in children with known hypercoagulable diseases and in those who fail to respond to more conventional medical treatments such as rehydration and antibiotic administration.[34–36]

Children who continue to deteriorate after the institution of anticoagulation therapy may be candidates for endovascular treatment. Such treatment is performed only if patients fail to demonstrate evidence of intracranial hemorrhage. Those manifesting intracranial hemorrhage, either subarachnoid or parenchymal, have a significantly higher risk of further hemorrhage and subsequent neurological decline.[32,37,38] The endovascular management of dural sinus thrombosis consists of two techniques: mechanical clot disruption and direct transvenous infusion of thrombolytics. Again, the relative safety of these techniques is well demonstrated in adults but only sporadically reported in small case studies of children.[32,37,38]

As in cases of intra-arterial thrombolysis, intrasinus thrombolysis theoretically provides intense, direct thrombolytic delivery to the site of the clot without disrupting the systemic coagulation cascade.[32,37,38] Nonetheless, several authors have documented hemorrhagic complications, including groin and retroperitoneal hematomas, associated with this selective route of administration.[32,37,38] The enlargement of preexisting cerebral hemorrhages and the development of new intracranial hematomas are rare complications. The use of intrasinus urokinase has been successful, and the results in children, although representing a small number of the total cases, are generally favorable in terms of neurological outcome.[32,37,38] Wasay et al[37] reported that patients administered urokinase locally had better outcomes than those treated with systemic heparinization.[37] This study included 40 patients, three of whom were children.[37] t-PA also has been used locally to treat sinus thrombosis and appears to be associated with similar risks and to provide similar beneficial outcomes. Again, however, the number of pediatric patients treated in this fashion has been small.

> **PEARL** For venous sinus thrombolysis mechanical disruptive techniques such as clot snaring and balloon angioplasty can augment the efficacy of thrombolytic agents.

Microcatheterization of the cerebral sinuses is performed in a standard fashion after the guide catheter is positioned in the jugular bulb. Unilateral sinus thrombosis may necessitate approaching the clot site from the contralateral transverse sinus. We prefer embedding the tip of the microcatheter directly into the thrombus. Mechanical disruptive techniques such as clot snaring and balloon angioplasty of the thrombosed segment of the sinus can further fragment the lesion and increase the surface area of thrombus exposed to the later delivery of thrombolytic agents. Typically, we employ a t-PA dosing regimen of 0.11 mg/kg body weight. If the clot fails to dissolve and involves a long segment of the sinus, we often leave the microcatheter in place for 24 hours for continuous infusion of 0.5 to 1 mg t-PA per hour. This technique mandates frequent assessment of fibrinogen and fibrin split product levels to avoid catastrophic hemorrhage from uncontrolled coagulopathy.

■ Complications of Endovascular Therapy

Complications associated with endovascular therapy for the treatment of pediatric stroke are related to access problems and to the effects of the pharmacological agents employed. In both circumstances, a young age and small size are predisposing factors for such complications.

Most such cases are derived from the cardiothoracic literature, which represents a much larger population than children undergoing endovascular treatment for stroke. In a study of 64 children undergoing transfemoral angioplasty for disease of the thoracic aorta or aortic valve, 29 (45.3%) manifested acute iliofemoral complications, including thromboses, complete transections, incomplete transections, and arterial tears.[33] Most of these injuries required operative repair.[33] The authors elucidated a significant correlation between groin complications and patient weight of less than 20 kg.[33] Such complications can produce acute groin and retroperitoneal hematomas and can result in chronic disturbances of lower extremity growth. The patients in this series were catheterized with 8 or 9 French sheaths.[33] Therefore, it is reasonable to assume that the rate of similar complications in the pediatric stroke population, in which smaller sheaths can be used, would be significantly smaller. Indeed, in neonates and infants, the femoral artery can be catheterized with an 18 gauge angiocatheter. Navigation to the intracranial circulation can be accomplished by directly employing a microcatheter inserted through this small angiocatheter.

> **PEARL** Preliminary data suggest that smaller and younger patients, especially neonates, have a higher complication rate with intravenous t-PA therapy.

Again, it is difficult to derive the rate of complications resulting from thrombolytic use in the setting of pediatric stroke because this population is decidedly small. Extrapolation from the pediatric literature, however, suggests that such complications are more likely to occur in smaller and younger patients, especially neonates, as well as in those who have a longer duration of thrombolytic therapy and a greater decrease in fibrinogen levels.[24,33] In a review of the safety of intravenous t-PA administration in 80 children treated for a variety of systemic intravascular thromboses, Gupta et al[24] reported major complications in 40% and minor complications in 30%.[24] Of the former, two patients had cerebral ischemia as a result of systemic hemorrhages that produced secondary hypotension.[24] Another two patients had intracerebral hemorrhages. Most hemorrhages were at the site of intravenous access.[24] Theoretically, local intra-arterial delivery of thrombolytic agents may be safer than systemic delivery because of the proximity of the embolus and because smaller doses of thrombolytics are typically employed. Nonetheless, it would seem rational to use such therapy only in refractory cases after more conventional techniques have failed.

REFERENCES

1. Roach ES. Stroke in children. Curr Treat Options Neurol 2000;2: 295–303
2. Lanzino G, Andreoli A, Di Pasquale G, et al. Etiopathogenesis and prognosis of cerebral ischemia in young adults: a survey of 155 treated patients. Acta Neurol Scand 1991;84:321–325
3. Karnik R, Valentin A, Ammerer HP, et al. Cerebral ischemia in children and young adults. Neurosurg Rev 1987;10:221–227
4. Schoenberg BS, Mellinger JF, Schoenberg DG. Cerebrovascular disease in infants and children: a study of incidence, clinical features, and survival. Neurology 1978;28:763–768
5. Lynch JK, Hirtz DG, DeVeber G, Nelson KB. Report of the National Institute of Neurological Disorders and Stroke workshop on perinatal and childhood stroke. Pediatrics 2002;109:116–123
6. Walsh LE, Garg BP. Ischemic strokes in children. Indian J Pediatr 1997;64:613–623
7. Camacho A, Villarejo A, de Aragón AM, Simón R, Mateos F. Spontaneous carotid and vertebral artery dissection in children. Pediatr Neurol 2001;25:250–253
8. Sarnaik SA, Ballas SK. Molecular characteristics of pediatric patients with sickle cell anemia and stroke. Am J Hematol 2001;67: 179–182
9. Pavlakis SG, Kingsley PB, Bialer MG. Stroke in children: genetic and metabolic issues. J Child Neurol 2000;15:308–315
10. Askalan R, Laughlin S, Mayank S, et al. Chickenpox and stroke in childhood: a study of frequency and causation. Stroke 2001;32: 1257–1262
11. Zimmerman RA. Pediatric cerebrovascular disease. JBR-BTR 2000; 83:245–252
12. Kaste SC, Rodriguez-Galindo C, Furman WL, Langston J, Thompson SJ. Imaging aspects of neurologic emergencies in children treated for non-CNS malignancies. Pediatr Radiol 2000;30:558–565
13. Caldarelli M, Di Rocco C, Gaglini P. Surgical treatment of moyamoya disease in pediatric age. J Neurosurg Sci 2001;45:83–91
14. Qureshi AI, Suri MF, Shatla AA, et al. Intraarterial recombinant tissue plasminogen activator for ischemic stroke: an accelerating dosing regimen. Neurosurgery 2000;47:473–479
15. Cognard C, Weill A, Lindgren S, Piotin M, Castaings L, Moret J. Basilar artery occlusion in a child: "clot angioplasty" followed by thrombolysis. Childs Nerv Syst 2000;16:496–500
16. Gruber A, Nasel C, Lang W, Kitzmüller E, Bavinzski G, Czech T. Intra-arterial thrombolysis for the treatment of perioperative childhood cardioembolic stroke. Neurology 2000;54:1684–1686
17. Gönner F, Remonda L, Mattle H, et al. Local intra-arterial thrombolysis in acute ischemic stroke. Stroke 1998;29:1894–1900
18. Iglesia KA, Fellows KE. Contemporary interventional procedures for vascular disorders in children. Semin Pediatr Surg 1994;3:87–96
19. Morris P. Interventional and Endovascular Therapy of the Nervous System: A Practical Guide. New York: Springer-Verlag; 2002
20. Dillon PW, Fox PS, Berg CJ, Cardella JF, Krummel TM. Recombinant tissue plasminogen activator for neonatal and pediatric vascular thrombolytic therapy. J Pediatr Surg 1993;28:1264–1269
21. Klinge J, Scharf J, Rupprecht T, Böswald M, Hofbeck M. Selective thrombolysis in a newborn with bilateral renal venous and cerebral thrombosis and heterozygous APC resistance. Nephrol Dial Transplant 1998;13:3205–3207
22. Thirumalai SS, Shubin RA. Successful treatment for stroke in a child using recombinant tissue plasminogen activator. J Child Neurol 2000;15:558
23. Carlson MD, Leber S, Deveikis J, Silverstein FS. Successful use of rt-PA in pediatric stroke. Neurology 2001;57:157–158
24. Gupta AA, Leaker M, Andrew M, et al. Safety and outcomes of thrombolysis with tissue plasminogen activator for treatment of intravascular thrombosis in children. J Pediatr 2001;139:682–688
25. The National Institute of Neurologic Disorders and Stroke rt-PA Stroke Study Group. Tissue plasminogen activator for acute ischemic stroke. N Engl J Med 1995;333:1581–1587
26. Qureshi AI, Siddiqui AM, Suri MF, et al. Aggressive mechanical clot disruption and low-dose intra-arterial third-generation thrombolytic agent for ischemic stroke: a prospective study. Neurosurgery 2002;51:1319–1329
27. deVeber GA, MacGregor D, Curtis R, Mayank S. Neurologic outcome in survivors of childhood arterial ischemic stroke and sinovenous thrombosis. J Child Neurol 2000;15:316–324
28. Carvalho KS, Bodensteiner JB, Connolly PJ, Garg BP. Cerebral venous thrombosis in children. J Child Neurol 2001;16:574–580
29. Lancon JA, Killough KR, Tibbs RE, Lewis AI, Parent AD. Spontaneous dural sinus thrombosis in children. Pediatr Neurosurg 1999;30:23–29
30. DeVeber G, Andrew M. Cerebral sinovenous thrombosis in children. N Engl J Med 2001;345:417–423
31. Einhaupl KM, Villringer A, Meister W, et al. Heparin treatment in sinus venous thrombosis. Lancet 1991;338:597–600
32. Philips MF, Bagley LJ, Sinson GP, et al. Endovascular thrombolysis for symptomatic cerebral venous thrombosis. J Neurosurg 1999;90: 65–71
33. Burrows PE, Benson LN, Williams WG, et al. Iliofemoral arterial complications of balloon angioplasty for systemic obstructions in infants and children. Circulation 1990;82:1697–1704
34. Barron TF, Gusnard DA, Zimmerman RA, Clancy RR. Cerebral venous thrombosis in neonates and children. Pediatr Neurol 1992; 8:112–116
35. Medlock MD, Olivero WC, Hanigan WC, Wright RM, Winek SJ. Children with cerebral venous thrombosis diagnosed with magnetic resonance imaging and magnetic resonance angiography. Neurosurgery 1992;31:870–876
36. Reddingius RE, Patte C, Couanet D, Kalifa C, Lemerle J. Dural sinus thrombosis in children with cancer. Med Pediatr Oncol 1997; 29:296–302
37. Wasay M, Bakshi R, Kojan S, Bobustuc G, Dubey N, Unwin DH. Nonrandomized comparison of local urokinase thrombolysis versus systematic heparin anticoagulation for superior sagittal sinus thrombosis. Stroke 2001;32:2310–2317
38. Horowitz M, Purdy P, Unwin H, et al. Treatment of dural sinus thrombosis using selective catheterization and urokinase. Ann Neurol 1995;38:58–67

19
###

Angioplasty and Stents in Children

TONY P. SMITH AND MICHAEL J. ALEXANDER

Percutaneous transluminal angioplasty has been successfully applied to the pediatric population for vessel narrowing in several peripheral anatomical areas, including the aorta for coarctation and the renal arteries. Although the indications are rare, transluminal angioplasty of the cervical and intracranial vessels may be performed to prevent or treat cerebral ischemia in narrowed or acutely occluded arteries. Endovascular stenting may be performed in the neurovascular circulation to reconstruct an arterial wall such as in dissection or traumatic pseudoaneurysm, or to help keep a narrowed artery or venous sinus open.

Although atherosclerotic disease is the most common indication for angioplasty of the cephalic arteries in the adult in the United States, this pathology virtually never presents in the pediatric population. Except in very rare circumstances such as the dyslipidemic states, atherosclerosis does not occur in the pediatric population. Although angioplasty has also been performed for other disease entities such as fibromuscular disease, these numbers are dwarfed in comparison.

The etiologies for ischemic stroke in this population are legion and a single one does not predominate. As a generalization, ischemic stroke in the pediatric population can be divided into thrombotic and embolic states. The list of possible causes for thrombotic stroke is extensive and includes infection, hematologic disorders including most predominantly sickle cell disease, prothrombotic states, and metabolic disorders. The most common identifiable etiology for embolic stroke is congenital cardiac disease. Unfortunately, the etiology for ischemic arterial stroke in the pediatric population is often unknown. Chabrier et al described 59 patients between 3 months and 16 years of age and found the pathophysiological process could be determined in 78%, although others placed the number at less than 50%.[1,2]

■ Neurovascular Diseases

Several pediatric disease entities lead to neurovascular arterial stenosis or acute occlusion that is potentially amenable to angioplasty (**Table 19–1**). Whether the patient should be treated medically or with angioplasty depends upon several factors, including degree of stenosis, symptomatology, and response to medical therapy. Listed following here are the neurovascular pathologies that may be amenable to either or both angioplasty and stenting.

Thromboembolic Disease

Ischemia due to thromboembolic disease may be seen in children with hypercoagulable states, particularly in patients with associated heart problems such as a patent foramen ovale or an atrial septal defect. In cases where there is severe narrowing or acute occlusion of one of the proximal cerebral arteries by clot, transluminal balloon angioplasty may be used in coordination with thrombolytic medications (tissue plasminogen activator or urokinase), IIbIIIa inhibitors, or clot retrieval

**TABLE 19–1 Etiology of Craniocervical Stenosis/
Occlusion in the Pediatric Population**

Thromboembolic disease
Systemic vasculitis
Takayasu's arteritis
Kawasaki disease
Vasculopathy
Fibromuscular dysplasia
Moyamoya disease
Arterial dissection
Postirradiation vasculopathy
Congenital narrowing of the great vessels
Pseudoaneurysm

devices. Qureshi et al have shown that aggressive mechanical clot disruption by balloon angioplasty in combination with intra-arterial reteplase is more effective in reaching a higher thrombolysis in myocardial infarction (TIMI) grade than intra-arterial reteplase alone.[3] When a short segment of cerebral artery is occluded by fresh thrombus, balloon angioplasty with a small, compliant balloon may break up the clot and lead to revascularization of the affected territory (**Fig. 19–1A–C**). Once the clot is broken up, adjuvant medical therapy is frequently necessary to prevent reformation of the clot with return of ischemic symptoms.

> **PEARL**   Balloon angioplasty with a small, compliant balloon may break up a clot and lead to revascularization.

Particularly remarkable results have been reported in pediatric patients who received balloon angioplasty for

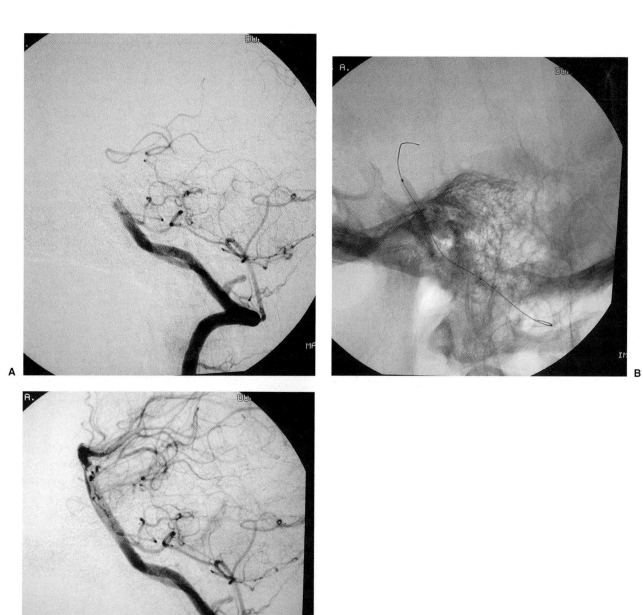

FIGURE 19–1 (A) Left vertebral angiogram in a 15-year-old boy with hypercoagulopathy who developed a locked-in syndrome from basilar trunk occlusion from a fresh thrombus. **(B)** A highly compliant 4 × 20 mm Hyperglide balloon (Micro Therapeutics, Inc., Irvine, CA) was used to break up the clot in coordination with intra-arterial tissue plasminogen activator. **(C)** Postangioplasty angiography demonstrates recanalization of the basilar artery.

basilar artery thrombosis. Kirton et al[4] reported the case of a pediatric patient with idiopathic basilar artery thrombosis who was clinically locked in for at least 20 hours, who underwent balloon angioplasty of the basilar artery and intra-arterial alteplase. The patient subsequently obtained a complete neurological recovery. Cognard et al[5] reported the case of an 8-year-old child who developed progressive neurological deficit over 30 hours leading to decerebrate rigidity and coma. The basilar artery was found to be occluded and balloon angioplasty was performed in the clot, followed by intra-arterial medical thrombolysis. The patient progressively improved and was neurologically normal by 3 months.

Balloon angioplasty with a compliant balloon may also be used to break up a clot in venous sinus thrombosis. Chaloupka and coworkers[6] reported balloon angioplasty and clot disruption in the superior sagittal sinus and transverse sinuses in combination with urokinase. Malek and coworkers[7] described the case of a 13-year-old boy with multiple dural arteriovenous fistulae who developed sinus thrombosis of the occipital and left transverse sinus as well as the right internal jugular vein and subsequent hydrocephalus. The sinus occlusions were successfully treated with balloon angioplasty; however, 3 days later he deteriorated and reocclusion of the occipital sinus was diagnosed. This was treated with repeat angioplasty and the placement of a stent in the occipital sinus. The patient did well and was neurologically intact at 12-month follow-up.

Systemic Vasculitis

Although virtually any vasculitis may involve arteries large enough to treat with angioplasty, it is for the most part limited in the neurovascular arena to Takayasu's arteritis, which frequently involves the proximal great vessels in young adults (type 1) (**Figs. 19–2** and **19–3**). However, symptoms due to limb and central nervous system ischemia are seldom reported in children. Muranjan et al reviewed their experience with 17 children ages 5 to 11 and found only one case with a neurological deficit that was secondary to hypertensive encephalopathy.[8] The presentation of Takayasu's arteritis in children is most often of the type 2 variety, which involves the abdominal aorta clinically resulting in hypertension. Percutaneous transluminal angioplasty of the aorta or the renal arteries has been safely performed in this group of children, although the results are only somewhat encouraging. Muranjan et al treated 15 subjects with percutaneous angioplasty after control of acute phase inflammatory state.[8] The procedure was partially beneficial in six subjects (40%); however, total withdrawal of antihypertensive drugs could not be achieved in any.

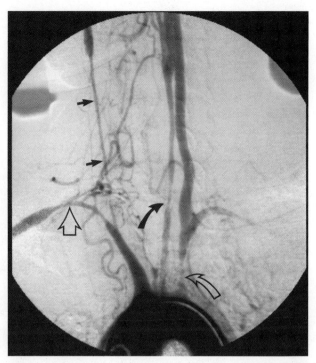

FIGURE 19–2 Angiography demonstrating classic findings of type 1 Takayasu's arteritis. Note the narrowing beginning in the distal right brachiocephalic artery with the long segment smooth narrowing extending into the right common carotid (small closed arrows) and right subclavian (open arrow) arteries. There is also narrowing of the left common carotid (curved closed arrow) and left subclavian (curved open arrow) arteries. Patient improved with an anti-inflammatory regimen and did not require angioplasty.

Angioplasty of Takayasu's arteritis in the brachiocephalic vessels has been reported to be successful in the adult population. Tyagi et al reported success equivalent to atherosclerotic disease in the subclavian arteries.[9] Carotid angioplasty with stenting has also been reported to be successful in the adult patient.[10] Sharma et al reported 20 patients who underwent angioplasty and stenting, five in the carotid artery distribution.[11] However, on follow-up, two (40%) of the carotid patients had restenosis. Based on limited adult data, angioplasty in the pediatric patient with Takayasu's arteritis of the great vessels is a treatment option if the patient has exhausted medical therapy and the symptoms warrant intervention. However, no data are available to determine the potential for success, failure, or complications in this patient population.

Kawasaki syndrome is an acute, febrile illness of infants and toddlers that results in an extensive vasculitis. The etiology is unknown. The disease is dramatically characterized by coronary involvement, particularly coronary artery aneurysms. Carotid artery involvement has been reported with Kawasaki syndrome, particularly regarding thrombosis.[12,13] There is also a reported loss of elasticity of the carotid arteries in patients with known coronary

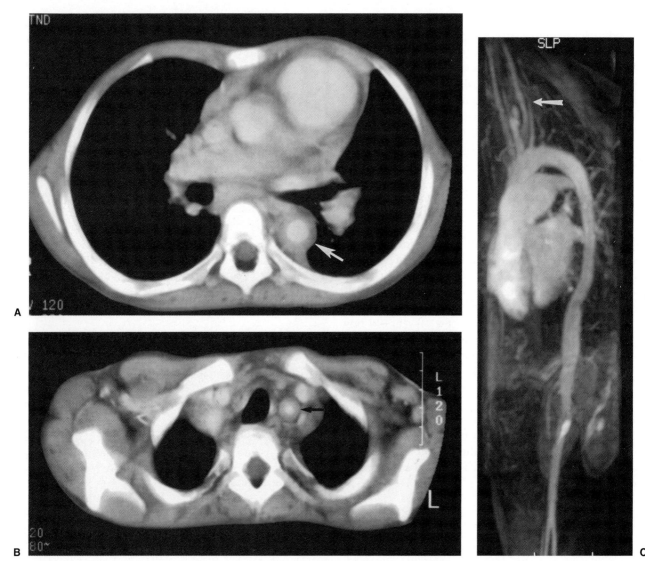

FIGURE 19–3 A 12-year-old with Takayasu's arteritis. Cross-sectional computed tomographic (CT) imaging demonstrates thickening of **(A)** the aorta (arrow) and **(B)** great vessels (arrow), which is a basic feature of the disease process. **(C)** Magnetic resonance angiography of the arch and great vessels shows areas of narrowing (arrow), but they are much less striking than with CT.

involvement.[14] Therapy is currently based on medical treatment regimens, usually with intravenous immunoglobulins.[15] Just as with Takayasu's arteritis, late-stage involvement refractory to medical therapy could conceivably be treated using endovascular means.

Vasculopathy

Fibromuscular dysplasia (FMD) is a nonatheromatous angiopathy that occurs in several arteries, most prominently the renal and carotid arteries. Transluminal angioplasty is well regarded as the treatment of choice for renal FMD. Carotid involvement is far less common. Schievink and Bjornsson reviewed all patients with a histologic diagnosis of FMD affecting the internal carotid artery over a 25-year interval in a single large medical center.[16] FMD of the internal carotid artery was a very rare autopsy finding detected in only four of 20,244 consecutive autopsies (0.02%), with an additional six identified in surgical specimens. All patients were adult females (mean age 53 years). Nine had the medial form of FMD and one the intimal form. By immunohistochemistry the lesions consist of proliferations of smooth muscle with a minor fibroblastic component. FMD was rarely limited to one carotid artery, and multivessel involvement was the rule.

FMD of the craniocervical vessels can lead to both embolic or ischemic symptoms and is a well-recognized predisposing factor to dissection. FMD is also known to occur in craniocervical vessels in children, although it is

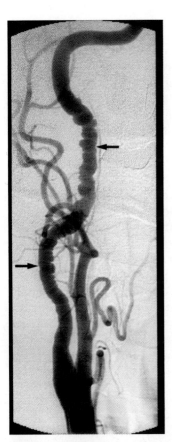

FIGURE 19–4 Fibromuscular dysplasia in a young adult. Note the typical string of beads appearance (arrows). The lesion is difficult surgically due to its distal extent but is highly amenable to angioplasty. Angioplasty alone without stenting is usually adequate. This patient was asymptomatic and was treated with antiplatelet therapy only.

very rarely symptomatic. Stroke from FMD, however, has been reported in both the carotid and vertebral artery distributions in children.[17,18] Potential treatments consist of medication, surgery, or angioplasty. Due to extensive and anatomically distal involvement of the cervical internal carotid artery, surgery can be difficult (**Fig. 19–4**). Angioplasty has been successfully performed in the adult carotid artery, although no large series are available. As in the adult, angioplasty would probably be the treatment of choice for symptomatic carotid or vertebral artery FMD refractory to medical therapy or when such therapy is not possible. One of the advantages of angioplasty for FMD is it often does not require stenting. The balloon is often opening webs rather than having to deal with atherosclerotic plaque, which often dissects and possesses elastic recoil following angioplasty.

> **PEARL** One of the advantages of angioplasty for FMD is it often does not require stenting.

Moyamoya disease is a vaso-occlusive process of the distal internal carotid artery, which may extend into the middle and anterior cerebral arteries.[19] Its name is derived from the angiographic appearance and its etiology is still unknown. The vessels are often occluded but may in fact be highly stenotic. Moyamoya can be debilitating with continued transient ischemic attacks, strokes, and hemorrhage. Surgery is controversial, including which procedures should be performed. There are studies that suggest surgery decreases the symptoms and increases activities of daily living, but the results are equivocal.[20–22] Revascularization of incompletely occluded vessels by endovascular means is a theoretical treatment option but has not been reported. Histopathologically, the involved arteries demonstrate fibrocellular thickening of the intima with proliferated smooth muscle cells and a prominently tortuous and often duplicated internal elastic lamina.[23]

Arterial Dissection

Dissection of the carotid and vertebral arteries can be the result of trauma, iatrogenic or otherwise, or may occur spontaneously with or without evidence of fibromuscular disease or other predisposing factors.[24] As in the adult population, treatment should consist of anticoagulation, initially with heparin, followed by coumadin for up to 6 months if possible. Dissection can be eloquently followed by computed tomographic (CT) or magnetic resonance (MR) angiography to determine healing or progression. If healing does not occur with anticoagulant therapy, if the patient cannot undergo anticoagulation, or if the patient is demonstrating symptoms despite adequate anticoagulant therapy, then endovascular treatment is an option, at least in the adult population. Endovascular therapy consists of angioplasty with stent placement to seal the dissection flap. This endovascular therapy has been successfully performed in the adult and has been the subject of case reports and small series.[25,26] Albuquerque et al reported successful treatment in 11 of 13 patients with carotid artery dissections; the other two could not be completely catheterized for stent placement.[26] The type of stent depends on the location of the dissection as well as the extent (length). Long dissections, particularly if located in the mid-cervical carotid artery (zone 2) are best treated with self-expanding stents. Short segment dissections in the carotid within the thorax (zone 1) or above the mandible (zone 3) or in the vertebral artery may be treated with either self-expandable or balloon-expandable stents as discussed later in this chapter. Although angioplasty with stenting for carotid or vertebral artery dissection has not been widely reported for the pediatric population, it is a reasonable therapeutic option in highly selected patients.

Postirradiation Vasculopathy

Postirradiation vasculopathy presents as large vessel disease in children several years following radiation therapy, usually for tumors. There are several types of radiation damage to arteries, but the most frequent is the accelerated development of an atherosclerotic variant. Radiation not only causes alterations to the artery but induces perivascular scar tissue formation, making surgical approaches to the artery difficult. In addition, although rare in the pediatric population, these patients may also have had previous tumor surgery in the same region that also resulted in scarring.

Postirradiation vasculopathy is one of the indications in the adult for entrance into high-risk carotid artery angioplasty and stenting trials. Unfortunately, in the pediatric population much of the radiation therapy is directed intracranially, resulting in much smaller vessel stenoses. Although intracranial angioplasty is becoming more widespread in the adult for atherosclerotic disease, in the pediatric population these are very small vessels and technical success and long-term patency rates are unknown. Cervical carotid stenting for radiation-induced stenoses has been reported to be successful in the adult population. Houdart et al reported seven patients with 10 radiation-induced stenoses of the carotid artery who underwent successful intervention.[27] Al-Mubarak et al reported 14 patients who underwent percutaneous stenting of 15 carotid arteries for severe radiation-induced extracranial stenoses.[28] In addition two patients underwent ipsilateral vertebral artery stenting concomitantly. One patient had a minor stroke after the procedure but recovered fully in 2 days. No other complications were encountered. Nine (64%) patients had 6-month follow-up imaging (angiography or duplex scanning) that showed no evidence of restenoses, and no repeat carotid artery interventions were required in the remaining patients.

Congenital Narrowing of the Great Vessels

It is extremely rare to have complex congenital heart disease with involvement of the great vessels amenable to angioplasty. A young patient carrying the diagnosis of Williams syndrome has been treated in our center (**Fig. 19–5A–C**). Congenitally acquired rubella could theoretically possess great vessel narrowing. Alagille syndrome (arteriohepatic dysplasia) does involve vessels of the central nervous system, but involvement is most often intracranial and resembles moyamoya angiographically.[29] However, with most of these diseases, craniocervical vessel involvement is extremely rare and would be amenable to percutaneous angioplasty techniques on a highly individualized basis, taking into account therapeutic alternatives in a particular patient.

Pseudoaneurysm

With the development of more flexible stent platforms and ultrathin expanded polytetrafluoroethylene (ePTFE) covering, with increased porosity, covered stent grafts are evolving for possible neurovascular use. Several reports have shown that stent grafts may be used in cases of traumatic pseudoaneurysms and fistulae.[30,31]

In traumatic pseudoaneurysms, stent grafts provide an attractive alternative to parent artery occlusion, particularly in the face of an enlarging pseudoaneurysm (**Fig. 19–6A–C**). Aneurysms and pseudoaneurysms at the skull base are difficult to treat by direct surgical intervention. The primary treatment options in the past have been either parent artery occlusion with either a surgical clip or endovascular detachable silicone balloons or coils versus occluding the parent artery in coordination with a bypass procedure. The risk of ischemia or embolic complications with parent artery occlusion in this scenario is relatively high, estimated at 5% or higher. The concept of a covered stent graft is to reconstruct the inner lumen via endovascular means to immediately seal the arterial wall defect, and to maintain patency of the parent artery.

> **PEARL**   In traumatic pseudoaneurysms, stent grafts provide an attractive alternative to parent artery occlusion.

Long-term studies are needed to evaluate the efficacy of ePTFE stent grafts in the neurovascular circulation and their risks for emboli and stent-associated stenosis. This treatment does not preclude the possible treatment of bypass at a later date, if necessary. In effect, it may function as either a definitive or temporizing measure in acute trauma.

■ Tools and Techniques

The tools and techniques for angioplasty and stenting are improving at a rapid rate; what one uses today may be obsolete tomorrow. Fortunately, for the pediatric population especially, one of the advances has been to decrease the size of the devices so as to limit the necessary arterial access sites and easily cross severe arterial stenoses. Angiography and angioplasty in the very young necessitate general anesthesia. In our experience, if at all in doubt, obtain the assistance of the department of anesthesiology for even older patients. The interventionist has enough to worry about without having to deal with sedation issues, and a motionless patient is key to a safe and technically successful procedure. In addition, the anesthesiologist will monitor all vital signs, give any

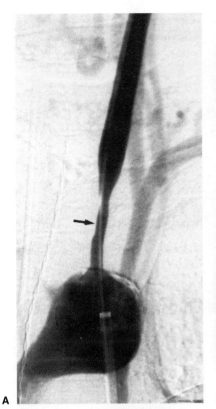

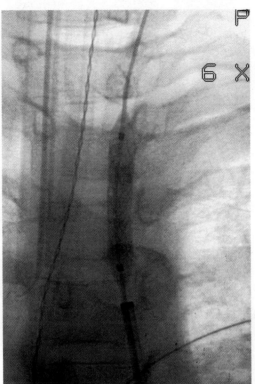

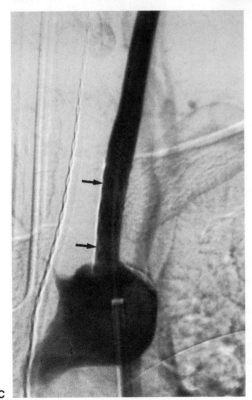

FIGURE 19–5 A 14-year-old male with Williams syndrome and narrowing of the great vessels. **(A)** Arch angiogram demonstrating narrowing of the proximal left common carotid artery (arrow). **(B)** Balloon expandable stent being placed at the area of narrowing in the left common carotid artery. **(C)** Postangioplasty and stenting of the left common carotid artery. Stenting produced an excellent radiographic result (arrows).

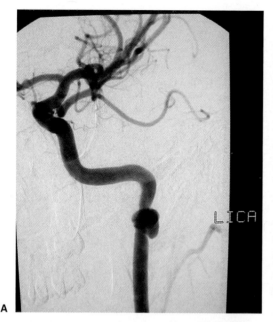

A

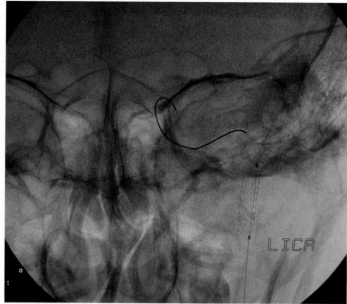

B

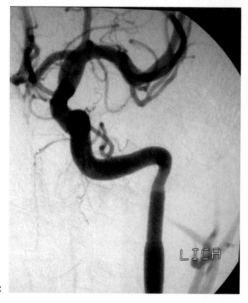

C

FIGURE 19–6 (A) Anteroposterior (AP) arteriogram of a 15-year-old boy following a knife wound to the left ear and skull base. Sequential arteriograms demonstrated an enlarging internal carotid artery pseudoaneurysm. **(B)** Placement of a covered balloon expandable stent graft (Jomed, Helsingborg, Sweden). **(C)** Immediate poststent AP arteriogram demonstrates exclusion of the pseudoaneurysm with endovascular reconstruction of the internal carotid artery.

necessary blood products, and be of invaluable assistance during acute recovery.

Antithrombosis

In the adult, anticoagulation and antiplatelet agents are an essential part of arterial angioplasty and stenting both to decrease acute thrombosis and to prevent restenosis. If not otherwise contraindicated, patients should be anticoagulated for the angioplasty procedure. In the adult catheterization laboratory, we strive for an activated clotting time of either twice baseline value or values of 200 to 300 seconds depending upon the site of the angioplasty and lesion morphology. If we are in a smaller vessel and if the balloon catheter is occlusive, or

for prolonged procedures, we prefer to have the patient at a greater level of anticoagulation based on activated clotting times obtained in the laboratory. In the pediatric population, dosing of heparin is most convenient if based on patient weight and an intravenous loading dose of 75 U/kg is a reasonable starting point. Monitoring can then be based on activated clotting times with the same prolongation schemes as for the adult. However, remember the activated clotting times require up to several milliliters of blood, which is not problematic in the adult or older child, but if repeated multiple times, can result in a fair amount of blood loss in the infant.

In the adult population, all patients undergoing cephalic angioplasty in our center are given aspirin and an oral platelet inhibitor prior to the procedure. Adult cardiac studies do tend to favor the patient receiving aspirin, which should be on board before the angioplasty, and the patient should be kept on this agent for a minimum of 6 months following the procedure if possible. Aspirin can be given to children and is routinely a part of angioplasty and stenting protocols in congenital cardiac laboratories. Aspirin has been used effectively in children with stroke. Strater et al performed a prospective multicenter follow-up study of 135 children with a first ischemic stroke who were randomized to receive prophylactic antithrombotic therapy consisting of low-molecular-weight heparin versus aspirin.[32] There was evidence that low-dose low-molecular-weight heparin is not superior to aspirin and vice versa in preventing recurrent stroke in white pediatric stroke patients. However, further adequately sized, randomized trials are required to obtain reliable information on safety and efficacy with respect to the antithrombotic medications used. One must, however, be cognizant of the problems with the use of aspirin in children.

All carotid stenting protocols currently in the United States require patients to be able to tolerate and to receive clopidogrel or ticlopidine before the procedure and up to 6 weeks following the angioplasty and stenting. Although neither of these drugs is approved for use in the pediatric population, weight-based dosing extrapolated from the adult doses is conceivable, but there are no data to support their use at this time in the pediatric population, although studies are ongoing.

Many pediatric cardiac centers place patients on warfarin with or without aspirin following stent placement. Warfarin doses have been well delineated for the pediatric patient and are easily administered orally. However, warfarin has been superseded in the adult population where studies with oral platelet inhibitors have unequivocally demonstrated benefit from the antiplatelet approach.[33] Six-month protocols for warfarin have shown no advantage over aspirin alone following coronary stenting.[34] An alternative would be to keep the patient on low-molecular-weight heparin for a time following angioplasty; the time frame, dosing, and risks/benefits would of course be empirical at best, especially in the pediatric population. Suffice it to say anticoagulation for the procedure and antiplatelet therapy postprocedure should be the goal but must be tailored to the individual pediatric patient until further data are available.

Equipment

The equipment for angioplasty consists of the best choice of guide wire, guiding catheters and sheaths, angioplasty balloons, and stents. Based originally on coronary technology, balloon systems adequate in size to dilate cephalic vessels, including the great vessels, can be placed over 0.018 in. or even smaller guide wires. A large variety of guide wires are available for both coronary and interventional neuroradiology. Because one often does not have the tortuosity of the great vessels in a child as compared with an adult, choice of guide wire will be based mostly on its response to torquing and the characteristics of the guide wire tip for crossing a particular stenosis rather than shaft stiffness. For example, if one has to place the tip of the guide wire well into the intracranial vessels, a soft-tip neurointerventional wire would be the best choice.

Most 0.018 in.-based angioplasty balloons for the cervical great vessels are manufactured for the peripheral circulation such as the renal or iliac arteries. These balloons have a relatively low uninflated (wrapped) profile even at inflated diameters of 8 mm or greater due to the small shaft sizes and tight balloon wrapping on the shaft. Most small vessel angioplasty balloons are manufactured for the coronary system and are available in sizes ranging from 1.5 to 5 mm in inflated balloon diameter. Depending on lesion morphology, balloon compliance may be an issue. A more compliant balloon will allow more precise sizing, which is particularly helpful in smaller vessels. For example, a particular balloon may reach its nominal size at a particular atmospheric inflation pressure (usually 6 or 8 atmospheres depending on the particular balloon), but will gradually "grow" as much as another millimeter based on an increase in inflation pressure. The downside of compliant balloons is of course that very resistant lesions may not be dilated with these balloons and will require noncompliant balloons, which do not grow with inflation pressures but will more readily open a very resistant lesion. The choice of balloon is based on a particular lesion's characteristics, its location, and the experience of the interventionist.

Although there are a large variety of stents now available, the choice of stents still remains either balloon expandable or self-expandable (**Fig. 19–7**). As a general rule, for cephalic angioplasty, self-expanding stents are used in the areas at danger of being crushed such as the cervical (zone 2) carotid artery. Currently available self-expanding stents are usually not as trackable as highly polished balloon-expandable varieties and are more difficult to place precisely; however, they are more flexible once in place if stenting over arterial bends is required. A few self-expanding ePTFE-covered stents are being manufactured currently, although at the time of this printing, they were not approved by the Food and Drug Administration for routine neurovascular use.

Balloon expandable stents come in a variety of lengths and diameters. They are usually considered to be more precise for placement. Stenting in the pediatric population is different from that in the adult in one main aspect: In the pediatric population one needs to account for somatic growth. For example, if one stents the carotid

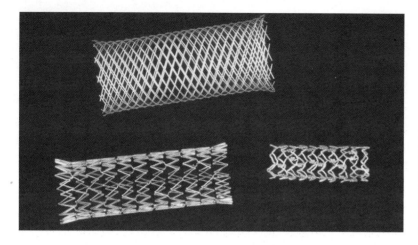

FIGURE 19–7 Three small vessel coronary stents. Magic Wallstent (top) and Radius (bottom left) stents (Boston Scientific, Natick, MA) are both self-expanding stents. The S660 (Medtronic, Inc., Minneapolis, MN) (bottom right) is one of several small vessel, low-profile balloon expandable stents. Note the difference in the configuration of the struts making up the stents.

artery in the child at 5 mm, when an adult, the vessel may be 8 mm in diameter. No data are currently available regarding dealing with this problem in the cephalic vessels, but it is being encountered for stenting of aortic coarctation and pulmonary vessel stenoses.[35] The best strategy in children is to perform angioplasty alone without stenting if possible. The lesion can then be redilated or even stented later as necessary. If stenting is required, the current recommendation is placement of stents that can be reexpanded as the patient grows. Therefore stents must be originally sized such that they can be expanded to larger diameters. Balloon expandable stents must be able to be redilated and must not foreshorten tremendously, and self-expandable stents must be oversized for the same reasons. In addition, depending on stent type, a larger diameter self-expanding stent may result in a much longer stented area initially, shortening with redilation at a later time. Stents for both aortic coarctation and pulmonary stenosis have been successfully redilated after significant growth in the swine model.[36] McMahon et al reported on 368 patients who had 752 stents implanted in a variety of locations for congenital heart disease, 220 of which were recatheterized.[37] Of those 220 patients, 103 underwent stent redilation. Indications for stent redilation included somatic growth ($n = 67$), serial dilation ($n = 27$), and development of neointimal proliferation or restenosis or both ($n = 9$). Interestingly, there was a low incidence of neointimal proliferation (1.8%) and restenosis (2%).

The arterial access site should be kept to the smallest possible size, which is based on the necessary guiding catheter or sheath utilized. The introducer system must be large enough to accommodate the balloons and stents and still allow free injection of contrast material for angioplasty and device placement. Very small diameter balloons can be placed through a guiding catheter as small as 4F, but larger balloons will require up to a 7F guiding catheter. In addition, stents require larger introduction systems, usually a minimum of a 6F guiding

catheter. One must always keep in mind that, although the initial plan may be to perform angioplasty alone, if a stent is required and the access device is too small, changing for a larger catheter may be problematic at that stage. Alternatively, one can work through an introducer sheath, which are available in lengths up to 90 cm. Because of the thin-walled nature of these sheaths, much larger devices can be placed. Virtually all of the stents and balloons for small vessels can be placed through a 5F introducer sheath and only the largest of stents in the pediatric population will require a 6F. These sheaths are somewhat prone to kinking in tortuous vessels, which should not be problematic in the pediatric population. Before every procedure, one should review the tools to be used such that an appropriate decision can be reached regarding the selection of an access catheter or sheath.

Interventional procedures require, particularly if difficult or problematic, larger amounts of contrast material than diagnostic angiographic procedures alone. This necessary contrast dosage is not usually problematic in older children but may be an issue in infants. There is no definite upper limit to contrast dosage because it varies regarding the time frame over which it is administered, usually in small boluses over a longer period of time for interventional procedures, as well as the basic constitution of individual patients and their fluid status and ability to rid the body of the contrast material. One needs to use the necessary amount of contrast to perform the procedure as well, as expediently and as safely as possible, but the operator must be cognizant of the total contrast dosage. We keep a running list of all contrast material injections throughout the entire case when dealing with the pediatric group. This allows the interventionist to gauge the procedure against the contrast material administered. Although there are no definite data regarding maximum contrast dosage, most radiology groups limit a single angiographic study to less than 5 mL/kg body weight when using low osmolar, nonionic contrast agents. The interventionist can safely exceed this dosage for long procedures where the contrast material is administered in small boluses over a longer period of time in an otherwise healthy infant. However, one must always strive to use the least possible amount of contrast material.

■ Complications

The major complication of craniocervical angioplasty is stroke. Ischemic stroke occurs from either embolization during or after the procedure or vessel thrombosis. Very little data are available in the pediatric population. Embolic stroke is the major concern for carotid angioplasty and stenting in the adult and has led to the popularity of distal protection devices. It is unknown if such devices are needed, particularly in the treatment of nonatherosclerotic disease, as is present in the pediatric population. Intracranial hemorrhage following angioplasty and stenting has occurred in adults and is believed to be related to anticoagulant therapy and disruption of the blood–brain barrier by ischemic events. Intracranial vessels are extremely thin and even minimal oversizing of the balloon can result in rupture and subarachnoid hemorrhage. Subarachnoid hemorrhage can also occur from perforation of an intracranial vessel with a guide wire.

Careful patient selection and meticulous technique are key to the safety of the procedure. Undersizing the balloon and stents and being willing to live with a less than perfect result is acceptable. Most carotid angioplasty and stenting protocols consider success to be less than or equal to 30% residual stenosis.

Procedures should be performed only by very experienced neurointerventionists. The lack of data makes one rely entirely on adult experience in dealing with pediatric patients. One must also be prepared to use rescue techniques including thrombolytic therapy for embolic disease or acute vessel thrombosis.

■ Conclusions

Craniocervical arterial angioplasty and stenting are becoming accepted techniques in the adult population as preventative and treatment measures for cerebral ischemia. Stroke is an unusual but difficult problem in the pediatric population. Angioplasty and stenting may also be applicable to the pediatric patient, but there are limitations based mostly on differences in the disease process etiologies and the population as a whole. There are virtually no data available regarding this type of endovascular therapy in children. However, as equipment and techniques continue to be refined in the adult, they will certainly find a role in the pediatric age group.

REFERENCES

1. Trescher WH. Ischemic stroke syndromes in childhood. Pediatr Ann 1992;21:374–383
2. Chabrier S, Husson B, Lasjaunias P, Landrieu P, Tardieu M. Stroke in childhood: outcome and recurrence risk by mechanism in 59 patients. J Child Neurol 2000;15:290–294
3. Qureshi AI, Siddiqui AM, Suri MF, et al. Aggressive mechanical clot disruption and low-dose intra-arterial third generation thrombolytic agent for ischemic stroke: a prospective study. Neurosurgery 2002;51:1319–1327
4. Kirton A, Wong JH, Mah J, et al. Successful endovascular therapy for acute basilar thrombosis in an adolescent. Pediatrics 2003;112:e248–e251
5. Cognard C, Weill A, Lindgren S, Piotin M, Castaings L, Moret J. Basilar artery occlusion in a child: "clot angioplasty" followed by thrombolysis. Childs Nerv Syst 2000;16:496–500
6. Chaloupka JC, Mangla S, Huddle DC. Use of mechanical thrombolysis via microballoon percutaneous transluminal angioplasty for the treatment of acute dural sinus thrombosis: case presentation and technical report. Neurosurgery 1999;45:650–656
7. Malek AM, Higashida RT, Balousek PA, et al. Endovascular recanalization with balloon angioplasty and stenting of an occluded occipital sinus for treatment of intracranial venous hypertension: technical case report. Neurosurgery 1999;44:896–901
8. Muranjan MN, Bavdekar SB, More V, Deshmukh H, Tripathi M, Vaswani R. Study of Takayasu's arteritis in children: clinical profile and management. J Postgrad Med 2000;46:3–8
9. Tyagi S, Verma PK, Gambhir DS, Kaul UA, Saha R, Arora R. Early and long-term results of subclavian angioplasty in aortoarteritis (Takayasu disease): comparison with atherosclerosis. Cardiovasc Intervent Radiol 1998;21:219–224
10. Murakami R, Korogi Y, Matsuno Y, Matsukawa T, Hirai T, Takahashi M. Percutaneous transluminal angioplasty for carotid artery stenosis in Takayasu arteritis: persistent benefit over 10 years. Cardiovasc Intervent Radiol 1997;20:219–221
11. Sharma BK, Jain S, Bali HK, Jain A, Kumari S. A follow-up study of balloon angioplasty and de-novo stenting in Takayasu arteritis. Int J Cardiol 2000;75(Suppl 1):S147–S152
12. Lauret P, Lecointre C, Billard JL. Kawasaki disease complicated by thrombosis of the internal carotid artery. Ann Dermatol Venereol 1979;106:901–905
13. Amano S, Hazama F, Hamashima Y. Pathology of Kawasaki disease, II: Distribution and incidence of the vascular lesions. Jpn Circ J 1979;43:741–748
14. Noto N, Okada T, Yamasuge M, et al. Noninvasive assessment of the early progression of atherosclerosis in adolescents with Kawasaki disease and coronary artery lesions. Pediatrics 2001;107:1095–1099
15. Sundel RP, Baker AL, Fulton DR, Newburger JW. Corticosteroids in the initial treatment of Kawasaki disease: report of a randomized trial. J Pediatr 2003;142:611–616
16. Schievink WI, Bjornsson J. Fibromuscular dysplasia of the internal carotid artery: a clinicopathological study. Clin Neuropathol 1996;15:2–6
17. Puri V, Riggs G. Case report of fibromuscular dysplasia presenting as stroke in 16-year-old boy. J Child Neurol 1999;14:233–238
18. Perez-Higueras A, Alvarez-Ruiz F, Martinez-Bermejo A, et al. Cerebellar infarction from fibromuscular dysplasia and dissecting aneurysm of the vertebral artery: report of a child. Stroke 1988;19:521–524
19. Numaguchi Y, Gonzalez CF, Davis PC, et al. Moyamoya disease in the United States. Clin Neurol Neurosurg 1997;99(Suppl 2):S26–S30

20. Caldarelli M, Di Rocco C, Gaglini P. Surgical treatment of moyamoya disease in pediatric age. J Neurosurg Sci 2001;45:83–91

21. Isono M, Ishii K, Kamida T, Inoue R, Fujiki M, Kobayashi H. Long-term outcomes of pediatric moyamoya disease treated by encephalo-duro-arterio-synangiosis. Pediatr Neurosurg 2002;36:14–21

22. Yilmaz EY, Pritz MB, Bruno A, Lopez-Yunez A, Biller J. Moyamoya: Indiana Medical Center experience. Arch Neurol 2001;58: 1274–1278

23. Fukui M, Kono S, Sueishi K, Ikezaki K. Moyamoya disease. Neuropathology 2000;20:S61–S64

24. Chabrier S, Lasjaunias P, Husson B, Landrieu P, Tardieu M. Ischaemic stroke from dissection of the craniocervical arteries in childhood: report of 12 patients. Eur J Paediatr Neurol 2003;7:39–42

25. Lee DH, Hur SH, Kim HG, Jung SM, Ryu DS, Park MS. Treatment of internal carotid artery dissections with endovascular stent placement: report of two cases. Korean J Radiol 2001;2:52–56

26. Albuquerque FC, Han PP, Spetzler RF, Zambramski JM, Mcdougall CG. Carotid dissection: technical factors affecting endovascular therapy. Can J Neurol Sci 2002;29:54–60

27. Houdart E, Mounayer C, Chapot R, Saint-Maurice J-P, Merland J-J. Carotid stenting for radiation-induced stenoses. Stroke 2001;32: 118–121

28. Al-Mubarak N, Roubin GS, Iyer SS, Gomez CR, Liu MW, Vitek JJ. Carotid stenting for severe radiation-induced extracranial carotid artery occlusive disease. J Endovasc Ther 2000;7:36–40

29. Connor SE, Hewes D, Ball C, Jarosz JM. Alagille syndrome associated with angiographic moyamoya. Childs Nerv Syst 2002;18:186–190

30. Alexander MJ, Smith TP, Tucci DL. Treatment of an iatrogenic petrous carotid artery pseudoaneurysm with a Symbiot covered stent: technical case report. Neurosurgery 2002;50:658–662

31. Redekop G, Marotta T, Weill A. Treatment of traumatic aneurysms and arteriovenous fistulas of the skull base using endovascular stents. J Neurosurg 2001;95:412–419

32. Strater R, Kurnik K, Heller C, Schobess R, Luigs P, Nowak-Gottl U. Aspirin versus low-dose low-molecular-weight heparin: antithrombotic therapy in pediatric ischemic stroke patients: a prospective follow-up study. Stroke 2001;32:2554–2558

33. Schomig A, Neumann FJ, Kastrati A, et al. A randomized comparison of antiplatelet and anticoagulant therapy after the placement of coronary artery stents. N Engl J Med 1996;334:1084–1089

34. Garachemani AR, Fleisch M, Windecker S, Pfiffner D, Meier B. Heparin and coumadin versus acetylsalicylic acid for prevention of restenosis after coronary angioplasty. Catheter Cardiovasc Interv 2002;55:315–320

35. O'Laughlin MP, Slack MC, Grifka RG, Perry SB, Lock JE, Mullins CE. Implantation and intermediate-term follow-up of stents in congenital heart disease. Circulation 1993;88:605–614

36. Morrow WR, Palmaz JC, Tio FO, Ehler WJ, VanDellen AF, Mullins CE. Re-expansion of balloon-expandable stents after growth. J Am Coll Cardiol 1993;22:2007–2013

37. McMahon CJ, El-Said HG, Grifka RG, Fraley JK, Nihill MR, Mullins CE. Redilation of endovascular stents in congenital heart disease: factors implicated in the development of restenosis and neointimal proliferation. J Am Coll Cardiol 2001;38:521–526

Index

Please note that page numbers followed by f and t indicate figures and tables, respectively.